Women, Children, and HIV/AIDS

Felissa Lashley Cohen, R.N., Ph.D., F.A.A.N., is Professor and Head, Department of Medical-Surgical Nursing, College of Nursing, and Clinical Chief for Medical-Surgical Nursing at the University of Illinois Hospital and Clinics, University of Illinois at Chicago. She is a Diplomate of the American Board of Medical Genetics and has a practice in genetic counseling. Dr. Cohen received a B.S. in nursing from Adelphi College, an M.A. (medical-surgical nursing, higher education) from New York University, and a Ph.D. (human genetics) from Illinois State University. She was selected as a member of Priority Expert Panel B for the National Center for Nursing Research, National Institutes of Health, to determine priority areas for AIDS-related research. Dr. Cohen has been selected as a distinguished lecturer for Sigma Theta Tau International for the 1990–1991 and the 1992–1993 bienniums. Her book, *Clinical Genetics in Nursing Practice*, won an *American Journal of Nursing* Book of the Year Award in two categories in 1984. With Dr. Durham she was coeditor of *The Person with AIDS: Nursing Perspectives*, which received Book of the Year Award in two categories in 1987. She has conducted many research studies in AIDS, including those on hospital policies and practices regarding AIDS, foster care of HIV-infected children, families of HIV-infected children, and quality of life in HIV-infected women. She is a member of the Association of Nurses in AIDS Care and recently served on the National League for Nursing HIV/AIDS Guidelines Revision Task Force for Schools of Nursing.

Jerry D. Durham, R.N., Ph.D., F.A.A.N., is Professor and Executive Associate Dean for Educational Service at Indiana University School of Nursing, Indianapolis. Dr. Durham holds six degrees: B.S. in Education, Southeast Missouri State University; M.A. in English, Bradley University; B.S.N., M.S.N. (medical-surgical nursing); Ph.D. (higher education administration), Saint Louis University; and M.S. (psychiatric nursing), University of Illinois at Chicago. In addition to his recognition as a Fellow of the American Academy of Nursing, Dr. Durham is a member of numerous professional organizations. He has worked as a nurse clinician, educator, researcher, writer, and consultant for almost 20 years. He has received two fellowships in ethics from the National Endowment for the Humanities. Books he coedited have received three *American Journal of Nursing* Book of the Year Awards. Along with Dr. Cohen, he is coeditor of *The Person with AIDS: Nursing Perspectives.*

Women, Children, — and — HIV/AIDS

Felissa L. Cohen, RN, PhD, FAAN

Jerry D. Durham, RN, PhD, FAAN

Editors

 Springer Publishing Company • New York

Copyright © 1993 by Springer Publishing Company, Inc.

Springer Publishing Company, Inc.
536 Broadway
New York, NY 10012-3955

93 94 95 96 97 / 5 4 3 2 1

Library of Congress Cataloging-in-Publication Data

Women, children, and HIV/AIDS / Felissa L. Cohen, Jerry D. Durham,
    editors.
        p. cm.
    Includes bibliographical references and index.
    ISBN 0-8261-7880-4
    1. AIDS (Disease) 2. Women—Diseases. 3. AIDS (Disease) in
children. 4. AIDS (Disease) in adolescence. I. Cohen, Felissa L.
II. Durham, Jerry D.
    [DNLM: 1. Acquired Immunodeficiency Syndrome—epidemiology.
2. Acquired Immunodeficiency Syndrome—prevention & control. 3. HIV
Infections—epidemiology. 4. HIV Infections—prevention & control.
WD 308 W8724]
RA644.A25W654   1993
614.5'993—dc20
DNLM/DLC
for Library of Congress   92-48971
                                                              CIP

Printed in the United States of America

With love to my children, Peter, Heather, Neal, and now Julie, who will always hold special places in my heart; and to big Tony O., my special "pal" and protector

and

To women in all cultures who are the caretakers and caregivers for their families and especially to the professional nurses who are caring for people affected by HIV infection.

—Felissa L. Cohen

To people everywhere whose struggle with HIV and AIDS lends eloquent testimony to the dignity of humanity.

—Jerry D. Durham

Contents

Preface

In fiction or in the movies, when there is an emergency and evacuation is necessary, the familiar cry is "women and children first!" In the case of AIDS that cry has seemed to be "women and children last."

Although AIDS was reported in women as early as 1981—the first year the Centers for Disease Control and Prevention (CDC) recognized AIDS—women have mostly been invisible in the AIDS epidemic. This is partly because many HIV-infected women did not—and still do not—meet the CDC definition of AIDS-defining illnesses because these were developed largely from data from males in whom AIDS was first reported. HIV-infected women tend to be poor, nonwhite, and less powerful than their male counterparts. Initially, attention was paid to the male majority with AIDS who tended to be white, middle-class, better educated and more politically active.

HIV-infection is increasing rapidly in women. In the last calendar year, even without a changed AIDS definition, more than 13% of the reported adult AIDS cases were in women. However, attention in the form of prevention, symptom recognition, disease detection, care, and treatment and support for women has only recently become evident, and due in large part to pressure from women's advocates. Some have viewed the issue of HIV infection and women mainly in the light of the effect on the children of infected women. While no one will deny the importance and magnitude of that problem, attention and services must be given to the HIV-infected woman in her own right. Moreover, while the greatest percentage of women with AIDS is in the category of injecting drug users, heterosexual contact is the only one in which women outnumber men in raw numbers—a dubious distinction. Since it is assumed that women who inject drugs and have AIDS contracted the virus from the drug use (and are counted in that category), the real magnitude of risk of heterosexual contact for women is not fully realized. As discussed in this book, women as a group may be unknowingly or unwillingly exposed to HIV infection. We must continue to address meaningful prevention efforts to *all* women regardless of their social, cultural, or economic status.

Women have been, and continue to be, both HIV-infected and HIV-affected. In most societies women are usually the ones who take care of family members across the lifespan, particularly children and the elderly. This caretaking role often means that women, whether healthy or ill, neglect their own needs in order to care for others. For women who are health care workers this caregiving role is magnified.

Women continue to fall through the cracks of the health care system. Female-specific conditions associated with HIV infection (e.g., chronic vaginal candidiasis) often go unrecognized as to their significance in regard to HIV/AIDS in women. Many health care professionals still do not maintain a high index of suspicion regarding HIV infection when the client is female, especially if she is married, middle-class, and white. Consequently women may be misdiagnosed, not diagnosed at all, or diagnosed later in their disease, leading to an unfavorable impact on survival. There are few health and social services that truly meet the needs of women in a broad sense.

The first reports of AIDS in children appeared in the literature in late 1982. Clinicians had actually been treating children with AIDS in the United States since the late 1970s. Despite the relatively small number of reported pediatric AIDS cases in the United States, AIDS has become the ninth leading cause of death among U.S. children between the ages of 1 and 4. In areas of high HIV prevalence it may be the leading cause for some subgroups. In developing countries the problem is even more serious: pediatric AIDS may account for 15 to 20% of the total number of AIDS cases in many of these nations, and the World Health Organization estimates that there are at least 500,000 pediatric AIDS cases worldwide. In the U.S. and elsewhere, the vast majority of cases of pediatric AIDS is perinatally acquired, meaning that each of these children has a mother who is also HIV-infected and a family that is or will soon be disrupted, thereby affecting family members who are themselves HIV-infected and those who are not.

HIV-infected mothers in developing countries face a cruel choice. Breast-feeding poses a risk for HIV-transmission to the breastfed infant, but in areas where malnutrition, unsafe water, and infectious diseases are present, breast-feeding may be the least risky path to infant survival. Street children in many developing countries are particularly vulnerable to drug use and sexual abuse and do not have the means (emotional, economic, or physical) to protect themselves against many life events, including AIDS. Yet, even in this country, the CDC does not publish statistics on AIDS acquired in a sexual manner or through direct injecting drug use in children under 13 years of age.

Adolescents constitute another group that is especially vulnerable to the acquisition of HIV infection. In the United States adolescent cases comprise less than a half percent of all cases of AIDS. However, the rate of reported

AIDS cases in adolescents is doubling about every 14 months, especially in females. Furthermore, based on what is known about the incubation period of HIV, it is apparent that the larger number of persons with AIDS in the 20 to 29 years of age group became infected in adolescence. Adolescents, with their propensity to experiment, take risks in their search for identity and love, resulting in behaviors that make them particularly vulnerable to HIV acquisition. Many children and adolescents can be reached for AIDS prevention efforts through the schools, but this is not enough. Other efforts in other settings are needed. Moreover, many school districts are not direct in their approaches to sensitive and controversial topics, particularly those related to HIV transmission by sexual behaviors and drug use, making education and prevention less effective.

The challenges of poverty, inadequate education, and nontraditional family structures must shape America's future HIV/AIDS prevention and intervention activities if this epidemic is to be effectively addressed. Access to decent health care for all Americans, but particularly for women (who currently earn only about 70% of their male counterparts), is an increasingly urgent concern. The underlying phenomena of racism and sexism, both of which shape opportunities and choices for women, has a profound influence on the HIV/AIDS epidemic in the United States and throughout the world. The lack of a family policy in this country—the only industrialized nation without such a policy—further limits opportunities and choices for women and their families.

This book provides readers with information and perspectives aimed at improving their knowledge about HIV/AIDS among women and children and at encouraging responsible advocacy on behalf of those living with HIV/AIDS. The problems and issues discussed in this book challenge nurses to assume leadership roles as practitioners, managers, educators, and participants in policy shaping. As the face of the epidemic shifts in the years ahead to include more women and children, nursing's proactive approach to new challenges and responses to individuals, family, and community needs must also change. Nurses must not only continue to assume their legitimate roles as knowledgeable, compassionate, and effective care providers, but also become fuller participants in HIV/AIDS policy developments that ultimately influence the lives of all Americans.

Contributors

Margaret Beaman, R.N., Ph.D., is associate professor, School of Nursing, Southern Illinois University, Edwardsville, Illinois. She is certified as an adult nurse practitioner. She is principal investigator of a National Center for Nursing Research project on persuading adolescents to use condoms and has also served as Southern Illinois site staff for the Midwest AIDS Education Training Center.

Barbara Berger, R.N., M.S., is a doctoral candidate, College of Nursing, University of Illinois at Chicago. She has worked as a research nurse in AIDS Prevention Services at Cook County Hospital, Chicago.

Carolyn Burr, R.N., M.S., is coordinator, National Pediatric HIV Resource Center, New Jersey Medical School, Newark. Ms. Burr is an ANA-certified pediatric nurse practitioner. She codeveloped the National Pediatric HIV Resource Center.

Risa Denenberg, R.N., M.S.N., F.N.P., is a family nurse practitioner and women's health specialist at the infectious disease clinic at Bronx Lebanon Hospital, New York. She has written and spoken widely on AIDS-related topics and is a member of ACT UP, New York.

John Douard, Ph.D., is assistant professor of philosophy and health policy at the Institute for the Medical Humanities, University of Texas Medical Branch, Galveston.

Katherine Foos, M.C.J., is employed by the City of Arvada, Colorado, as a commissioned police officer assigned to special investigations. She is the aunt and adoptive parent of a child with perinatally acquired AIDS.

Donna M. Harris, R.N., M.S., C.S., is a pediatric nurse practitioner in the neonatology division of Children's Hospital, Milwaukee, Wisconsin. She was clinical coordinator and clinical specialist at the Special Infectious Disease Clinic at Children's Memorial Hospital, Chicago. She holds ANA certification as both a pediatric nurse and family practitioner therapist. Ms. Harris consults and presents widely in regard to pediatric AIDS and has assisted in the development of the pediatric HIV infection program at Children's Memorial Hospital.

Carol Ren Kneisl, R.N., M.S., C.S., is president and educational director of Nursing Transitions, Inc., Williamsville, New York. She is ANA-certified in adult psychiatric nursing. Ms. Kneisl has served as an HIV-AIDS consultant for the New York State Office of Mental Health, for whom she authored an AIDS nursing manual.

Ann E. Kurth, R.N., M.S.N., M.P.H., C.N.M., is currently the clinical research director of the Division of Acquired Diseases, Indiana State Department of Health. As HIV-AIDS Program Coordinator at Methodist Hospital of Indiana, Inc., she assisted in the development of one of the first HIV clinics in the Midwest. She has been involved with HIV-related research/education projects in both clinical and public health settings in the U.S. and in East Africa. She is active in both the American College of Nurse-Midwifery and the Association of Nurses in AIDS Care.

Katherine Cavallari Malm, R.N., M.S., is educational coordinator, Children's Memorial Hospital, Chicago. She is coinvestigator on a funded research project examining the impact of perinatal AIDS on families.

Wendy M. Nehring, R.N., Ph.D., is assistant professor in the Department of Maternal Child Nursing, College of Nursing, University of Illinois at Chicago. She is coprincipal investigator on two funded AIDS research projects—one on foster care and one on the impact of perinatal AIDS on families.

Kathleen Fordham Norr, Ph.D., is assistant professor in the Department of Maternal-Child Nursing, College of Nursing, University of Illinois at Chicago and a medical sociologist. She is principal investigator of a funded research project using peer education models for AIDS prevention among Botswana women.

James L. Norr, Ph.D., is associate head, Department of Sociology, University of Illinois at Chicago. He has expertise in comparative political economy and is currently engaged in a comparative cross-national study of health.

Sheila D. Tlou, R.N., Ph.D., is lecturer, Faculty of Nursing, University of Botswana, Gaborone, Botswana. She is coinvestigator on a funded project examining peer education as a means of AIDS prevention among women in Botswana.

Vida M. Vizgirda, R.N., B.S.N., is a doctoral student at the College of Nursing, University of Illinois at Chicago. She is a part-time staff nurse at the University of Illinois Hospital and Clinics on a unit with many AIDS patients and has provided home health care to patients with AIDS.

Part I
Introduction

1

HIV Infection and AIDS: An Overview

Felissa L. Cohen

It now seems incredible that a little more than a decade ago, the terms *acquired immunodeficiency syndrome* (AIDS) and *human immunodeficiency virus* (HIV) were in neither our vocabulary nor our consciousness. While this book focuses primarily on women and children in relation to HIV infection and AIDS, this chapter presents a brief overview of essential information about HIV infection in general for readers to understand later material better. Detailed general information about HIV infection and AIDS not specific to women and children may be found elsewhere (Durham & Cohen, 1991).

ETIOLOGY

There is scientific consensus that the etiologic agent of AIDS is the human immunodeficiency virus (HIV), a human retrovirus belonging to the lentivirus subfamily (Mak & Wigzell, 1991). HIV is currently known to have at least two subtypes, type 1 (HIV-1) and type 2 (HIV-2), each of which may have many strains. Genetic variation may be seen within a single person over time and within populations (Johnson & Cann, 1992). HIV-1 is responsible for most of the AIDS cases in the world at this time, except in West Africa where HIV-2 is prevalent. Recently a few cases of acquired immunodeficiency without evidence of HIV-1 or -2 have been identified raising questions about whether their etiology is from another agent, another type of HIV, or was caused by HIV-1 or -2 but was not detectable by current techniques (Laurence, Siegal, Schattner, Gelman, & Morse, 1992; "Unexplained CD4+ T-lymphocyte . . .", 1992). Unless otherwise specified, HIV means HIV-1 in this chapter.

Several factors may play a role in the acquisition of HIV infection, its transmission efficiency, development of specific clinical manifestations, disease progression, and ultimate survival. Such cofactors may act with HIV, with each other, or with unknown factors to modulate clinical expression. Cofactors have been proposed that relate to the host (such as genetic factors), the organism (such as the virulence of a strain), the environment (such as stress), and interaction effects. In addition, some scientists have proposed that other agents (e.g., mycoplasmas) may play a facilitating role for HIV.

TRANSMISSION

The major documented transmission modes for HIV are those in which individuals are exposed to HIV-containing blood or body fluid (1) through intimate sexual contact, homosexual or heterosexual; (2) through blood or parenteral exposure through transfusions, injecting drug use (IDU), needlestick or the like; and (3) from mother to infant, prenatally, perinatally, or postnatally. HIV has been isolated from a variety of body fluids, cells, and tissues such as blood, blood products, semen, cervical and vaginal secretions, breast milk, lymph nodes, tears, brain tissue, saliva, urine, retina, cornea, ear secretions, bronchial fluid, Langerhans cells of the skin and mucous membranes, synovial fluid, and amniotic cells and fluid. The importance of these fluids, cells, and tissues in transmission varies, as does the concentration of HIV within them (Levy, 1989; Levy, 1990). Receptive oral intercourse with ejaculation has been reported to carry a risk of HIV transmission (Lifson et al., 1990). Horizontal transmission to household contacts or transmission through vectors such as insects has not been documented (Friedland et al., 1990). Transmission from an HIV-infected health-care worker to patients is considered in Chapter 16.

Other factors may influence the efficiency of HIV transmission. Some that have been identified include (1) certain risky behaviors such as receptive anal intercourse and numerous sexual encounters, particularly with high-risk partners; (2) increased plasma concentrations of HIV; (3) the presence of other sexually transmitted diseases, especially genital and anorectal ulcers, often caused by syphilis or herpes simplex virus infection, and endocervical infections, often caused by *Chlamydia trachomatis* or gonorrhea (Holmes, 1991; Hook et al., 1992). Risky behaviors are important in acquiring HIV.

HOW HIV INFECTS CELLS

When HIV encounters a cell with a specific receptor for it, primarily the CD4 molecule (a surface glycoprotein), a binding reaction occurs, and the virus enters the cell through fusion of the virus and cell membranes. After HIV enters the cell, the viral ribonucleic acid (RNA) is transcribed by means of an enzyme known as reverse transcriptase into proviral deoxyribonucleic acid (DNA), which may accumulate in the cell cytoplasm or become integrated into the DNA of the host cell's chromosomes. There may then be a latent phase. Viral expression begins when there is transcription of viral RNA leading to protein synthesis, processing, viral assembly, and release of mature HIV from the cell surface by budding (Bednarik & Folks, 1992).

Preferentially infected cells include T-helper lymphocytes (T4 cells, CD4+ lymphocytes), monocytes, macrophages, and antigen-presenting dendritic cells (Haseltine, 1991; Smith, 1990). Other cells, such as fibroblasts and glial cells, can also become infected (Levy, 1989).

After HIV infection occurs, there is a period during which the person does not demonstrate antibodies to HIV. This period is known as the "window period." Usually antibodies to HIV appear by three to six weeks after infection and are nearly always present by three months post-HIV infection, although in some cases seroconversion may take six months or even longer (Imagawa et al., 1989; VanDevanter, 1991). HIV is persistent even if quiescent, allowing for its transmission years after the initial infection even if the infected person is asymptomatic (Cohen, 1991b; Greenberg, 1992; Lifson, Rutherford, & Jaffe, 1988).

HIV infection results in (1) quantitative and qualitative immune impairment (largely through effects on T4 lymphocytes); (2) increased susceptibility to opportunistic infections; (3) direct infection of the central nervous system; and (4) an increased incidence of neoplasias (Rosenberg & Fauci, 1991; Wong-Staal, 1991). The clinical spectrum of HIV infection is discussed later in this chapter.

DEFINITIONS AND CLASSIFICATION

Infection with HIV can result in a wide variety of manifestations, ranging from asymptomatic infection to such life-threatening immunodeficiency-linked conditions as serious opportunistic infections and cancers. The Centers for Disease Control (CDC) has proposed expanding its 1987 surveillance case definition for AIDS in adults and revising its HIV classification system for adolescents and adults for expected implementation in 1992 ("Revision of the CDC," 1987; Centers for Disease Control, 1991). These updates are based on the following criteria for HIV infection:

> Persons aged 13 years or older with repeatedly reactive screening tests for HIV-1 antibody (e.g., enzyme immunoassay) who also have specific antibody identified by the use of supplemental tests (e.g., Western blot, immunofluorescence assay) are considered to be infected.

Other specific tests for HIV-1 diagnosis are specified.

This definition of AIDS includes all adolescents and adults with HIV infection who have laboratory evidence of severe immunosuppression, defined as an

TABLE 1.1 Clinical Categories of the Proposed Revision of the HIV Classification System for Adults and Adolescents

Category A One or more of the conditions listed below occurring in an adolescent or adult with documented HIV infection. Conditions listed in categories B and C must not have occurred.
- Asymptomatic HIV infection
- Persistent generalized lymphadenopathy (PGL)
- Acute (primary) HIV infection with accompanying illness or history of acute HIV infection

Category B Symptomatic conditions occurring in an HIV-infected adolescent or adult which are not included among conditions listed in clinical category C and which meet at least one of the following criteria: (a) the conditions are attributed to HIV infection and/or are indicative of a defect in cell-mediated immunity; or (b) the conditions are considered by physicians to have a clinical course or management that is complicated by HIV infection. Examples of conditions in clinical category B include, but are not limited to:
- Bacterial endocarditis, meningitis, pneumonia, or sepsis
- Candidiasis, vulvovaginal; persistent (> 1 month duration), or poorly responsive to therapy
- Candidiasis, oropharyngeal (thrush)
- Cervical dysplasia, severe; or carcinoma
- Constitutional symptoms, such as fever ($\geq$38.5°C) or diarrhea lasting >1 month
- Hairy leukoplakia, oral
- Herpes zoster (shingles), involving at least two distinct episodes or more than one dermatome
- Idiopathic thrombocytopenic purpura
- Listeriosis
- *Mycobacterium tuberculosis*, pulmonary
- Nocardiosis
- Pelvic inflammatory disease
- Peripheral neuropathy

Category C Any condition listed in the 1987 surveillance case definition for AIDS and affecting an adolescent or adult (Table 1.3). The conditions in clinical category C are strongly associated with severe immunodeficiency, occur frequently in HIV-infected individuals, and cause serious morbidity or mortality.

HIV-infected persons should be classified based on both the lowest accurate (but not necessarily the most recent) CD4+ lymphocyte determination and the most severe clinical condition diagnosed regardless of the patients' current clinical condition (e.g., someone previously treated for oral or persistent vaginal candidiasis but who is now asymptomatic should be classified in clinical category B). The classification system is based on the absolute number of CD4+ cells but allows for the use of the CD4+ percent when the counts cannot be obtained or are outdated in view of the patients current clinical condition.

Source: Centers for Disease Control. 1992 revised classification system for HIV infection and expanded AIDS surveillance case definition for adolescents and adults (Draft) November 15, 1991.

TABLE 1.2 1992 Proposed Revision of the Classification System for HIV Infection and Expanded AIDS Surveillance Case Definition for Adolescents and Adults*

	CLINICAL CATEGORIES		
CD4+ Cell categories	(A) Asymptomatic, or persistent generalized lymphadenopathy, acute infection	(B) Symptomatic, not (A) or (C) conditions	(C) AIDS-indicator conditions**
≥ 500/mm³	A1	B1	C1
200-499/mm³	A2	B2	C2
<200/mm³ AIDS-indicator cell count	A3	B3	C3

*The shaded cells illustrate the expansion of the AIDS surveillance case definition. People with AIDS-indicator conditions (category C) are currently reportable to health department in every state and U.S territory. In addition to people with clinical category C conditions (categories C1, C2, and C3), persons with lymphocyte counts of less than 200/mm³ (categories A3 or B3) also will be reportable as AIDS cases.
**See Table 1.3

Source: Centers for Disease Control. 1992 revised classification system for HIV infection and expanded AIDS surveillance case definition for adolescents and adults (Draft) November 15, 1991.

absolute CD4+ lymphocyte count of less than 200/mm³ (0.2×10^9/L or 200/microliter) or a CD4+ percent of total lymphocytes of less than 14 if the absolute count is not available. The expanded surveillance case definition is consistent with the proposed 1992 revised HIV classification system. In this classification system, three laboratory categories are combined with three clinical categories (Table 1.1) to create nine combined subcategories (Table 1.2). Subcategories A3, B3, C1, C2, and C3 will be defined as actual AIDS for surveillance purposes. Thus, the clinical conditions specified in Categories A or B are not sufficient for an AIDS diagnosis unless the CD4+ count is below 200/mm³. The AIDS-indicator conditions of Category C are shown in Table 1.3. The expanded definition also includes people with the clinical conditions listed in the current definition. Implementation of the new AIDS surveillance case definition has been delayed because of controversy. For example, among voiced concerns are that the new definition may exclude conditions causing serious morbidity in HIV-infected women, and that CD4+ counts can vary widely even from day to day and laboratory to laboratory ("CDC's expanded case . . .", 1992).

TABLE 1.3 AIDS: Indicator Conditions in Adults/Adolescents

Candidiasis of bronchi, trachea, or lungs
Candidiasis, esophageal
Coccidioidomycosis, disseminated or extrapulmonary
Cryptococcosis, extrapulmonary
Cryptosporidiosis, chronic intestinal (> 1 month duration)
Cytomegalovirus disease (other than liver, spleen or nodes)
Cytomegalovirus retinitis (with loss of vision)
HIV encephalopathy
Herpes simplex: chronic ulcer(s) (> 1 month duration); or bronchitis, pneumonitis or esophagitis
Histoplasmosis, disseminated or extrapulmonary
Invasive cervical cancer
Isosporiasis, chronic intestinal (> 1 month duration)
Kaposi's sarcoma
Lymphoma, Burkitt's (or equivalent term)
Lymphoma, immunoblastic (or equivalent term)
Lymphoma, primary in brain
Mycobacterium avium complex or *M. kansasii*, disseminated or extrapulmonary
Mycobacterium tuberculosis, disseminated or extrapulmonary
Mycobacterium, other species or unidentified species, disseminated or extrapulmonary
Pneumocystis carinii pneumonia
Progressive multifocal leukoencephalopathy
Pulmonary tuberculosis
Recurrent pneumonia
Salmonella septicemia, recurrent
Toxoplasmosis of brain
Wasting syndrome due to HIV

Source: Centers for Disease Control. 1992 revised classification system for HIV infection and expanded AIDS surveillance case definition for adolescents and adults. (Draft) November 15, 1991: Centers for Disease Control (1992c). Addendum to the proposed expansion of the AIDS surveillance case definition, October 22, 1992.

STATISTICS AND PATTERNS IN THE UNITED STATES

The numbers of AIDS cases in the United States and the world continue to increase in adults, adolescents, and children. At the end of June 1992, a total of 230,179 AIDS cases in adults, adolescents and children had been reported in the United States, and of these 152,153 (66.1%) had died (Centers for Disease Control, 1992). An additional 125,000 persons in the United States estimated to have a CD4+ count <200 cells/microliter have not been counted as AIDS cases ("The second 100,000 cases," 1992). It is estimated that about 1 million persons in the United States have been infected with HIV and have antibodies to it. HIV seroprevalence varies according to the population that has been examined, such as applicants to the military, Job Corps participants, STD clinic attendees, potential blood donors, and so forth.

The CDC has analyzed characteristics of the first 100,000 cases of AIDS in this country, reported by August 1989, compared to the second 100,000 cases, reported through November 1991 ("The second 100,000 cases," 1992). The magnitude of the HIV epidemic is illustrated by the fact that the first 100,000 cases were reported in an approximate eight-year period, the second 100,000 cases in a two-year period. When comparing the first to the second 100,000 persons with AIDS the following can be observed:

1. The percentage of cases among homosexual-bisexual males decreased, while the percentage in heterosexual males and female injecting drug users increased;
2. There was a 44% increase in cases attributed to heterosexual transmission (5% to 7%);
3. The percentage of cases in women increased (9% to 12%);
4. The percentage of perinatally acquired pediatric cases increased (81% to 87%);
5. The percentage of cases among blacks and Hispanics increased (blacks, 27% to 31%; Hispanics, 15% to 17%);
6. The percentage of cases due to blood transfusions decreased in both adults (2.5% to 1.9%) and children (11% to 5.6%) ("The second 100,000 cases," 1992).

Those states having the highest numbers of adult AIDS cases are New York, California, Florida, Texas, and New Jersey. Those states reporting the fewest cases of AIDS in adults are North Dakota, South Dakota, Montana, Wyoming, and Vermont. Metropolitan areas having AIDS case rates of 50 or higher per 100,000 population in the one-year period of July 1991 to June 1992 were San Francisco, Miami, New York City, Jersey City, San Juan (Puerto Rico), Ft. Lauderdale, and Newark (Centers for Disease Control, 1992).

WORLDWIDE STATISTICS AND PATTERNS

For many countries, the reporting of AIDS cases is still less than reliable. As of July 1992, 501,272 cases of AIDS were reported worldwide (World Health Organization, 1992a). Because of underreporting, however, it is believed that at least 1.5 million adults and more than 500,000 pediatric cases of AIDS may have occurred. At least 9 to 11 million adults and about 1 million children are believed to have been infected with HIV worldwide. The World Health Organization projects that worldwide by the year 2000, there will be 30 million HIV-infected adults and 10 million HIV-infected children (Holmes, 1991; World Health Organization, 1992b). Countries with the largest number of AIDS cases (not taking into account the rate per population) are the United States, Tanzania, Uganda, Brazil, and France (World Health Organization, 1992a).

In geographic areas such as sub-Saharan Africa and some areas of the Caribbean, HIV transmission is predominately heterosexual and the male-to-female sex ratio is about 1:1, with perinatal transmission common. Countries with this pattern are known as Pattern II countries. HIV is also spreading rapidly through heterosexual transmission in many Latin American countries such as Brazil, Chile, and Honduras, and in Thailand and India. The worldwide patterns are described in detail elsewhere (Holmes, 1991).

HIV-2 appears endemic in such African countries as Senegal, Guinea-Bissau, Mali, Burkina Faso, Ivory Coast, Angola, and Mozambique. At this time, its primary means of transmission is through heterosexual contact (Holmes, 1991).

EXPOSURE CATEGORIES

Exposure categories are epidemiological groupings of data about AIDS cases. The CDC orders these categories in a hierarchical, mutually exclusive manner; thus cases with multiple characteristics that belong in more than one exposure category are assigned to the category listed first. In hierarchical order for adults and adolescents, these are

1. Men who have sex with men (formerly male homosexual-bisexual contact);
2. Injecting drug use (formerly intravenous drug use);
3. Men who have sex with men and use injecting drugs;
4. Hemophilia/coagulation disorder;
5. Heterosexual contact;
6. Recipient of transfusion of blood, blood components, or tissue;
7. Other/undetermined.

The number and percentage distribution of adult AIDS cases in the United States by exposure category are shown in Table 1.4 (Centers for Disease Control, 1992). Those specific to pediatric AIDS are discussed in Chapter 7.

TABLE 1.4 United States Adult/Adolescent AIDS Cases by Exposure Category as Reported to the CDC through June, 1992

Category	No.	Percent
Men who have sex with men	130,822	57.8
Injecting drug use	51,477	22.8
Men who have sex with men and inject drugs	14,487	6.4
Hemophilia/coagulation disorder	1,875	0.8
Heterosexual contact	14,045	6.2
Recipient of blood transfusion, blood components, or tissue	4,659	2.1
Other/undetermined	8,916	3.9
Total:	226,281	100

Source: Centers for Disease Control (1992). HIV/AIDS Surveillance, July, 1992, p. 1–18.

Men Who Have Sex With Men (MSWM)

AIDS was first identified among homosexual men presenting with Kaposi's sarcoma and *Pneumocystis carinii* pneumonia (Centers for Disease Control, 1981a, 1981b). Persons in the exposure category, men who report sexual contact with other men (MSWM), still comprise the largest percentage of cases of adult AIDS in the United States, accounting for about 58% alone and about 64% if those who also inject drugs are included (Centers for Disease Control, 1992). The vast majority of cases classified in this exposure category occurs in white males. There appears to be a plateau in reported cases in this category in New York, San Francisco, and Los Angeles; however, this trend is not observed in other areas with populations of 1 million or more (Karon & Berkelman, 1991). It is estimated that approximately 20% of males in this country may have at least one same-sex encounter during their lifetime (Lifson, 1992). Chu and coworkers (1992) point out that bisexual men differ from homosexual men in behavioral and epidemiological aspects of HIV infection. Among MSWM, more black* (41%) and Hispanic (31%) than white (21%) men with AIDS reported bisexual behavior, thus exposing their female partners to HIV. Nearly 25% of bisexual males with AIDS who died were married at the time of death. Bisexual men reported more IDU than homosexual men (20% vs. 9%). Bisexual males may be harder to reach with education and intervention programs as they are less likely to identify with gay organizations and may be less likely to perceive that they are at risk of HIV infection (Chu, Peterman, Doll, Buehler, & Curran, 1992).

Injecting Drug Use

This category was formerly known as intravenous drug use (IVDU). In 1991, the CDC changed the terminology to "injecting drug user" (IDU), or "drug injector" to describe those persons who use needles for self-injection of drugs not prescribed by a physician. This terminology would include those who "skin pop" and those who take such unprescribed drugs as anabolic steroids or vitamins by injection (Centers for Disease Control, 1991). IDU in females and heterosexual males accounts for about 22% of adult AIDS cases in the United States, and the combined category of MWSM and IDU accounts for another 6%. HIV may enter the blood of an IDU through use of a contaminated needle or syringe, through sharing drug apparatus of others, through multiple use of "cookers" to prepare syringes, or through drawing blood up into the syringe when preparing an injection (Page, 1990). There is a disproportionate overrepresentation of blacks and Hispanics in this exposure category when compared with their percentage

---

*The terms *black* rather than *African American* and *Hispanic* rather than *Latina* are used because of their epidemiological meaning.

in the United States at large. IDU is an important exposure category for women, as discussed in Chapter 3. Sex partners of IDUs who are not themselves IDUs are at risk for contracting HIV infection if they engage in unsafe sex, although they are not counted in this category (see Chapter 4).

Hemophilia/Coagulation Disorder

Most of the HIV-infected persons who have hemophilia or another blood-coagulation disorder acquired the infection through transfusion of factor concentrates used in treatment (Cohen, 1991b). The majority of persons with hemophilia in the United States became HIV seropositive between 1979 and 1982 (Hilgartner, 1987). While the spectrum of HIV infection has been seen in persons with hemophilia, the onset of HIV-associated clinical abnormalities and progression to AIDS has been slow (Alexander, Gabelnick, & Spieler, 1990).

Heterosexual Contact

Heterosexual contact includes all persons who do not fit into one of the exposure categories listed first in the hierarchy shown above and fit into the subcategories shown in Table 1.5. Worldwide, current estimates suggest that 75% of all HIV infection in adults have resulted from heterosexual transmission. It is believed that this will increase to over 90% by the year 2000 (World Health Organization, 1991). HIV transmission is more efficient from male to female than vice versa. Some persons are infected via this route after just one or a few unprotected sexual encounters; others remain uninfected after hundreds of such encounters with HIV-positive partners, thereby suggesting that cofactors influence HIV acquisition.

Duration of relationship in steady HIV-infected partners is of importance. Women in relationships of one to five years with HIV-infected partners are more

Table 1.5 Subcategories of the Adult/Adolescent AIDS Exposure Category "Heterosexual Contact," as Reported to the CDC through June 1992

Subcategory	N	% Of Subcategory
Sex with injecting drug user	7,451	53.1
Sex with bisexual male	743	5
Sex with person with hemophilia	113	0.8
Born in Pattern-II country	2,737	19.4
Sex with person born in Pattern-II country	190	1.4
Sex with transfusion recipient with HIV infection	274	2.0
Sex with HIV infected person, risk not specified	2,537	18.1
Subcategory Total:	14,045	

Source: Centers for Disease Control (1992) HIV/AIDS Surveillance, July, 1992; p. 1–18.

at risk than those so engaged for less than one year (Lazzarin, Saracco, Musicco, Nicolosi, & Italian Study Group on HIV Heterosexual Transmission, 1991). Latex condoms, used properly, are essential for prevention of HIV transmission (see Chapter 4). Heterosexual partners of IDUs who are not themselves IDUs are classified into the heterosexual-contact category. The number of cases reported to CDC in 1990 that occurred among sex partners of IDUs reflected an increase of nearly 32% from 1989 (Centers for Disease Control, 1991). In 1990, nearly two-thirds of the females and half of the males who had gotten AIDS through heterosexual contact had had a sex partner who was an IDU. Persons who use noninjecting drugs such as alcohol or crack cocaine often have impaired judgement leading to riskier sexual behavior (Centers for Disease Control, 1991). Heterosexual contact is an important exposure route for women and is discussed in detail in Chapter 3, as are the subcategories of this category.

Receipt of Transfusion of Blood, Blood Components or Tissue

Since routine screening of blood and blood products used for transfusion was instituted, the risk of acquisition of HIV through this route is now very low in the United States. It is estimated that the national average for the risk of acquiring HIV from a blood transfusion is .02%. This figure may be higher in areas such as San Francisco and New York and lower in low-HIV-prevalence areas (Perkins, 1989; Salzberg, Dolins, & Ruser, 1988). This is an important mode of HIV acquisition in persons over 55 years (Ferro & Salit, 1992).

Other/Undetermined

The category "other/undetermined" includes persons with no reported history of HIV exposure through any of the routes listed in the hierarchy of exposure categories. This category includes persons who are currently under investigation; those lost to follow-up through death, refusal to be interviewed, or other means; and those for whom investigation is complete but no exposure mode was identified. "Other" refers to persons who developed AIDS after exposure to HIV-infected blood within the health-care setting. Upon identification of an exposure mode, these cases are reclassified into the appropriate ones (Centers for Disease Control, 1992).

HIV TESTING AND COUNSELING

Tests to detect HIV include those to detect HIV antibodies (e.g., enzyme-linked immunosorbent assay [ELISA] and Western blot), HIV nucleic acids (e.g., polymerase chain reaction [PCR]), HIV antigens (e.g., antigen capture test), and HIV culture methods. The PCR can detect tiny amounts of HIV-1 DNA, and is proving useful in testing infants of HIV-positive mothers to distinguish between actual infection and maternal antibodies (see Chapters 7 and 10). In the United States at present, most testing involves the ELISA for screening and the Western blot as a confirmatory test for HIV-1. Both are usually performed on blood specimens. Testing for HIV antibodies will not detect those who are in the window period, as defined earlier. (Phair & Wolinsky, 1992; Sloand, Pitt, Chiarello, & Nemo, 1991). Pre- and post-test counseling preceded by informed consent are considered integral to the procedure of HIV testing. Partner notification of HIV-positive persons has engendered some controversy; however, with the advent of early treatment options such notification assumes new urgency ("Partner notification for preventing," 1991). (See VanDevanter, 1991 for an indepth discussion of testing and counseling.)

CLINICAL SPECTRUM

Overview and Classification

The effects of HIV on the immune system render the infected person susceptible to a variety of opportunistic infections and neoplasms. HIV-infected persons can show a broad spectrum of effects, ranging from acute infection through an asymptomatic phase through full-blown AIDS. The CDC has revised and expanded its classification system for HIV infection, largely based on the recommended clinical standard of obtaining CD4+ counts. Its rationale is that the CD4+ count consistently correlates with HIV-related immune dysfunction and disease progression and therefore is needed to guide medical management along with other parameters. Under this system, manifestations of HIV infection are classified into nine mutually exclusive groups, summarized in Table 1.2.

Natural History

The time period from infection with HIV to the development of symptoms or of CDC-defined AIDS can vary considerably. In some persons, the time between initial HIV infection and the development of AIDS can be as much as 10 years or more (Rosenberg & Fauci, 1991). A variety of factors may affect this period, including age, HLA type, viral strain, and more (Itescu et al., 1992). At this time, for the vast majority of HIV-infected persons, the ultimate outcome of AIDS is death (Lifson, Hessol, & Rutherford, 1992). However, the longer that persons with HIV infection can survive without progressing to AIDS and the longer persons can survive once they develop AIDS, the greater the hope for postponement of a fatal outcome (Cohen, 1991a).

In a detailed autopsy series of patients who died with AIDS, both disease processes and organ-system failures were analyzed. Opportunistic infections were found in 96% of patients and neoplasms in 65%. Cytomegalovirus (CMV) disease was found in 81%, candidiasis in 69%, *Pneumocystis carinii* pneumonia in 68%, herpes simplex virus disease in 39%, mycobacterial infection in 35%, and cryptococcal disease in 13%. More than half the patients died from respiratory failure followed by hypotension, neurologic disease, cardiac dysfunction, and others. Pneumonias due to *P. carinii*, bacteria, and CMV were the most frequent specific fatal processes in this series (McKenzie et al., 1991). In another autopsy series, the lung was also the most common site of infections, being affected in 90% of patients (Afessa et al., 1992).

Primary Infection

Primary infection with HIV may result in an acute flulike illness that is recognizable in about 10–15% of cases. While the time from infection to the onset of acute illness can be five days to three months, the most common is two to four weeks (Pinching, 1988; Tindall & Cooper, 1991). Symptoms typically include fever, malaise, sweating, sore throat, headache, joint pain, muscle pain, rash, and lymphadenopathy, although others may occur, including other neurological features (Tindall & Cooper, 1991).

Other Manifestations

Following initial infection, the most usual clinical course for the HIV-infected person is to enter an essentially asymptomatic phase. Some develop persistent generalized lymphadenopathy (PGL) before other symptoms develop. PGL may be seen alone or in conjunction with systemic symptoms such as fevers, fatigue, or night sweats (Cohen, 1991a). The most frequent lymph nodes involved are cervical, axillary, inguinal, supraclavicular, infraclavicular, and popliteal (Levine, 1988). Autoimmune thrombocytopenic purpura (AITP) may also be seen. AITP, in which easy bruisability with ecchymoses, petechiae, and platelet counts below 100,000/mm occur, has been observed in all exposure categories and may be a precursor to the imminent development of full-blown AIDS (Landonio et al., 1990).

Constitutional symptoms (including the HIV wasting syndrome) is a grouping that describes many persons who formerly would have been classified as having AIDS-related complex. HIV wasting syndrome is defined as "findings of profound involuntary weight loss >10% of baseline body weight plus either chronic diarrhea (at least two loose stools per day for 30 days or more) or chronic weakness and documented fever for 30 days or more, intermittent or constant in the absence of a concurrent illness or condition other than HIV infection that could explain the finding" ("Revision of the CDC," 1987, p. 12S).

Opportunistic Infections

Opportunistic infections, which have become hallmarks in persons with HIV infection, were not commonly seen in humans before the AIDS epidemic. Many infections are reactivations of previously acquired latent infections or infections with organisms that usually cause little or no pathogenicity in the immunocompetent person. Moreover, in persons with AIDS, these infections may have atypical locations, show more rapid progression, be more severe, be more likely to be disseminated, have a different disease presentation, and have a high density of organisms (Fishman, 1988; Glatt, Chirgwin, & Landesman, 1988). It is common for the HIV-infected person to have multiple infections. The fungal, parasitic, and viral infections are frequently not curable. Treatment usually aims at controlling the acute episode and providing long-term suppressive therapy. A brief overview of the most important infections seen in persons with AIDS will be presented below.

Pneumocystis carinii pneumonia (PCP).   PCP is generally self-limiting in healthy persons and is seen in those who are immunosuppressed by HIV or receiving chemotherapy or immunosuppressive therapy. *Pneumocystis carinii* is classified as a protozoan, but some believe it should be classified as a fungus. In persons with AIDS, PCP is the most common presenting opportunistic infection seen. The most common symptoms are relatively nonspecific and include fever, nonproductive cough, tachypnea, and shortness of breath (Glatt et al., 1988).

Standard therapy has included trimethoprim-sulfamethoxazole (TMP-SMX, co-trimoxazole, Bactrim, or Septra), pentamidine, and dapsone, while trimetrexate, piritexim, fansidar, difluoromethylornithine, and clindamycin plus primaquine have also been tried (Hughes, 1991). Pentamidine has been used increasingly in aerosol form, especially for prophylaxis, but is not effective against extrapulmonary *P. carinii* infection, which is rare but increasing (Cotton, 1991). In compliant patients, aerosol pentamidine can be 90% effective in preventing a first PCP occurrence. Corticosteroids are being explored as adjunctive therapy for PCP, particularly for those with severe hypoxemia (McGowan, Chesney, Crossley, & LaForce, 1992). A hydroxynaphthoquinone compound, 566C80, has received investigational new drug status from the FDA for treatment of mild to moderately severe PCP (Hughes, 1992).

Toxoplasmosis.   Toxoplasmosis is caused by the protozoan *Toxoplasma gondii* and is the most common cause of focal encephalitis in persons with AIDS. This encephalitis is the second most common neurological disease in AIDS. In HIV-infected persons, toxoplasmosis most often results from reactivation of previously acquired latent infection (Dannemann et al., 1992). The major signs and symptoms include fever, headache, hemiparesis, seizures, ataxia, aphasia, movement disorders, visual field loss, confusion, lethargy, psychosis, global cognitive impairment, delusions, and coma. Multiorgan involvement is common. Standard treatment is accomplished with pyrimethamine and sulfadiazine, but there is a high frequency of complications and relapse (Israelski & Remington, 1988; Lee & Safrin, 1992). Promising new therapies include the hydroxynaphthoquinone 566-C80, clindamycin, doxycycline, and interferon gamma (Cotton, 1991; Dannemann et al., 1992; Sweeney, Peters, & Main, 1991).

Cryptosporidiosis. Cryptosporidiosis is caused by the protozoan parasite *Cryptosporidium* spp. In persons with AIDS, it causes choleralike diarrhea with bowel movements of up to 20 or more per day with fluid volume losses of as much as 10 to 15 liters per day (Rolston & Fainstein, 1986). While diarrhea is the major effect, lung colonization and involvement of the gall bladder and biliary tree have been seen. Therapy, largely ineffective, has consisted of spiramycin, eflornithine, and standard antidiarrheic agents. Potential new therapies are hyperimmune bovine colostrum, oral paromomycin, diclazuril, and somatostatin analogues such as octreotide, vapreotide or sandostatin (Romeu et al., 1991).

Isospora belli. This protozoan parasite causes isosporiasis with symptoms very similar to those of cryptosporidiosis. While recurrences are common and prophylactic regimens may be needed, isosporiasis does respond to treatment with oral trimethoprim-sulfamethoxazole (TMP-SMX) (Glatt et al., 1988).

Microsporidiosis. Microsporidia are obligate intracellular spore-forming protozoa that are extremely rare in persons who are not HIV-infected (Weber et al., 1992). Microsporidiosis is not currently considered an AIDS-defining disease but is being increasingly recognized as responsible for persistent diarrhea in HIV-infected persons and affecting other tissues such as muscle and the eye. Different microsporidia species appear to be responsible for various clinical manifestations (Shadduck, 1989; Weber et al., 1992). Recent treatment approaches include metronidazole and albendazole (a broad-spectrum antiparasitic agent) (Cotton, 1991).

Cryptococcosis. *Cryptococcus neoformans* is classified under the fungi and is the fourth most commonly recognized cause of life-threatening infections in the person with AIDS, developing in an estimated 6% to 13% (Murray & Mills, 1990). The lung is the usual primary infection site. Meningitis is the most frequent life-threatening manifestation, developing in up to 90% of patients with AIDS who are infected with *C. neoformans* (Levitz, 1991; Powderly, 1992). Pneumonia is another frequent consequence, although virtually any organ system may be affected, and disease may be disseminated. Manifestations are often subtle and may be overlooked (Levitz, 1991). Antifungal agents such as amphotericin B, 5-flucytosine, and fluconazole compose the major therapeutic approaches. Long-term maintenance is necessary, and relapses are common (Powderly, 1992).

Candidiasis. Candidiasis of the oral cavity and esophagus are the most common fungal infection of HIV-infected persons (80–95%) and is caused by *Candida albicans* (Stevens, Greene, & Lang, 1991). Oropharyngeal candidiasis may be seen in several forms, the most common usually synonymous with thrush, and white removable plaques can be seen on the oral mucosa (Greenspan,

Greenspan, & Winkler, 1990). Oral candidiasis is considered a prognostic indicator of progressive disease. Esophageal candidiasis meets criteria for an AIDS diagnosis. Esophageal candidiasis is a major cause of dysphagia, painful swallowing, and retrosternal pain, leading to impaired nutrition (Diamond, 1991). Treatment for oral candidiasis can include topical treatment with nystatin or clotrimazole, or systemic therapy with ketoconazole or fluconazole and usually responds well to therapy (Bagdades, 1991; Diamond, 1991). Esophageal candidiasis is more difficult to treat, and currently ketoconazole or fluconazole are agents of choice (Bagdades, 1991; Galgiani, 1990). Daily doses of fluconazole may prevent recurrent episodes (Stevens et al., 1991).

Tuberculosis (TB).   In the United States, tuberculosis (caused by *Mycobacterium tuberculosis*) had declined over a period of more than 30 years, but by 1986, the number of cases began to increase. This increase is attributed to the increasing numbers of HIV-infected persons. CDC recommendations for a definition of purified protein derivative (PPD) tuberculin positivity may underestimate the true TB infection rate in HIV-positive persons (Graham et al., 1992). In one study of patients with tuberculosis in 20 clinics, subjects had an HIV-seroprevalence ranging from 0% to 46.3%. Most HIV-infected patients in the study had pulmonary TB, but HIV infection was more frequent in patients with extrapulmonary TB (Onorato, McCray, & the Field Services Branch, 1992). The increase in TB in this country poses an additional risk to health-care workers. Multidrug-resistant strains have become common. Combinations of chemoprophylaxis have been suggested for TB control in persons with HIV infection, such as rifampin, pyra-zinamide, isoniazid, and ethambutol. Additionally, long-term drug therapy with isoniazid has been suggested for at least 12 months and may be needed throughout the life of patients (Barnes, Bloch, Davidson, & Snider, 1991).

Mycobacterium Avium Complex.   *Mycobacterium avium* complex (MAC) consists of two organisms, *M. avium* and *M. intracellulare*, although some nonclassified strains may also be included (Wolinsky, 1992). Disseminated MAC infection is considered the most common AIDS-associated systemic bacterial infection (Ellner, Goldberger, & Parenti, 1991; Hornsburgh, 1991). At first it was thought that MAC was merely an opportunistic colonizer, but now it is recognized as making a substantial contribution to morbidity and mortality in persons with AIDS (Ellner, Goldberger, & Parenti, 1991; Hornsburgh, 1991). The most prevalent symptoms of MAC infection are fever, night sweats, anorexia, malaise, weight loss, and weakness. Cough, headache, diarrhea, and lymphadenopathy may be seen. Single-agent therapy is rarely successful. Multidrug combinations of ambutol, rifabutin, ciprofloxacin, amikacin, or clofazamine are often used. Agents being evaluated include azithromycin, clarithromycin, rifapentine, WIN57273, and sparfloxacin (Cohen, 1991c; Ellner et al., 1991; Smith, Quinn, Strober, Janoff, & Masur, 1992).

Cytomegalovirus. Active cytomegalovirus (CMV) infection develops in about 90% of persons with AIDS. While CMV infection may involve multiple organs simultaneously or be systemic, predilection is for the eye, gastrointestinal tract, lung, brain, and adrenal glands (Drew, 1992). CMV retinitis is the leading cause of vision loss in persons with AIDS, occurring in about 20% of patients with AIDS. Ganciclovir (DHPG, Cytovene) produces stabilization or improvement in up to 80%, with long-term maintenance therapy being necessary for the rest of the patient's life. It does, however, produce significant side effects in patients, particularly since its toxicity overlaps with zidovudine. At present, ganciclovir is widely used as the first-line treatment. Foscarnet (trisodium phosphonoformate, Foscavir), inhibits specific enzymes in CMV and also in HIV. AZT and foscarnet have little overlap and may have additive benefits. Recent studies show that foscarnet may be superior to ganciclovir for initial therapy. New approaches, such as BW 256-U87 and anti-CMV monoclonal antibodies, continue to be evaluated (Hirsch, 1992; "Studies of Ocular Complications," 1992).

Herpes Simplex Virus (HSV), Types 1 and 2. Although overlap exists, HSV-1 is responsible for oral-facial lesions, visceral infections, and encephalitis, while HSV-2 is associated with genital-tract infections and neonatal disease. Primary infection is often acquired during the first decade of life, after which the virus lies dormant until it is reactivated following stress, including decreased cellular immunity ("Herpes simplex virus," 1989). HIV-infected persons have a high prevalence of infection with the herpes simplex virus, which may cause perianal infections, esophageal lesions and ulcerations, proctitis, oral lesions, and keratitis. The lesions can be painful, and the resultant complications depend upon the site and extent of infection. Standard treatment is with acyclovir (Zovirax) (Drew, Buhles, & Erlich, 1988; Safrin, Ashley, Houlihan, Cusick, & Mills, 1991; Smith et al., 1992).

Neoplasms

Neoplasms are frequent in many congenital and acquired immunodeficiency states, as well as in AIDS. The malignancies most frequently associated with HIV infection are Kaposi's sarcoma and malignant lymphomas, particularly of the central nervous system. Other malignancies seen with increased frequency in AIDS include oral cancer, anorectal carcinoma, testicular cancer, and small-cell carcinoma of the lung (Biggar, 1991; Cohen, 1991a).

Kaposi's Sarcoma (KS). KS is the most frequently observed malignancy among persons with AIDS. While the proportion of persons with AIDS who develop KS has decreased, the total number of cases has increased (Cotton, 1991; Friedman-Kien, 1988). KS continues to be most prevalent among homosexual males with AIDS. Within this group, the percentage with KS was twice as high for whites as for blacks and higher for those between 25 and 44 years than any other age group (Beral et al., 1990). It has been postulated that KS may be due to an infectious sexually transmitted agent other than HIV or that cofactors such as amyl nitrite may play a role (Beral et al., 1990). Recently it has been suggested that human papillomavirus (HPV) may play a role (Huang et al., 1992).

The type of KS seen in connection with HIV infection, unlike those that had been previously recognized, is more epidemic. Lesions may range from flat macular patches to papules, plaques, and elevated nodules ranging in color from faint pink to dark purple to bluish brown, growing quickly in size and number (Friedman-Kien, 1988). Lymphatic obstruction leading to lymphedema can cause discomfort. Other organ systems and sites can be affected, such as the oral cavity, lymph nodes, gastrointestinal (GI) tract, lung, liver, and heart. GI involvement may be seen in as many as 75% of AIDS-related KS at autopsy, and respiratory tract lesions occur in about 40% of cases (Schwartz, 1988). Systemic signs and symptoms such as fever, weight loss, diarrhea, and intermittent fevers may be seen (Friedman-Kien, 1988). Treatment has been by surgical removal of lesions and drug therapy, such as with the vinca alkaloids. Alpha interferon has shown decreases in both tumor size and number. Other therapies being investigated include fumagillin analogues and pentasan polysulfate (Cotton, 1991; Lane et al., 1990).

Lymphomas. An increased incidence of non-Hodgkin's lymphomas is frequently observed in association with HIV infection. Most frequently seen are primary central nervous system (CNS) lymphomas and systemic lymphomas, including immuno-blastic lymphoma and Burkitt's lymphoma ("Epstein-Barr virus," 1991). The Epstein-Barr virus (EBV) is known to be associated with many lympho-proliferative disorders and appears to be consistently present in primary CNS lymphomas in persons with AIDS and in 30–50% of systemic lymphomas associated with AIDS (MacMahon et al., 1991). Additionally lymphomas may develop subsequent to long-term antiviral therapy for HIV infection (Raub, 1990).

Primary lymphoma of the CNS has been considered a defining criterion for AIDS since the beginning of the epidemic. Patients often present with confusion, lethargy, memory loss, cranial nerve palsies, hemiparesis, headache, or seizures, although onset may be more subtle (Levy, Bredesen, & Rosenblum, 1990). Systemic lymphomas may present with symptoms such as fever, night sweats, or weight loss. Other specific symptoms depend on the sites involved (Cohen, 1991a). Treatment is generally unsatisfactory.

Nervous System Effects

It was not until about 1985 that the impact of HIV on the nervous system began to be fully appreciated. With advanced HIV disease, progressive and global involvement of the nervous system is seen (Ruttimann, Hilti, Spinas, & Dubach, 1991). Rosenberg and Fauci (1991) note that HIV is present in the central nervous system of all HIV-infected individuals, regardless of the state of infection. The macrophage or microglial cell is the key cell associated with HIV infection in the brain. The exact mechanisms remain elusive but may involve damage from toxic factors such as cytokines, through suppression of neuronal cell function or other mechanisms (Mak & Wigzell, 1991; Rosenberg & Fauci, 1991). HIV-associated neurological dysfunction can result from

1. direct infection with HIV
2. opportunistic infections
3. primary or metastatic neoplasms
4. cerebrovascular etiologies
5. metabolic encephalopathies
6. complications secondary to therapy (Cohen, 1991a).

The most common cause of neurological dysfunction in persons who are HIV-infected is AIDS dementia complex (ADC) or HIV encephalopathy (Dalakas, Wichman, & Sever, 1989). Cognitive impairment is generally seen first and may be manifested as forgetfulness, difficulty in maintaining attention, memory retrieval problems, and confusion. Behavioral aspects may include personality changes, apathy, and depression. Later, motor functioning may be impaired (Dalakas, Wichman, & Sever, 1989; Krikorian & Wrobel, 1991). A recent report suggests that executive function deficit may also occur and that attentional disorders are prevalent, providing rationale for treatment with psychostimulant medication (Krikorian & Wrobel, 1991). HIV infection may be an important cause of dementia in the older person (Ferro & Salit, 1992).

Vacuolar myopathy, predominately affecting the lateral and posterior columns of the thoracic spinal cord; progressive multifocal leukoencephalopathy, caused by the JC virus; neuromuscular dysfunctions; peripheral neuropathies; and myopathies may also be seen in the person with AIDS, contributing to various types of dysfunction (Cohen, 1991a; Collier et al., 1992). A recent study demonstrated CNS involvement in most of the participants with early HIV infection but found clinically significant impairment uncommon, although this issue is far from settled (Collier et al., 1992).

In one report, autonomic dysfunction was identified in 60% of HIV-infected patients. Thus, some nonspecific symptoms, such as dizziness, sweating, bladder dysfunction, and altered gastrointestinal motility, may, at least in part, be due to autonomic alterations (Ruttimann et al., 1991).

TREATMENT

Pharmacologic treatment of HIV infection and AIDS includes both direct and indirect approaches. In-depth discussion of potential and current therapeutic agents is found elsewhere (see Cohen, 1991a; Cohen, 1991b). Approaches to the treatment of HIV infection/AIDS may be conceptualized as follows:

1. therapy aimed at combating HIV
2. modifying the biologic response of the host and modulating the immune response
3. therapy aimed at the treatment or prevention of opportunistic infections and their reoccurrence
4. therapy aimed at the treatment of neoplasms
5. combinations of these (Cohen, 1991a; Cohen, 1991b)

Only the first two approaches are discussed below since the others have been previously discussed in this chapter.

Therapy Aimed at Combating HIV

Knowledge obtained from basic science research about the life cycle of HIV has led to the development of agents that could have activity in blocking HIV at specific points in that cycle. Currently, a major approach is to use multiple combinations of drugs and therapies to attack simultaneously multiple sites in the HIV replication cycle, to overcome viral resistance, reduce toxic effects, and deliver the drug to multiple cell types (Cohen, 1991a, Cohen, 1991b). Unfortunately, little of the drug research and few of the clinical trials have included women and children until very recently.

As of November 1992, only three drugs had been specifically licensed by the Food and Drug Administration for activity against HIV. Zidovudine (3'-azido-3'deoxythymidine, azidothymidine, AZT, Retrovir, ZDV) was the first antiviral agent approved for AIDS treatment in adults, only three years after AIDS was recognized to be caused by HIV. While available under certain conditions for treatment in children with AIDS, it was not licensed for such use until 1990. On October 9, 1991, ddI (dideoxyinosine, didanosine, Videx) was approved simultaneously for use in children and adults (Fauci, 1992). In 1992, zalcitabine (HIVID), formerly known as dideoxycytidine or ddC was approved as a treatment option for adults with advanced HIV infection (Nightingale, 1992).

Zidovudine is a nucleoside analogue resembling thymidine that preferentially binds to HIV reverse transcriptase, leading to both competetive inhibition and chain termination of HIV deoxyribonucleic acid (DNA) (Cohen, 1991b; Yarchoan, Mitsuya, & Broder, 1988). Although initially zidovudine was FDA-approved only for use in persons with CD4+ cell counts of less than 200/mm³, the use has broadened, and it is now available to those with CD4+ cell counts of less than 500/mm³. It has been recognized that lower dosages can be used for efficacy with less toxicity (Volberding et al., 1990). The most severe adverse effects of zidovudine are the result of hematologic and myopathic effects that may require the temporary or permanent cessation of zidovudine therapy, although constitutional symptoms such as nausea are frequently complaints. Diminished effects and resistance may be seen after prolonged use (Fauci, 1992; Nightingale, 1991). The clinical benefits are well documented, and zidovudine reduces morbidity for both asymptomatic patients and those who are already symptomatic. However, the best time to begin zidovudine therapy has not been determined. A recently reported controlled study comparing early and late therapy over a four-year period indicated that early zidovudine therapy reduced the rate of development of clinical AIDS substantially. However, it did not improve survival. If the benefits of zidovudine are time limited, it might be better to delay the start of therapy, switch to another drug or use a combination of therapies (Corey & Fleming, 1992; Hamilton et al., 1992).

Study of zidovudine in HIV-infected pregnant women and newborns to examine its safety and tolerance has begun. A second goal of AZT studies involving pregnant women is to try to prevent transmission of HIV from the mother to infant (National Institute of Allergy and Infectious Diseases, 1991).

The drug ddI is indicated for both children (over six months) and adults with advanced HIV infection who have developed deterioration during zidovudine therapy or have become intolerant to zidovudine (Nightingale, 1991). It also is a nucleoside analogue that acts against HIV by inhibiting the enzyme reverse transcriptase. The major toxic effects have been pancreatitis and peripheral neuropathy, although others have been noted (Cohen, 1991b; Lee & Safrin, 1992; Nightingale, 1991). Zidovudine and ddI as combination therapy may be even more effective than either used alone (Fauci, 1992).

Zalcitabine is indicated for use in adult patients with advanced HIV infection (CD4+ cell counts at or below 300/mm^3) who show signs of clinical or immunological deterioration. It is currently meant to be used in combination with zidovudine. The major clinical toxic effects are peripheral neuropathy, stomatitis, constitutional symptoms, and pancreatitis (to a lesser degree than with ddI) (Nightingale, 1992; Saag, 1992).

Biologic Response Modification

Modification of the biologic response to HIV infection includes efforts to restore, improve, or modify the response of the immune system of hosts who are affected by HIV. Theoretically, this modification would protect against the development of HIV-related opportunistic infections and neoplasms (Cohen, 1991c). Agents such as the interferons, interleukins, isoprinosine, and Imreg are all being examined alone or in combination with zidovudine and/or ddI.

Others

New agents continue to be evaluated alone and in combination. For a review of the major drugs in clinical trials, please see J. Cohen (1991). At present, about 88 drugs are in testing ("AIDS research intensifies," 1992). Other, less traditional therapies are often used by HIV-infected persons. Well-designed studies of their effectiveness have not yet been published. However, as for any person, it is important to maximize the best possible overall mental and physical health through health-promoting activities such as good nutrition, adequate rest, exercise, and stress reduction.

VACCINE DEVELOPMENT

One of the requirements for a successful vaccine against HIV is that it will have the ability to induce protection against most or all of the strains of HIV (Wigzell, 1991). In 1989, it was demonstrated that a vaccine can protect rhesus monkeys against simian immunodeficiency virus. A vaccine is desired that will both prevent HIV infection in unifected people and slow or stop disease progression in those who are already HIV-infected. Most of the studies to date have focused on safety and the capacity to evoke an immune response, but effectiveness has not been examined. There is urgency in examining efficacy, particularly in populations at greatest risk. The present strategy appears to be that multiple vaccines will be tested at multiple sites in the United States and elsewhere to answer questions regarding safety and effectiveness of an HIV vaccine in humans (Taylor, 1992).

SUMMARY

This chapter has presented a brief overview of the major information necessary to understand HIV infection and AIDS in general before the issues in women, adolescents, and children are explored. Behaviors such as risky sexual contacts and injecting drug use continue to be the major source of HIV acquisition and transmission. Clinically, many types of opportunistic infections tend to be difficult to treat. There may be a relatively long asymptomatic period for those infected, and careful early selection of therapies are making longer lifespans more of a reality. Prevention continues to hinge on education for behavioral change, safer sexual contacts, screening of blood donations and changing indications for blood transfusion, research into ways of interfering with perinatal transmission, and development of prophylactic medication and/or vaccines.

REFERENCES

Afessa, B., Greaves, W., Green, W., Olopoenia, L., Delapenha, R., Saxinger, C., & Frederick, W. (1992). Autopsy findings in HIV-infected inner-city patients. *Journal of Acquired Immune Deficiency Syndromes, 5*, 132–136.
AIDS research intensifies: 88 drugs in testing, 14 approved. (1992, January). *Pharmacist*, 14.
Alexander, N. J., Gabelnick, H. L., & Spieler, J. M. (Eds.) (1990). *Heterosexual transmission of AIDS*. New York: Wiley-Liss.

Bagdades, E. K. (1991). Current treatment of opportunistic infections in HIV disease. *AIDS Care, 3,* 461–456.

Barnes, P. F., Bloch, A. B., Davidson, P. T., & Snider, D. E., Jr. (1991). Tuberculosis and HIV infection. *New England Journal of Medicine, 323,* 1884.

Bednarik, D. P., & Folks, T. M. (1992). Mechanisms of HIV-1 latency. *AIDS, 6,* 3–16.

Beral, V., Peterman, T. A., Berkelman, R. L., & Jaffe, H. W. (1990). Kaposi's sarcoma among persons with AIDS: a sexually transmitted infection? *Lancet, 335,* 123–128.

Biggar, R. J. (1990). Cancer in acquired immunodeficiency syndrome: An epidemiological assessment. *Seminars in Oncology, 17,* 251–260.

CDC's expanded AIDS case definition sparks controversy. *AIDS Alert, 7*(5), 65–71.

Centers for Disease Control. (1985). Provisional public health inter-agency recommendations for screening blood and plasma for antibody to the virus causing acquired immunodeficiency syndrome. *Morbidity and Mortality Weekly Report, 34,* 1–5.

Centers for Disease Control. (1985). Revision of the case definition of acquired immunodeficiency syndrome for national reporting—United States. *Morbidity and Mortality Weekly Report, 34,* 373–375.

Centers for Disease Control. (1988). Update: Serological testing for antibody to human immunodeficiency virus. *Morbidity and Mortality Weekly Report, 36,* 833–840.

Centers for Disease Control. (1989). MMWR interpretation and use of the Western blot assay for serodiagnosis of human immunodeficiency virus type 1 infections. *Morbidity and Mortality Weekly Report, 38,* 1–7.

Centers for Disease Control. (1981a). Kaposi's sarcoma and pneumocystis pneumonia among homosexual men—New York and California. *Morbidity and Mortality Weekly Report, 31,* 507–515.

Centers for Disease Control. (1991a). *HIV/AIDS prevention, 2*(2), 1–8.

Centers for Disease Control. (1991b). Drug use and sexual behaviors among sex partners of injecting-drug users—United States, 1988–1990. *Morbidity and Mortality Weekly Reports, 40,* 855–860.

Centers for Disease Control. (15 November 1991). 1992 revised classification system for HIV infection and expanded AIDS survillance case definition for adolescents and adults. Draft (unpaginated).

Centers for Disease Control. (1992a, July). *HIV/AIDS surveillance report,* 1–22.

Centers for Disease Control. (1992b). Pneumocystis pneumonia-Los Angeles. *Morbidity and Mortality Weekly Reports, 30,* 250–252.

Centers for Disease Control. (1992c). Addendum to the proposed expansion of the AIDS surveillance case definition, October 22, 1992.

Chu, S. Y., Peterman, T. A., Doll, L. S., Buehler, J. W., & Curran, J. (1992). AIDS in bisexual men in the United States: Epidemiology and transmission to women. *American Journal of Public Health, 82,* 220–224.

Classification system for human T-lymphotropic virus type-III/lymphadenopathy-associated virus infections. (1986). *Morbidity and Mortality Weekly Report, 35,* 334–339.

Cohen, F. L. (1991a). The clinical spectrum of HIV infection and its treatment. In J. D. Durham & F. L. Cohen (Eds.), *The person with AIDS: Nursing perspectives* (2nd ed.) (pp. 135–205). New York: Springer.

Cohen, F. L. (1991b). The etiology and epidemiology of HIV infection and AIDS. In J. D. Durham & F. L. Cohen (Eds.), *The person with AIDS: Nursing perspectives* (2nd ed.) (pp. 1–59). New York: Springer.

Cohen, F. L. (1991c). The pharmacologic treatment of HIV infection and AIDS in adults. *Nursing Clinics of North America, 26*(2), 315–329.

Cohen, J. (1991). AIDS vaccine meeting: International trials soon. *Science, 254,* 647.

Collier, A. C., Marra, C., Coombs, R. W., Claypoole, K., Cohen, W., Longstreth, W. T., Jr., et al. (1992). Central nervous system manifestations in human immunodeficiency virus infection without AIDS. *Journal of Acquired Immune Deficiency Syndromes, 5*, 229–241.

Corey, L., & Fleming, T. R. (1992). Treatment of HIV infection—progress in perspective. *New England Journal of Medicine, 326*, 484–486.

Cotton, P. (1991). Medicine's arsenal in battling "dominant dozen," other AIDS-associated opportunistic infections. *Journal of the American Medical Association, 266*, 1476–1481.

Dalakas, M. C., Illa, I., Pezeshkpour, G. H., Laukaitis, J. P., Cohen, B., & Griffin, J. L. (1990). Mitochondrial myopathy caused by long-term zidovudine therapy. *New England Journal of Medicine, 322*, 1098–1105.

Dalakas, M., Wichman, A., & Sever, J. (1989). AIDS and the nervous system. *Journal of the American Medical Association, 261*, 2396–2399.

Dannemann, B., McCutchan, J. A., Israelski, P., Antoniskis, D., Leport, C., Luft, B., Nussbaum, J., Clumeck, N., Morlat, P., Chiu, J., Vilde, J-L, Orellana, M., Feigal, D., Bartok, A., Heseltine, P., Leedom, J., Remington, J., and the California Collaborative Treatment Group. (1992). Treatment of toxoplasmic encephalitis in patients with AIDS. *Annals of Internal Medicine, 116*, 33–43.

Diamond, D. D. (1991). The growing problem of mycoses in patients infected with the human immunodeficiency virus. *Reviews of Infectious Diseases, 13*, 480–486.

Drew, W. L. (1992). Cytomegalovirus infection in patients with AIDS. *Clinical Infectious Diseases, 14*, 608–615.

Drew, W. L., Buhles, W., & Erlich, K. S. (1988). Herpesvirus infections (Cytomegalovirus, herpes simplex virus, varicella-zoster virus) *Infectious Disease Clinics of North America, 2*(2), 495–509.

Durham, J. D., & Cohen, F. L. (1991). *The person with AIDS: Nursing perspectives* (2nd ed.). New York: Springer.

Ellner, J. J., Goldberger, M. J., & Parenti, D. M. (1991). *Mycobacterium avium* infection and AIDS: A therapeutic dilemma in rapid evolution. *Journal of Infectious Diseases, 163*, 1326–1335.

Epstein-Barr virus and AIDS-associated lymphomas. (1991). *Lancet, 338*, 979–981.

Fauci, A. S. (1992). Combination therapy for HIV infection: Getting closer. *Annals of Internal Medicine, 116*, 85–86.

Ferro, S. & Salit, I. E. (1992). HIV infection in patients over 55 years of age. *Journal of Acquired Immune Deficiency Syndromes, 5*, 348–355.

Fishman, J. A. (1988). An approach to pulmonary infection in AIDS. *Hospital Practice, 23*(4), 196–204.

Friedland, G., Kahl, P., Saltzman, B., Rogers, M., Feiner, C., Mayers, M., Schable, C., & Klein, R. S. (1990). Additional evidence for lack of transmission of HIV infection by close interpersonal (casual) contact. *AIDS, 4*, 639–644.

Friedman-Kien, A. E. (1988). AIDS-related Kaposi's sarcoma. *Recent Results in Cancer Research, 112*, 27–36.

Galgiani, J. N. (1990). Fluconazole, a new antifungal agent. *Annals of Internal Medicine, 110*, 937–940.

Glatt, A. E., Chirgwin, K., & Landesman, S. H. (1988). Treatment of infections associated with human immunodeficiency virus. *New England Journal of Medicine, 318*, 1439–1448.

Graham, N. M. H., Nelson, K. E., Solomon, L., Bonds, M., Rizzo, R. T., Scavotto, J., Astemborski, J., & Vlahov, D. (1992). Prevalence of tuberculin positivity and skin test anergy in HIV-1-seropositive and -seronegative intravenous drug users. *Journal of the American Medical Association, 267*, 369–373.

Greenberg, P. (1992). Immunopathogenesis of HIV infection. *Hospital Practice, 27*(2), 109–124.

Greenspan, J. S., Greenspan, D., & Winkler, J. R. (1990). Diagnosis and management of the oral manifestations of HIV infection and AIDS. In M. A. Sande & P. A. Volberding (Eds.), *The medical management of AIDS* (2nd ed.) (pp. 131–144). Philadelphia: Saunders.

Hamilton, J. D., Hartigan, P. M., Simberkoff, M. S., Day, P. L., Diamond, G. R., Dickinson, M. D., et al. (1992). A controlled trial of early versus late treatment with zidovudine in symptomatic human immunodeficiency virus infection. *New England Journal of Medicine, 326*, 437–443.

Haseltine, W. A. (1991). Molecular biology of the human immunodeficiency virus type 1. *FASEB Journal, 5*, 2349–2360.

Herpes simplex virus latency. (1989). *Lancet 1*, 194–195.

Higgins, D. L., Galavotti, C., O'Reilly, K. R., Schnell, D. J., Moore, M., Rugg, D. L., & Johnson, R. (1991). Evidence for the effects of HIV antibody counseling and testing on risk behaviors. *Journal of the American Medical Association, 266*, 2419–2429.

Hilgartner, M. W. (1987). AIDS and hemophilia. *New England Journal of Medicine, 317*, 1153–1154.

Hirsch, M. (1992). The treatment of cytomegalovirus in AIDS—more than meets the eye. *New England Journal of Medicine, 326*, 264–266.

Holmes, K. K. (1991). The changing epidemiology of HIV transmission. *Hospital Practice, 26*(11), 153–178.

Hook, E. W., III, Cannon, R. O., Nahmias, A. J., Lee, F. F., Campbell, C. H., Jr., Glasser, D. & Quinn, T. C. (1992). Herpes simplex virus infection as a risk factor for human immunodeficiency virus infection in heterosexuals. *Journal of Infectious Diseases, 165*, 251–255.

Horsburgh, C. R., Jr. 1991). *Mycobacterium avium* complex infection in the acquired immunodeficiency syndrome. *New England Journal of Medicine, 324*, 1332–1338.

Huang, Y. Q., Li, J. J., Rush, M. G., Poiesz, B. J., Nicolaides, A., Jacobson, M., et al. (1992). HPV-16-related DNA sequences in Kaposi's sarcoma. *Lancet, 339*, 515–518.

Hughes, W. T. (1991). Prevention and treatment of *Pneumocystis carinii* pneumonia. *Annual Review of Medicine, 42*, 287–295.

Hughes, W. T. (1992). A new drug (566C80) for the treatment of *Pneumocystis carinii* pneumonia. *Annals of Internal Medicine, 116*, 953–954.

Imagawa, D. T., Lee, M. H., Wolinsky, S. M., Sano, K., Morales, F., Kwok, B. S., Sninsky, J. J., Nishanian, P. G., Giorgi, J., Fahey, J. L., Dudley, J., Visscher, B. R. & Detels, R. (1989). Human immunodeficiency virus type 1 infection in homosexual men who remain seronegative for prolonged periods. *New England Journal of Medicine, 320*, 1458–1462.

Israelski, D. M., & Remington, J. S. (1988). Toxoplasmic encephalitis in patients with AIDS. *Infectious Disease Clinics of North America, 2*(2), 429–445.

Itescu, S., Mathur-Wagh, U., Skovron, M. L., Brancato, L. J., Marmor, M., Zeleniuch-Jacquotte, A., & Winchester, R. (1992). HLA-B35 is associated with accelerated progression to AIDS. *Journal of Acquired Immune Deficiency Syndromes, 5*, 37–45.

Johnson, M. A., & Cann, A. J. (1992). Molecular determination of cell tropism of human immunodeficiency virus. *Clinical Infectious Diseases, 14*, 747–755.

Karon, J. M., & Berkelman, R. (1991). The geographic and ethnic diversity of AIDS incidence trends in homosexual/bisexual men in the United States. *Journal of Acquired Immune Deficiency Syndromes, 4*, 1179–1189.

Krikorian, R., & Wrobel, A. J. (1991). Cognitive impairment in HIV infection. *AIDS, 5*, 1501–1507.

Landonio, G., Galli, M., Nosari, A., Lazzarin, A., Cipriani, D., Crocchiolo, P., Coltolin, L., Giannelli, F., Irato, L., De Cataldo, F., & Moroni, M. (1990). HIV-related severe thrombocytopenia in intravenous drug users: Prevalence, response to therapy in a medium-term follow-up and pathogenetic evaluation. *AIDS, 4*, 29–34.

Lane, H. C., Davey, V., Kovacs, J. A., Feinberg, J., Metcalf, J. A., Herpin, B., et al. (1990). Interferon a in patients with asymptomatic human immunodeficency virus (HIV) infection. *Annals of Internal Medicine, 112*, 805–811.

Laurence, J., Siegal, F. P., Schattner, E., Gelman, I. H., & Morse, S. (1992). Acquired immunodeficiency without evidence of infection with human immunodeficiency virus types 1 and 2. *Lancet, 340*, 273–274.

Lazzarin, A., Saracco, A., Musicco, M., Nicolosi, A., & the Italian Study Group on HIV Heterosexual Transmission (1991). Man-to-woman sexual transmission of the human immunodeficiency virus. *Archives of Internal Medicine, 151*, 2411–2416.

Lee, B. L., & Safrin, S. (1992). Interactions and toxicities of drugs used in patients with AIDS. *Clinical Infectious Diseases, 14*, 773–779.

Levine, A. M. (1988). Reactive and neoplastic lymphoproliferative disorders and other miscellaneous cancers associated with HIV infection. In V. T. DeVita, Jr., S. Hellman, & S. A. Rosenberg (Eds.), *AIDS: Etiology, diagnosis, treatment and prevention* (2nd ed.) (pp. 263–275). Philadelphia: J. B. Lippincott.

Levitz, S. M. (1991). The ecology of *Cryptococcus neoformans* and the epidemiology of cryptococcosis. *Reviews of Infectious Diseases, 13*, 1163–1169.

Levy, J. A. (1990). Features of HIV and the host-response influence progression to disease. In M. A. Sande & P. A. Volberding (Eds.), *The medical management of AIDS* (2nd ed) (pp. 23–37). Philadelphia: W. B. Saunders.

Levy, J. A. (1989). Human immunodeficiency viruses and the pathogenesis of AIDS. *Journal of the American Medical Association, 261*, 2997–3006.

Levy, R. M., Bredesen, D. E., & Rosenblum, M. L. (1990). Neurologic complications of HIV infection. *American Family Physician, 41*, 517–536.

Lifson, A. (1992). Men who have sex with men: Continued challenges for preventing HIV infection and AIDS. *American Journal of Public Health, 82*, 166–167.

Lifson, A. R., Hessol, N. A., & Rutherford, G. W. (1992). Progression and clinical outcome of infection due to human immunodeficiency virus. *Clinical Infectious Diseases, 14*, 966–972.

Lifson, A. R., O'Malley, P. M., Hessol, N. A., Buchbinder, S. P., Cannon, L., & Rutherford, G. W. (1990). HIV seroconversion in two homosexual men after receptive oral intercourse with ejaculation: Implications for counseling concerning safe sexual practices. *American Journal of Public Health, 80*, 1509–1511.

Lifson, A. R., Rutherford, G. W., & Jaffe, H. W. (1988). The natural history of human immunodeficiency virus infection. *Journal of Infectious Diseases, 158*, 1360–1367.

MacMahon, E. M. E., Glass, J. D., Hayward, S. D., Mann, R. B., Becker, P. S., Charache, P., McArthur, J. C., & Ambinder, R. F. (1991). Epstein-Barr virus in AIDS-related primary central nervous system lymphoma. *Lancet, 338*, 969–973.

Mak, T. W., & Wigzell, H. (1991). AIDS: Ten years later. *The FASEB Journal, 5*, 2338–2339.

McGowan, J. E., Jr., Chesney, P J., Crossley, K. B., & LaForce, F. M. (1992). Guidelines for the use of systemic glucocorticosteroids in the management of selected infections. *Journal of Infectious Diseases, 165*, 1–13.

McKenzie, R., Travis, W. D., Dolan, S. A., Pittaluga, S., Feuerstein, I. M., Shelhamer, J., Yarchoan, R., & Masur, H. (1991). The causes of death in patients with AIDS: A clinical and pathologic study with emphasis on the role of pulmonary diseases. *Medicine, 70*, 326–343.

Meeker, T. C., Shiramizu, B., Kaplan, L., Herndier, B., Sanchez, H., Grimaldi, J. C., Baumgartner, J., Rachlin, J., Feigal, E., Rosenblum, M., & McGrath, M. S. (1992) Evidence for molecular subtypes of HIV-associated lymphoma: division into peripheral mono-clonal, polyclonal and central nervous system lymphoma. *AIDS, 5,* 669–674.

Moore, R. D., Hidalgo, J., Sugland, B. W., & Chaisson, R. E. (1991). Zidovudine and the natural history of the acquired immunodeficiency syndrome. *New England Journal of Medicine, 324,* 1412–1416.

Murray, F., & Mills, J. (1990). Pulmonary infectious complications of human immunodeficiency virus infection. *American Review of Respiratory Disease, 141,* 1356–1372.

National Institute of Allergy and Infectious Diseases. (1991, March 8). Statement. Study of AZT in HIV-infected pregnant women and their offspring to begin. *Backgrounder* (unpaginated).

Nightingale, S. L. (1991). Didanosine (DDI) approved for advanced HIV infection. *Journal of the American Medical Association, 266,* 2528.

Nightingale, S. L. (1992). Zalcitabine approved for use in combination with zidovudine for HIV infection. *Journal of the American Medical Association, 268,* 705.

Onorato, I. M., McCray, E., & the Field Services Branch (1992). Prevalence of human immunodeficiency virus infection among patients attending tuberculosis clinics in the United States. *Journal of Infectious Diseases, 165,* 87–92.

Page, J. B. (1990). Shooting scenarios and risk of HIV-1 infection. *American Behavioral Scientist, 33,* 478–490.

Partner notification for preventing HIV infection. (1991). *Lancet, 338,* 1112–1113.

Perkins, H. A. (1989). More on transmission of HIV by blood transfusion. *New England Journal of Medicine, 320,* 463.

Phair, J. P., & Wolinsky, S. (1992). Diagnosis of infection with the human immunodeficiency virus. *Clinical Infectious Diseases, 15,* 13–16.

Pinching, A. J. (1988). Clinical aspects of AIDS and HIV infection in the developed world. *British Medical Bulletin, 44*(1), 89–100.

Powderly, W. G. (1992). Therapy for cryptococcal meningitis in patients with AIDS. *Clinical Infectious Diseases, 14*(Suppl 1), S54–S59.

Raub, W. (1990). High probability of lymphoma found after long-term, anti-HIV therapy. *Journal of the American Medical Association, 264,* 2191.

Revision of the CDC surveillance case definition for acquired immunodeficiency syndrome. (1987). *Morbidity and Mortality Weekly Report, 36*(lS), 3S–15S.

Rolston, K. V. I., & Fainstein, V. (1986). Cryptosporidiosis. *European Journal of Clinical Microbiology, 5,* 135–137.

Romeu, J., Miro, J. M., Sirera, G., Mallolas, J., Arnal, J., Valls, M. E., Tortosa, F., Clotet, B., & Fox, M. (1991). Efficacy of octeotide in the management of chronic diarrhoea in AIDS. *AIDS, 5,* 1495–1499.

Rosenberg, Z. F., & Fauci, A. S. (1991). Immunopathogenesis of HIV infection. *FASEB Journal, 5,* 2382–2390.

Ruttimann, S., Hilti, P., Spinas, G. A., & Dubach, U. C. (1991). High frequency of human immunodeficiency virus-associated autonomic neuropathy and more severe involvement in advanced stages of human immunodeficiency virus disease. *Archives of Internal Medicine, 151,* 2441–2443.

Saag, M. S. (1992). Nucleoside analogues: Adverse effects. *Hospital Practice, 27* (Suppl. 2), 26–36.

Safrin, S., Ashley, R., Houlihan, C., Cusick, P. S., & Mills, J. (1991). Clinical and serologic features of herpes simplex virus infection in patients with AIDS. *AIDS, 5,* 1107–1110.

Salzberg, A. M., Dolins, S. L., & Runser, R. H. (1988). Transmission of HIV by blood transfusion. *New England Journal of Medicine, 319,* 515.

Schwartz, R. A. (1988). *Skin cancer.* New York: Springer-Verlag.

The second 100,000 cases of acquired immunodeficiency syndrome—United States, June 1981–December 1991. (1992). *Morbidity and Mortality Weekly Report, 41*, 28–29.

Seeing the way forward for treatment of CMV retinitis. (1991). *Lancet, 338*, 1494–1495.

Shadduck, J. A. (1989). Human microsporidiosis and AIDS. *Reviews of Infectious Diseases, 2*, 203–207.

Sloand, E. M., Pitt, E., Chiarello, R. J., & Nemo, G. J. (1991). HIV testing. *Journal of the American Medical Association, 266*, 2861–2866.

Smith, P. D., Quinn, T. C., Strober, W., Janoff, E. N., & Masur, H. (1992). Gastrointestinal infections in AIDS. *Annals of Internal Medicine, 116*, 63–77.

Smith, R. D. (1990). The pathobiology of HIV infection. *Archives of Pathology & Laboratory Medicine, 114*, 235–239.

Stevens, D. A., Greene, I., & Lang, O. S. (1991). Thrush can be prevented in patients with acquired immunodeficiency syndrome and the acquired immunodeficiency syndrome-related complex. *Archives of Internal Medicine, 151*, 2458–2464.

Studies of Ocular Complications of AIDS Research Group in Collaboration with the AIDS Clinical Trials Group. (1992). Mortality in patients with the acquired immunodeficiency syndrome treated with either foscarnet or ganciclovir for cytomegalovirus retinitis. *New England Journal of Medicine, 326*, 213–220.

Sweeney, J., Peters, B. S., & Main, J. (1991). Clinical care and management. *AIDS Care, 3*, 457–466.

Taylor, R. (1992). Hesitation blues: AIDS researchers struggle to prepare candidate HIV-1 vaccines for large-scale efficacy trials. *The Journal of NIH Research, 4*(7), 89–93.

Tindall, B., & Cooper, D. A. (1991). Primary HIV infection: Host responses and intervention strategies. *AIDS, 5*, 1–14.

Unexplained CD4+ T-lymphocyte depletion in persons without evident HIV infection—United States. (1992). *Morbidity and Mortality Weekly Report, 41*, 541–545.

Update: Acquired immunodeficiency syndrome—United States, 1991. (1992). *Morbidity and Mortality Weekly Report, 41*, 463–468.

VanDevanter, N. L. (1991). HIV testing and counseling. In J. D. Durham & F. L. Cohen (Eds.), *The person with AIDS: Nursing perspectives* (2nd ed.) (pp. 72–95). New York: Springer.

Volberding, P. A., Lagakos, S. W., Koch, M. A., et al. (1990). Zidovudine in asymptomatic human immunodeficiency virus infection. *New England Journal of Medicine, 322*, 941–949.

Weber, R., Bryan, R. T., Owen, R. L., Wilcox, C. M., Gorelkin, L., Visvesvara, G S., & Enteric Opportunistic Infections Working Group. (1992). Improved light-microscopical detection of microsporidia spores in stool and duodenal aspirates. *New England Journal of Medicine, 326*, 161–166.

Wigzell, H. (1991). Prospects for an HIV-vaccine. *The FASEB Journal, 5*, 2406–2411.

Wolinsky, S. (1992). Mycobacterial diseases other than tuberculosis. *Clinical Infectious Diseases, 15*, 1–12.

Wong-Staal, F. (1991). The AIDS virus. *Western Journal of Medicine, 155*, 481–487.

World Health Organization. (1991). Update on AIDS. *Weekly Epidemiological Record, 66*(48), 353–357.

World Health Organization. (1992a). Acquired immunodeficiency syndrome (AIDS)—data as at 1 July 1992. *Weekly Epidemiological Record, 67*(27), 201–204.

World Health Organization. (1992b, February 12). AIDS-over a million new infections in eight months. *WHO Press*, 1–2.

Yarchoan, R., Mitsuya, H., & Broder, S. (1988). AIDS therapies. *Scientific American, 259*(4), 110–119.

2

Caring for a Child with AIDS: Views of a Family Member

Katherine Foos

A person with AIDS is not the sole victim of the disease. AIDS has a rippling effect that touches and alters the lives of family, friends, and neighbors. Sixty percent of the children with AIDS are cared for by extended families, foster parents, or adoptive parents; single natural mothers care for another 40% of these children (Septimus 1989). I have come to realize that if AIDS can influence my life, it can impinge on anyone's life.

A FAMILY FACES AIDS

Our family is from a small community in western Nebraska with a population of approximately 3,000. My four siblings and I are of European descent. Upon reaching adulthood, each took a different direction in life. My younger sister, Emmy, moved to Lincoln, Nebraska, to complete her nursing degree. Emmy's light brown hair that looks almost blond and large blue eyes are beaming qualities, but her finest attribute is being a compassionate, caring person.

In 1983, while working in a retirement home as a nurse's aide to assist in paying for her education, Emmy met a man named Felix. Felix gave Emmy attention and a feeling of being needed; eventually Emmy and Felix moved in together. In 1986, Emmy became aware that Felix was using narcotics and possibly selling cocaine and marijuana. During the Christmas season of the same year, Emmy became pregnant.

As a close family, we all tried to give Emmy support during her pregnancy, even though we all lived miles away. On August 3, 1987, Emmy had the most beautiful little girl I have ever seen—Clarice. The moment I saw Clarice, I knew she was going to be very special. Emmy's delivery was not without problems. Clarice was delivered via cesarean section because of fetal distress due to ingestion of meconium-stained amniotic fluid. Within two weeks, both Emmy and Clarice were released from hospital care.

During the next eight months, Felix was ill off and on. Emmy told me that Felix had cancer of the stomach and that it was considered terminal. In May 1988, Clarice was hospitalized for hepatitis. Clarice's condition was very critical, so Mom and I drove to Omaha to give comfort. When we visited the hospital, there were signs posted on the outside of Clarice's isolated cubicle advising of needle precautions and mandatory use of gloves, gowns, and masks. I briefly thought it strange that so much attention was given to such precautions, but I quieted my concern by believing the precautions were used because hepatitis is contagious. Clarice went home a month later.

Throughout the summer of 1988, Clarice was in and out of the hospital so many times that I lost count. One evening in September 1988, Mom called and told me that Emmy's best girlfriend had called a few weeks earlier and told her that Emmy and Clarice had AIDS. The friend felt that Mom had the right to know her daughter's condition. My reply was "That was a horrible joke to pull on someone." I had no idea why Emmy's best friend would say such a thing. Mom explained that she would have asked me sooner but that she was afraid it might be true, adding that she had already been crying for two weeks. I reassured Mom that the friend had played a cruel joke and that I would call Emmy and find out what was really going on.

I immediately called Emmy, who was at the hospital in Omaha with Clarice. After a few minutes of small talk, I asked Emmy what was really going on with Clarice. Emmy told me to sit down as she explained that Felix had been an IV drug user in the early 1980s, heroin his drug of choice. Felix first experimented with heroin during a tour in the Vietnam War. Emmy further explained that Felix did not know he had HIV until three months after Clarice was born. Felix was diagnosed at that time with *Pneumocystis carinii* pneumonia (PCP) and full-blown AIDS. In December 1987, Emmy tested positive for HIV and in May 1988, when Clarice was hospitalized with hepatitis, she too tested positive. During this conversation, I learned that Emmy was being both verbally and physically abused by Felix and that she feared for her own and Clarice's safety. With such intolerable conditions, I explained to Emmy that she was always welcome in my house.

After I hung up, I sat down on my bed and cried for several hours, experiencing many of the same emotions I had felt when my father died ten years earlier. I did not call my mom back. I had decided that if Mom did not bring the subject up again, I would not bring it up. Emmy had also begged me not to tell Mom because she wanted to tell her in person.

Early in October 1988, my oldest sister, who lived in Omaha, called me to let me know she was buying Emmy and Clarice a plane ticket to Denver. Emmy had temporarily moved in with her since Clarice was in the hospital. While Emmy was staying there, Felix had called and threatened to kill Emmy and kidnap his daughter. My oldest sister had intercepted this conversation and gave Emmy the encouragement she needed to break away from the hostile environment Felix presented.

With only two suitcases of personal belongings and an ailing Clarice, Emmy boarded a plane for the first time in her life, bound for Denver where she knew only me and had only a referral to University Hospital. When I greeted Emmy and Clarice at the airport, I saw renewed strength and fight in my sister as she held a 13-month-old child who resembled a child of no more than 6 months. With all the love I felt for Emmy and Clarice, I forgot about their illness as I hugged them, relieved to have my sister with me. We immediately went to University Hospital, where a lethargic Clarice was admitted. I sat with Emmy for hours in Clarice's large hospital room while numerous doctors and nurses interviewed and reinterviewed Emmy.

The care and attention Clarice received at University Hospital was genuine and dramatically different from that of the hospital in Omaha. The nurses and doctors wore gloves when touching Clarice but used no gowns and masks. This gave a warmer and more personal atmosphere. (Masks are normally used by staff when they have colds or if they are working with numerous children who have respiratory diseases.)

I talked openly with doctors, nurses, and Emmy about precautions that needed to be taken at home. They described routines that were simple and should be done no matter who is living with you. For example, you should always wear plastic gloves when dealing with blood or bodily fluids. You may change diapers without gloves, but only if you feel comfortable and always wash your hands upon completion. Another precaution explained to me was not to handle the child if you are ill, but if you have to be around her and you are ill, wear a mask. (The child is at a greater risk of catching something from you than you are of becoming HIV-infected from her.) Otherwise, common sense about routine household cleaning and maintenance was all that I needed to know.

By the middle of October, Clarice's illness was diagnosed as an infection in the Hickman catheter that had been inserted in her chest; consequently, it was removed. By October 28, 1988, Clarice and Emmy were finally spending their first night in their new house, which they transformed into a home. At Thanksgiving, Emmy had told everyone in the immediate family about their illness.

CARING FOR A CHILD WITH AIDS

Clarice had won the affection of a hemophilia specialist, Dr. Marilyn Manco-Johnson, who sees approximately 300 male patients, compared to her four female patients. Many of these patients have AIDS. Dr. Manco-Johnson believes in an aggressive medical approach to AIDS but also believes in keeping the patient as comfortable and functional as possible. At this point, Clarice was clinically diagnosed as having AIDS-related complex. Dr. Manco-Johnson and Emmy talked about starting Clarice on zidovudine (ZDV, AZT, retrovir). Emmy informed me that Clarice's doctor in Omaha had not allowed Clarice to take

AZT, for two reasons: first, it was was too experimental for infants; second, he firmly believed that with AIDS, nature should take its course. This doctor had prescribed monthly intravenous immunoglobulin to boost Clarice's immune system, hoping to prevent other opportunistic infections, but this was the extent of his aggressive treatment.

When Clarice came home, she started taking AZT. Emmy was also taking the AZT capsule. For Clarice, she cut it in half, poured out the white powderlike medicine, and divided it into two equal portions. One-half of this metallic-tasting potion would then be given to Clarice by mixing it in her baby food four times a day. Clarice's initial ingesting of AZT was accompanied with weekly check-ups, which included blood tests from finger pricks. A remarkable difference was seen in Clarice in about two days. Clarice's lethargic state diminished. Over a six-month period, she became more alert and began sitting, crawling, talking, and trying to pull herself up. Even the yellow tint to the whites of her eyes from hepatitis disappeared. Eventually Clarice no longer attended her weekly check-ups, and she was limited to one admission a month for the intravenous immunoglobulin, which we termed "Clarice's tune-ups."

Clarice has always been a beautiful child with brown doelike eyes sheltered by extraordinary long eyelashes. Her button nose and small dimple resting in her chin complements her perfect little permanent tan. Her brown wispy hair makes her look a year younger. The addition of AZT brought personality to Clarice. She began learning to communicate with others without resorting to waiting or crying. I remember the time when Clarice was sitting at the break-fast counter in her booster chair playing. She had always heard me refer to her mother as Emmy, so one day I asked her who I was. Clarice responded, "Mama." I then pointed at Emmy and asked Clarice who she was. Clarice replied, "Emmy." Emmy spent the next hour explaining and reinforcing who was the aunt and who was the mom. I truly believe that Clarice knew who was who but was just playing around. Clarice may have been physically slow in motion and speech, but her intelligence matched her age.

Summer 1988 was a very productive one for Clarice. Any diaper rash was contained by simply using vaseline on her cleaned bottom. We also learned that Clarice was very sensitive to certain brands of diapers; for unexplained reasons, Luvs was the best type of diaper to use to minimize her rash. Clarice had a hardy appetite, eating practically everything put in front of her.

Clarice has four cousins ranging in age from 10 to 16. They were told about Clarice's condition and treated Clarice no differently than any other 2-year-old. That summer, they played with her in the wading pool, went swinging, read books, played dolls, and watched "Sesame Street." Clarice loved "Sesame Street," graduating from her favorite character, Grover, to her new favorite character, Big Bird. The movie *Batman* had just been released, and Clarice's cousins had taught her to sing along with the television series theme song.

Throughout the summer, Clarice continued with her "tune-ups" at University Hospital. The only other medicine Clarice took orally besides the AZT was Nilstat, to keep her thrush in check, and liquid children's vitamins. Emmy was getting comfortable riding the bus to the hospital and becoming very persistent and proficient in getting the financial (i.e., Social Security Insurance, Medicaid, and Social Security) and mental support she needed to get through each day (Clarice's father was considered 100% disabled). Emmy also worked on getting Clarice into a special county school for disabled children and scheduling regular visits to a physician to maintain her own health.

There was a babysitting issue that Emmy and I had to address. A 15-year-old neighbor girl would babysit for Clarice a couple of times a month. We had not told most of our neighbors about Clarice's and Emmy's condition, for fear of being ostracized. That summer, Rock Hudson's former lover sued Hudson's estate and successfully won because Hudson had not told his lover that he had AIDS. I feared that if we did not tell the babysitter and her parents of Clarice's condition, the ramifications from the Hudson case could apply to me. Even though I knew the babysitter was not exposed to the virus, we elected not to have anyone babysit Clarice except for those friends and neighbors who were aware of Clarice's condition.

We celebrated Clarice's second birthday by inviting the neighborhood children for a party. Numerous kids and adults attended and enjoyed the summer evening, celebrating with balloon animals, a clown, hot dogs, cake, and ice cream. The kids helped Clarice blow out her two candles and delighted in helping her open her presents.

August continued to be a busy month for Emmy. She was taking Clarice to the Margaret Walters School twice a week to attend a toddler program for disabled children. Clarice also began to reject attempts to give her the powdered AZT, and this had to be overcome. Clarice also started to sneeze to such an extent that it would make her throw up. The first week of September, Clarice was hospitalized for that continuous sneezing, which was revealed as a fungal infection in her lungs. In the meantime, Clarice had been taken off the AZT for fear that the sneezing was a reaction to its extended use. During the hospital stay, a concern arose between Dr. Manco-Johnson and the infectious-diseases personnel. Clarice had received all of her current childhood vaccinations except her measles-mumps-rubella shot. Dr. Manco-Johnson was concerned over Clarice's reaction to this shot, but the decision was to go ahead and give Clarice the shot because the reaction to the MMR shot certainly would not be as severe as her developing the disease.

While Clarice was in the hospital, I would walk into the empty bedroom she shared with her mom and feel a painful hollowness. I would sit on Emmy's bed staring at Clarice's crib and cry about how tragic their lives had been. I was afraid that Clarice would not return home. I was afraid that I would lose my new companions. I feared how empty my life would be without Clarice, the one person who was eager to welcome me home from work with outstretched arms. She was my little companion, and I was not ready to lose her.

Clarice did come home, but things were never the same. Emmy and I had talked about Clarice dying. I was concerned about how Emmy would handle the grief. Scenarios were rehearsed in which Emmy revealed some hidden thoughts of career options. Emmy was dealing with Clarice's deteriorating health throughout September, which we blamed on the MMR shot. Clarice was still off AZT, and all the progress she had made seemed lost. Clarice was listless and nonengaging, perking up for only short periods. Emmy complained only slightly about her own health and was hospitalized on October 27, 1989, for a hiatal hernia. Soon after Emmy's hospitization, all the immediate family flew into Denver to visit Emmy because the doctors had advised us that Emmy's condition was grave and they did not know what was wrong with her.

On the morning of November 13, 1989, at 5:30 A.M., Clarice penetrated the silence in her room, which was also being occupied by her grandmother, by crying out, "Mama, Mama." Clarice's voice woke up her grandmother, who now heard a voice that sounded like Emmy whimpering, "Mommy, Mommy." A couple of minutes later, we were telephoned by the hospital. Emmy had gone into cardiac arrest. Emmy's cause of death was adult respiratory distress syndrome, which was related to a liver dysfunction. She had been unable to clear fluids from her bloodstream, and the fluid then leaked into the lungs.

Clarice is a very perceptive child, and she knew that her mommy had died. In the morning, she would not eat or play. She cried more frequently and would look around the house as if she were searching for someone. Clarice had dropped from 25 to 21 pounds. The next tune-up resulted in at least a dozen "pokes," finally resulting in an IV being inserted in a scalp vein that protruded from her head because of her loss of weight. When the nurses brought Clarice to me, I just started to cry uncontrollably—I felt so bad for her. The nurses reassured me that Clarice did not mind the position of the IV because she could now use both hands. I rocked Clarice for the next four hours as the immunoglobulin dripped into her vein. Clarice rested peacefully in my arms as I counted the "boo-boos" on her hands, feet, and arms, in some places accompanied with bruising.

Clarice had been put back on AZT, but she was reluctant to eat anything. I had mistakenly put the AZT in some of her favorite foods. What worked out much better was to put the AZT in some ugly-looking strained plums and to tell Clarice that this was her medicine and that I would not put it in any other foods. Clarice would reluctantly take her plums because she knew that once they were eaten, none of her favorite foods would taste like metal again.

My mom had taken a leave of absence from her work and moved in with me to help raise Clarice. This was a difficult and unselfish decision for my mother, as she was leaving behind fifty years of friends and a job to become a full-time grandmother. My mom was a balm for the emptiness Clarice felt from the loss of Emmy, and in return Clarice has become very attached to her most favorite and only grandma.

The addition of my mother to my household has helped me forge ahead with my chosen profession. Clarice has not and will not hinder my life. Clarice is part of my life; she fits in perfectly.

The spring of 1990 involved the addition of aerosolized pentamidine mist (to prevent *Pneumocystis carinii* pneumonia) to Clarice's monthly tune-ups and the promised liquid AZT. The AZT dosage prescribed by Dr. Manco-Johnson was 5 ml, equivalent to one teaspoon, four times a day. Mom and I felt that this dosage was too much because we believed Emmy's high prescribed dosage of AZT caused her liver dysfunction. Within a month, we had decided to drop Clarice's dosage to 3 ml three times a day.

Gradually Clarice started to improve. Her solemn but inquisitive look became a smile and the few sign-language words that she had learned in school were coming back to her, or at least she was getting back the energy she needed to communicate.

Mom continued to take Clarice to toddler school till summer break. By June 1, 1990, we had moved to a bigger home, Clarice was going to Children's Hospital for her tune-ups, and she was getting physical therapy at home. Children's Hospital was a welcome change since the hospital is bright and cheery and the staff is accustomed to working with children. An infusion room is used for children who need outpatient IVs. No longer did Clarice have to go through Patient Admissions, nor did she have to experience half a dozen pokes before a vein was found to administer the immunoglobulin.

Clarice's fine, wispy brown hair had finally started to grow into soft flowing curls, causing her to resemble a little angel. Clarice lacked interest in eating foods, so her diet was supplemented by whole milk mixed with Carnation Instant Breakfast or Ensure, by bottle, to provide sufficient caloric intake. Clarice now weighed 24 pounds and was potty-trained. Clarice cannot walk or crawl to the potty chair, but she will sign that she needs to go potty and we will place her on the chair. She is usually successful at this task while jamming to music and looking at her kitty and doggy books.

A few weeks after Clarice's third birthday, she went back to toddler school. In September (I hate Septembers because Clarice always seems to get sick), Clarice was placed in the hospital for three days because of severe blood loss in her stools. Clarice was given a blood transfusion and Maalox to neutralize the thrush-related lesions present in her digestive tract. (Clarice had patches of thrush in her mouth. She had not been taking Nilstat for several months.) Clarice also managed to get a cold sore (herpes), which was confined to the inside of her mouth. Clarice's doctor was hesitant to prescribe another drug to dry up the herpes, so I would apply Crest toothpaste by Q-tip to the infected area. Within a week and a half, the sore had healed.

Clarice is a very touch-oriented child needing constant reassurance and hugs. Clarice very rarely sleeps through the night: she will awake at least twice each night. Her interrupted sleeping patterns are caused by hunger, night sweats, or the fear of being alone. As Clarice's grandmother states, "Caring for Clarice is a full-time job. I really enjoy it, and believe me, every day is never the same." When relatives recommend that Clarice be institutionalized, my mom responds, "She's a joy. Clarice knows when she is getting to me. She'll hold my face and give me a kiss or a big hug, and all my problems melt away. I've kept a calendar and a log of Clarice's daily activities, meds, and physical well-being—and yes, every day, more than once, I'll go in to see if she's still breathing. You see, I'm still learning how best to care for her and glad too I have her another day."

The school year was successful, with Clarice attending twice a week for one and a half hours. she is a very popular child at school. She has a special chair with wheels her classmates push to get her around. Several of Clarice's schoolmates can't hear; therefore, communication with them is through sign language. Clarice picks up signing quickly, as she can hear the words being spoken and finds it easier to sign than to speak. Clarice has cookie-and-milk breaks with her class, and her teacher proudly announced to me that the kids all share with Clarice, something unusual for children 3 years of age.

School has been very good for Clarice because of the socialization. We are not overly concerned about Clarice catching childhood diseases. The teachers and administration are aware of Clarice's condition. Clarice is not the only child with a suppressed immune system. Many of the more compromised children have weaker immune systems. Clarice's teachers also highlighted my day by telling me that Clarice has attended more regularly and has been healthier than most of her classmates.

In 1991, Clarice was taken off AZT since she was throwing up after it was administered, and her appetite again dwindled. Clarice was desensitized to Septra to terminate the aerosol pentamidine treatments that caused irritation to her throat. Once off AZT, Clarice added a couple of pounds, tipping the scale at 27 pounds. Dr. Manco-Johnson said that she thought Clarice would sustain for a year without any additional preventive treatment but thought it best if we tried ddI (dideoxyinosine). So for the month of May and part of June, Clarice was on ddI. Two days after being on ddI, Clarice started complaining about headaches, body aches, and fevers. She would not eat anything and was taking less of her milk supplement. I made the decision to take Clarice off ddI because it was sapping all her energy. She was losing her battle. As I write, Clarice is back to her normal self: loving, inquisitive, frustrating, impatient, mimicking—just her beautiful self.

Some weeks are good, some bad. The bad days can make you very anxious over the future. Some days you feel as if Clarice could live for years and years, and some days reality becomes so heavy, you wish it were over.

I get frightened by reading all the published articles on pediatric AIDS. It terrorizes me to think that the brain is a primary site of HIV infection in infants and children. It is likely that the central nervous system is infected early and that infection may occur in the majority of patients if not all. After initial infection of the brain, HIV may remain latent in an integrated proviral form or may be actively expressed and replicated (Epstein, Sharer, & Goudsmit, 1988).

The prognosis for children with AIDS is grim. Of children diagnosed under 1 year, many, perhaps half, die within six months after diagnosis. Of children over 1 year of age, half die within approximately 20 months after diagnosis (Rogers, 1988). Maybe, just maybe, Clarice will continue to be that miracle child. Besides, she is going to be her Uncle Billy's flower girl when he gets married in January 1992, even if the ring bearer has to pull her down the aisle in a decorated red wagon.

At one time, in a brief moment of defeated posture, I felt lucky to have a boyfriend who was supportive of my situation. I told myself that I should settle for this friend because most men would not want to get involved with a woman who has a special child. As I became more comfortable with Clarice's illness and more comfortable about sharing this information, I became more confident in my choice to raise Clarice. No longer did I feel lucky because I know I can mold my future no matter what is thrown my way by participating in it. I would not want my family to settle for someone who felt pity, sympathy, and partial love.

My friend and I eventually broke our bond. My life went on. Clarice has not prevented me from finishing my graduate degree, developing special relationships, and enjoying life. The truly *lucky* person would be the man I marry because he would be welcomed into a warm, close family with unconditional love.

GIFTS

If there were no suffering, this world would be very shallow. From suffering come heroes. There are no greater heroes than the courageous kids living with AIDS. Clarice is my hero. Her strength, spirit, and loving soul inspire me to continue on life's hard journey. Clarice has given me focus and purpose in my life.

Although my close family has become a part of the AIDS statistics, the bonds and struggles that we share bring us closer and make us stronger. In a letter Emmy dated July 8, 1989, to Felix, two days before he died, she wrote:

> You gave me the prettiest, most wonderful daughter I could ever dream of. She is the most important thing in my life. When I had her, I never dreamt that a child could make your life so wonderful and complete. For her I thank you very much.
>
> Thank you Felix for allowing me in your life. Although you're a troubled man, you're also a sensitive and loving man. Thank you for allowing me a glimpse of that man.
>
> I understand the circumstances that surrounded our split had a lot to do with pressures from financial to physical. Mental as well, because of the stress from de-

creased physical resistance to this disease. Believe me Felix, I don't blame you for this. We didn't ask for this disease, but it's here and we just have to learn how to live with it. Clarice and I will get the best of doctors and medical care possible because it is important to us and my family.

I'm sorry you're isolated and alone. But that was the lifestyle you led.

Now Felix, as you are almost gone from mine and Clarice's life forever, remember that we love you and think a lot about you. Again thank you for her.

Love, Emmy and Clarice

When I read this letter and discovered how forgiving and thankful my sister was, I learned that I had no right to feel anger or frustration over this situation. My hatred for Felix had subsided with Emmy's words of solace. In addition, I had learned that I had not lost a sister but had obtained wisdom from a friend.

Forgiveness, courage, and heroes are wonderful gifts from AIDS. One last note of encouragement for families raising children with AIDS: Clarice is a success story because of her loving environment and her aggressive medical treatment. Clarice is not a child dying from AIDS but a child living with AIDS.

REFERENCES

Epstein, L. G., Sharer, L. R., & Goudsmit, J. (1988). Neurological and neuropathological features of human immunodeficiency virus infection in children. *Annals of Neurology*, *23* (suppl.), S19–S23.

Rogers, M. F. (1988). Pediatric HIV infection: Epidemiology, etiopathogenesis and transmission. *Pediatric Annals*, *17*(5), 324–331.

Septimus, A. (1989). Psychosocial aspects of caring for families of infants infected with human immunodeficiency virus. *Seminars in Perinatology*, *13*, 49–54.

Part II
HIV Infection and AIDS in Women

3

Epidemiology of HIV Infection and AIDS in Women

Felissa L. Cohen

Although the first case of AIDS in a woman was reported in 1981, relatively little epidemiologic attention has been paid to women by the majority of researchers and practitioners (Centers for Disease Control, 1981). This neglect may stem partially from the fact that in the early period of the epidemic, women accounted for only a few cases of AIDS. This has changed. By 1987, AIDS was cited as the eighth leading cause of death in women 15 to 44 years of age (Chu, Buehler, & Berkelman, 1990). In New York City, AIDS has been the leading cause of death in women between the ages of 15 and 44 years since 1986. In some areas it has become the leading cause of death for black women in the United States (Anastos & Palleja, 1991).

STATISTICS AND PATTERNS IN THE UNITED STATES

By July 1992, of the 226,281 cases of AIDS in adults that had been reported to the CDC, 24,323 were in females. In 1981, the first year in which AIDS cases were reported to CDC, only 6 cases of AIDS were reported in women, representing 3.2% of the total. Since 1981, the cumulative percentage of adult females with AIDS has increased from 3.2% to more than 10%. In the year from July 1991 to June 1992, females constituted more than 13% of the adult cases of AIDS reported in that year (Centers for Disease Control, 1992; Update: Acquired Immunodeficiency Syndrome, 1992).

While causes of death among women 15 to 44 years other than HIV infection have remained relatively stable over the last 10 years, the death rate due to HIV infection quadrupled between 1985 and 1988 (Chu et al., 1990).

AIDS cases in females have now been reported in all 50 states and the District of Columbia. The last state to report an AIDS case in a female was North

Dakota (Centers for Disease Control, 1990). The cumulative incidence rates of AIDS cases in females per 100,000 female population are highest in New Jersey, New York, Florida, Rhode Island, Connecticut, Delaware, Maryland, Massachusetts, Washington, D.C., and Puerto Rico. These 10 areas have reported nearly 75% of all the AIDS cases in females (Ellerbrock & Rogers, 1990). This is in contrast to the geographical distribution in men, in which rates in western states such as California, Nevada, and Texas are similar to those along the East Coast (Cohen, 1991). Those states with the lowest rates of AIDS cases in females include North Dakota, South Dakota, West Virginia, Idaho, Wisconsin, Montana, Minnesota, Iowa, Kansas, Nebraska, and New Mexico (Ellerbrock & Rogers, 1990).

In female AIDS cases in states with high cumulative incidence rates, most affected women resided in urban counties. For example, in New Jersey, about 75% of the AIDS cases in females were reported from 4 of the state's 21 counties. These 4 counties all contained large urban areas but only about one-third of New Jersey's population. In Florida, about 67% of the cases have been reported from three counties. These three counties contain only about one-third of Florida's population but contain large urban areas (Ellerbrock & Rogers, 1990). Only about 5% of females with AIDS reported residences in towns with populations below 50,000 (Ellerbrock, Bush, Chamberland, & Oxtoby, 1991). Thus, at this time, AIDS in females has been described as primarily urban (Ellerbrock & Rogers, 1990). It should be pointed out, however, that at one time the geographic face of AIDS in general could have been described in the same manner.

The peak age range for reported AIDS cases cumulatively for males is 30–34 years of age with about 85% falling between 25 and 49. For females, the peak age range is also 30–34 years of age with about 83% falling between 25 and 49. Persons 60 years of age and older account for about 3% of male cases and more than 4% of female cases. These data are shown in Table 3.1.

The racial-ethnic distribution of adult cases of AIDS in the United States by age and gender is shown in Table 3.2. More than half of the adult AIDS cases reported in women occurred in black women, with about 21% occurring in Hispanics and about 25% in white women. Thus, while black and Hispanic women together account for about 19% of all women in the United States, they constitute about 73% of all cases of AIDS among adult women ("AIDS in women," 1991; Centers for Disease Control, 1992). This distribution is generally more similar to pediatric AIDS cases than to those of adult males. However, the point has been made that the distribution in women more closely parallels that found in heterosexual rather than homosexual males (Ellerbrock et al., 1991). Black and Hispanic women have also been found to be at greater statistical risk for acquiring HIV infection through sex with an infected IDU than are white women (Guinan & Hardy, 1987).

TABLE 3.1 Adult/Adolescent AIDS Cases by Age and Sex as Reported to CDC through June 1992

Age Range (in years)	Sex					
	Males			Females		
	No.	% Male Adults	% of Total Adults	No.	% Female Adults	% Total Adults
13–19	630	0.3	0.28	242	1.0	0.1
20–24	7,314	3.6	3.2	1,597	6.6	0.7
25–29	30,912	15.3	13.7	4,672	19.2	2.1
30–39	94,139	46.7	41.6	11,389	46.8	5.0
40–49	47,978	23.8	21.2	3,943	16.2	1.7
50–59	15,191	7.5	6.7	1,343	5.5	0.6
60–64	3,203	1.6	1.4	400	1.6	0.2
65 & over	2,591	1.3	1.1	743	3.1	0.3

Source: Centers for Disease Control, HIV/AIDS Surveillance, July 1992, pp. 1–18.

HIV SEROPREVALENCE

The prevalence of HIV infection in women is as important as, and perhaps even more important than, the number of AIDS cases in women. Unless improved treatment becomes available, most and probably all HIV infected women will eventually progress to AIDS, as discussed in Chapter 5. Moreover, many women who are HIV-infected do not know that they are infected and may find this out incidentally. Many of these women who are in their childbearing years will unknowingly pass the infection on to their infants. Upon their death, their families will be motherless.

Most HIV seroprevalence information comes from research studies conducted in specific groups. In the United States, many of these studies providing information about HIV infection in women have been conducted in the eastern part of the United States, especially New York. HIV seroprevalence studies were done in nearly 29,000 women attending family planning clinics in New York State that serve predominately women under 25 years of age. Overall, 21% were black, and 13% were Hispanic. (In New York State, approximately 14% of the population is black, 12% Hispanic.) The highest HIV seroprevalence was found in New York City (0.82%). One mobile clinic in the city had a rate of 3.9%. Without including New York City, the HIV seroprevalence rate was 0.15%, and the overall adjusted statewide rate was 0.31%. Women who were black or Hispanic had approximately six times the HIV seroprevalence rates of the non-Hispanic whites, and women between 35 and 39 years of age had approximately nine times the HIV seroprevalence rate of the 15–19-year-olds (Stricof, Nattell, & Novick, 1991).

Among females entering prison in New York State, the HIV seroprevalence rate was 18.8%, with the highest rates among women from 30 to 39 years of age (25%) in Hispanic women (29.4%) and among women who lived in New York City (23.8%). About 45% of these acknowledged that they were injecting drug users (IDUs) (Smith et al., 1991).

To estimate HIV seropositivity in childbearing women, newborns are tested because maternal antibodies are transferred across the placenta to the fetus, thus reflecting the HIV status of their mothers (see Chapter 6). The overall national average of HIV seroprevalence for childbearing women has been estimated at 0.15%. In a study in Durham, North Carolina, a supposedly low-incidence area for HIV infection, a surprising rate of 0.43% was found (Shih et al., 1990). In New York State, the overall HIV seroprevalence in newborns was 0.66%, with a rate of 0.16% in upstate New York and 1.25% in New York City. Rates for newborns whose mothers were 20–29 and 30–39 years of age had higher rates (1.30% and 1.35%, respectively) than those whose mothers were younger than 20 years of age (0.72%). HIV seropositivity was higher for black and Hispanic newborns (1.8% and 1.3%, respectively) than for white infants (0.13%) (Novick et al., 1989). In a national study, areas with the highest HIV seroprevalence rate in childbearing women were the District of Columbia (5.5 per 1,000), Florida (4.5 per 1,000), New Jersey (4.9 per 1,000), and New York (5.8 per 1,000). Race-specific HIV seroprevalence rates are substantially higher in black women (Gwinn et al., 1991).

TABLE 3.2 Adult AIDS Cases in the United States by Sex and Race/ Ethnic Group as Reported to CDC through June 1992

	Sex					
	Female			Male		
Race/Ethnic Group	N	% Ethnic Group (all)	% Female Cases	N	% Ethnic Group (all)	% Male Cases
White/NonHispanic	6,192	5.1	25.5	114,760	94.9	57.0
Black/NonHispanic	12,835	19.5	52.9	53,037	80.5	26.3
Hispanic	5,067	13.6	20.9	32,095	86.4	15.9
Asian/Pacific Islander	117	8.3	0.5	1,290	91.7	0.6
American Indian/Alaskan Native	54	14.3	0.2	323	85.7	0.2
Total*	24,265			201,505		

*excludes 453 males and 58 females whose race/ethnicity is unknown.

Source: Centers for Disease Control (1992). HIV/AIDS Surveillance, July 1992 pp. 1–18.

At the time that two states (Louisiana and Illinois) were mandating premarital serologic testing for HIV antibodies, prevalences for both males and females being tested ranged from 0% in Shreveport, Louisiana, to 0.9% at Charity Hospital in New Orleans. For females, the HIV seroprevalences ranged from 0 to 0.4% (Petersen, White, & Premarital Screening Study Group, 1990).

WORLDWIDE STATISTICS AND PATTERNS

Accurate world estimates of the prevalence of HIV infection are difficult to determine. At present, the World Health Organization believes that more than one-third of the approximately 10 to 12 million people infected with HIV worldwide are female (Kent, 1991; World Health Organization, 1992). Of these females, 80% are in sub-Saharan Africa ("Searching for women," 1991; also see Chapter 15). The geographic prevalence of HIV infection varies considerably across the world. HIV seroprevalence in females 15 to 49 years of age varies from about 2,500 per 100,000 in sub-Saharan Africa to fewer than 5 per 100,000 in most of Asia and Eastern Europe (Chin, 1990).

In a study of childbearing women in Kigali, Rwanda, the overall HIV seroprevalence rate was 32%. Rates were higher in those who were single, reported more than one lifetime sexual partner, or began a steady relationship after 1981. Other studies in Rwanda of HIV-1 infection in 1986, showed an overall seroprevalence of 18% in the urban sample with 30% among 26–40-year-olds. Other HIV seroprevalence studies done in targeted high-risk groups indicated that among prostitutes, 88% were infected in Butare, Rwanda; 67% in Nairobi, Kenya; and 27% in Kinshasha, Zaire (Allen et al., 1991).

AIDS has become the leading cause of death for women 20 to 40 years in most central African cities (Chin, 1990). Projections of HIV infections in females in pattern II countries (see Chapter 1) exceed 4,000,000 by the end of 1992. It is further projected that by the end of 1992, 3 million children will be born to HIV-infected women in pattern II countries, approximately 1 million of whom will themselves be infected with HIV (Chin, 1990).

When considering HIV infection in women from a worldwide perspective, it is important to realize the complex interplay of cultural differences among countries, for example in Africa, and of ethnic differences within countries. These differences are important when ascertaining risks and targeting prevention efforts (see Chapters 4 and 15).

TRANSMISSION

Adult women generally contract HIV infection through intimate sexual contact with an infected person involving exposure to HIV-infected secretions or fluids, or exposure to contaminated blood or blood products. Two specific exposure categories, injecting drug use and heterosexual contact with an HIV-infected male, encompass the vast majority of AIDS cases in adult females. Among injecting drug users, the risk for HIV infection is associated with both drug-using behaviors (e.g., sharing needles) and sexual behaviors (e.g., not using condoms). One of the major concerns about the acquisition of HIV infection in women relates to the risk of transmission to their infants. However, it is imperative that women with HIV infection be considered important persons in their own right and not merely as vessels for the fetus or caretakers for others. Perinatal transmission is considered in Chapters 6 and 7.

The overwhelming majority of cases of sexual transmission involving females occurs through heterosexual contact. For several reasons, females are at higher risk than males for encountering an HIV-infected heterosexual partner, as discussed later in this chapter. Male-to-female sexual transmission of HIV is more efficient than female-to-male transmission (Padian, Shiboski, & Jewell, 1991). This finding is consistent with observations made about transmission of other sexually transmitted diseases. For example, there is a 50% to 80% or higher risk of transmission of gonorrhea from males to females following a single exposure, while for female-to-male transmission, this is estimated at 20% to 25% (Handsfield, 1991). Structural reasons may be part of the reasons for the differences in transmission rates. For anatomical reasons, retention of secretions is common in women (Handsfield, 1988).

Menstrual Cycle

Relatively little has been reported about the influence of menstrual cycle on the transmission efficiency of HIV during sexual contact. Are male partners more likely to acquire infection from an HIV-positive menstruating female? For example, does menopause make a woman more or less vulnerable to HIV acquisition through vaginal intercourse? What is the influence of oral contraceptives and of estrogen replacement therapy?

Sexual Assault

One sexually transmitted means by which women may become HIV-infected is through sexual assault or rape by acquaintances or strangers. In the vast majority of rape cases (94–95%), women are the victims. Because this type of assault is also an expression of violence, physical trauma may occur, making the transmission of HIV and sexually transmitted diseases (STDs) even more likely than it would be for consensual sexual intercourse (Schwarcz & Whittington, 1990). In one study, traumatic injury had occurred in nearly 75% of the women who had been raped, and nearly 20% reported forced anal intercourse (Lacey, Roberts, Wooley, & Chandiok, 1991). In another study it was estimated that about 12% of victims of reported rapes contracted STDs other than HIV from that attack. Because HIV is transmitted less efficiently than many other STDs, theoretically, transmission would be less (Brownworth, 1990).

Women Who Have Sex with Women

A woman's perception of her sexual identity may not be the same as the health professional's definition. Women who identify themselves as lesbians may engage in sex with men. This liaison can be with men who identify themselves as gay, or with others. Women who identify themselves as heterosexual may engage in sex with other women.

Although relatively uncommon, female-to-female sexual transmission of HIV has been reported (Marmor et al., 1986; Monzon, & Capellan, 1987). Currently it is estimated that less than 1% of AIDS cases in adult women in the United States occur in lesbians. The majority of these appear to be related to injecting drug use rather than direct female-to-female sexual transmission (Chu, Buehler, Fleming, & Berkelman, 1990). In one CDC study, among the female participants, 5% reported sex with a female partner who injected drugs ("Drug use and sexual behaviors," 1991). However, relatively little is known about sexual practices among lesbians, and few preventive efforts address this group. Lesbians may acquire HIV in the same way as any other women and be at risk for transmitting HIV to their female sexual partner through sexual contact. Lesbians may also become HIV-infected through artificial insemination if the donor is HIV-infected. The role of sex toys, rough sex that damages tissue, exposure to menstrual blood, and practices such as cunnilingus in transmission of HIV between women is largely unexplored (Greenhouse, 1987). Thus, safe-sex information specifically addressing techniques between women is needed (Dicker, 1989). Some may be found in the text and references of *Women, AIDS & Activism* (The ACT UP/New York Women and AIDS Book Group, 1990).

Substance Use

Among injecting drug users, the risk for HIV infection is associated with both drug-using behaviors (e.g., sharing needles) and sexual behaviors (e.g., not using condoms). The use of both cocaine and crack (a smokeable form of cocaine that is relatively inexpensive and highly addictive) is thought to have increased the risk of HIV transmission through the exchange of sexual favors for the drug and decreased sexual inhibitions (Fullilove, Fullilove, Bowser, & Gross, 1990; McCoy & Khoury, 1990). In addition, the half-life of cocaine is short (about 12 minutes), and therefore users of this drug may inject it at more frequent intervals, increasing risk of HIV infection with each injection (Schoenbaum, 1990). The use of any mind-altering substances by any route can indirectly increase chances of HIV acquisition. Alcohol is the most commonly used mind-altering substance in the United States, and its use can result in impaired judgment and less self-protective and more high-risk sexual and drug-use behaviors (Weinstein, DeMaria, Jr., & Rosenthal, 1992).

EXPOSURE CATEGORIES

Exposure categories were developed in a hierarchical, mutually exclusive manner, as discussed in Chapter 1. The ones that apply to women are (in order)

1. injecting drug use
2. hemophilia/coagulation disorder
3. heterosexual contact
4. recipient of transfusion of blood, blood components, or tissue
5. other/undetermined.

A reported case of AIDS is assigned to the first category to which it pertains. A case with multiple characteristics that could fit into more than one exposure category is thus assigned to the group listed first. The first major category that applies to women is injecting drug use (IDU). A woman contracting AIDS who injects drugs and also has had sex with an injecting drug user would be classified for statistical reporting purposes under injecting drug use. Thus, the true role of heterosexual transmission in HIV acquisition in women might not be fully appreciated by the use of this categorization. A comparison of AIDS cases by exposure categories on the basis of gender is shown in Table 3.3.

TABLE 3.3 **United States Adult/Adolescent AIDS Cases by Exposure Category and Sex as Reported to the CDC through June, 1992**[*]

Adult/adolescent exposure categories	Male			Female		
	N	% of Male Adults	% of Total Adults	N	% of Female Adults	% of Total Adults
Men who have sex with men	130,822	64.8	57.8	—	—	—
Injecting drug use	39,364	19.5	17.4	12,113	49.8	5.3
Men who have sex with men and inject drugs	14,487	7.2	6.4	—	—	—
Hemophilia/coagulation disorder	1,834	0.9	0.8	41	0.2	0.02
Heterosexual contact	5,521	2.7	2.4	8,524	35.1	3.8
Recipient of blood transfusion, blood components, or tissue	2,843	1.4	1.3	1,816	7.5	0.8
Other/undertermined	7,087	3.5	3.1	1,829	7.5	0.8
Total:	201,958	100	89.2	24,323	100	10.8
Grand Total: 226,281						

[*]Totals may not add up precisely due to rounding error.

Source: Centers for Disease Control (1992) HIV/AIDS Surveillance, July 1992, pp. 1–18.

Injecting Drug Use

About 50% of all adult female cases of AIDS in the United States are classified by the CDC into this exposure category, representing more than 5% of the total adult cases of AIDS (see Table 3.3).

In regard to HIV infection, women may be affected by injecting drug use either by direct use of drugs themselves, sexual contact with someone who uses drugs in this way, or trading sex for drugs or money to purchase drugs. Only those women who inject drugs are classified into this exposure category. It is estimated that 500,000 women in the United States are IDUs (Wiener, 1991) and that an estimated 30–50% of these engage in prostitution (Shayne & Kaplan, 1991).

More than half of IDUs in the United States live in the New York metropolitan area, and most of the rest reside in urban areas of the East and Puerto Rico. HIV infection is believed to have entered this population in the mid to late 1970s (Friedland & Selwyn, 1990). The entry of HIV into the blood of an IDU might occur through the use or reuse of a contaminated needle or syringe, sharing other "works," "booting" or drawing blood back up into the syringe when preparing an injection, or shared use of "cookers" (containers in which drugs are mixed with water) (Page, 1990; see Chapter 4). Those using drugs in a "shooting gallery" (place where IDUs congregate to inject drugs, and where drug-related injection apparatus such as needles can be rented) may increase the chance of encountering equipment that is HIV-positive. In one study, those who reported always injectinq drugs in a shooting gallery had HIV seropositive rates of 52%, as compared with rates of 29% in those who had frequented shooting galleries less than one-half the time in the previous six months (McCoy & Khoury, 1990).

To ascertain a woman's risk for HIV infection because of injecting drug use, it is important to obtain a history as far back as 1977 when evidence of the existence of HIV infection in heterosexual women IDUs was demonstrated (Thomas, O'Donnell, Williams, & Chiasson, 1988). Further, it is important to ask questions at the level that the woman can understand. For example, it may be inappropriate to ask "Do you inject illegal drugs?" A more appropriate question may be "Have you ever shot up or used a needle when doing drugs?" (Lyons & Fahrner, 1990).

Differences may exist between those women who have entered treatment programs and those who have not. Nonetheless, some psychological characteristics that have been identified in women who are IDUs include low self-esteem, depression, anxiety, past history of abuse, risk-taking behaviors, and feelings of powerlessness (Lyons & Fahrner, 1990). For some of these women, being able to reproduce and to present their partner with a child may be a means of countering feelings of low self-esteem, isolation, depression, and powerlessness, and achieving a greater measure of status for themselves and their partners. Reproduction may be a means of positive self-identity, regardless of the HIV-related risk to themselves and their offspring. Moreover, those who might contemplate pregnancy termination could experience difficulty in obtaining Medicaid-funded abortions (Mitchell, 1989).

Women seeking treatment programs may encounter difficulties. Some programs do not accept women; still others may not deal with major needs of women IDUs (such as child care) or may not accept pregnant women.

In a study of IDUs in south Florida, 77% of the males and 69% of the females reported having multiple sexual partners in the preceding six months. Among those with multiple partners, only 8% of the males and 7% of the females stated that they always used a condom for sexual encounters (McCoy & Khoury, 1990). These data regarding condom drug use are similar to those reported by the CDC in a national study ("Drug use," 1991).

Hemophilia/Coagulation Disorder

This exposure category is a relatively minor one for females. About 0.2% of the female adult cases of AIDS can be classified into this category. Because hemophilia is transmitted in an X-linked recessive manner, very few females are afflicted with hemophilia. Females, however, may manifest other coagulation disorders which are either inherited in a different manner or acquired (Cohen, 1984). The major risk of acquisition in this category is by multiple transfusions, particularly of factor concentrates for treatment of coagulation disorders.

Heterosexual Contact

The exposure category of heterosexual contact is the only one in which females with AIDS in the United States outrank males. Of all the adult U.S. cases of AIDS, the percentage of males in this category is 2.4%; for females, 3.8%. Of all of the female adult cases of AIDS in the United States, more than one-third were classified into this exposure category; for males, 2.7% of the male adult cases were classified in this category (see Table 3.3). The subcategories of heterosexual contact for adult females with AIDS are shown in Table 3.4. More than 60% of the heterosexual contacts for females were with an IDU. Thus, particularly for women, injecting drug use poses direct and indirect threats.

The first report of females who developed AIDS through sexual contact with a male who had AIDS was made in January 1983. At that time, there were 13 females who had no risk factors for AIDS other than sexual contact with male partners who were either IDUs or who (as is now known) had symptoms of HIV infection (Centers for Disease Control, 1983).

Heterosexual transmission of HIV poses a number of issues for women. HIV transmission by sexual contact appears more efficient from men to women than vice versa. Second, women may be relatively powerless in their sexual relationships. Third, many women do not perceive that they are at risk for HIV

TABLE 3.4 Subcategories in Adult Females of the AIDS Exposure Category "Heterosexual Contact" as Reported to the CDC through June, 1992

Subcategory	N	% of Subcategory In Adult Females	% of AllFemales with AIDS
Sex with injecting drug user	5,212	61.2	21.4
Sex with bisexual male	743	8.7	3.1
Sex with person with hemophilia	102	1.2	0.4
Born in Pattern-II country	806	9.5	3.3
Sex with person born in Pattern-II country	86	1.0	0.35
Sex with transfusion recipient with HIV infection	182	2.1	0.8
Sex with infected HIV person, risk not specified	1,393	16.3	5.7
Total:	8,524	100	35.1

Source: Center for Disease Control. (1992). HIV/AIDS Surveillance, July 1992, pp, 1–18.

infection. Fourth, as discussed above, the women at greatest risk for HIV are of lower socioeconomic status, are black or Hispanic, and may live in urban areas where the level of HIV seropositivity is already high and drug use is common. Thus, the chance for their sexual partner to be HIV-positive is greater than for someone living in a rural community. For example, in one study of males 15 to 44 years of age in urban New York and New Jersey, prevalence rates for HIV infection were 18–20% (St. Louis et al., 1990). Fifth, HIV infection is more common in men than women, making it more likely that women would have an infected partner rather than vice versa.

It is not unusual for women to be unaware that they are at risk for HIV infection. Some women may be in what they believe to be a stable relationship or may be married. The woman may be monogamous and assume monogamy in her partner. This assumption is not always valid. Her male partner may engage in sexual activities outside this relationship. Even if this occurs only once or rarely, this contact is often likely to be with someone who carries a risk of HIV transmission. An Australian study examined men who frequented "beats" (places such as public toilets or parks) to meet men for sexual encounters; 12% of these men were married, and 82% stated that they had also had sexual contacts with women. Of the latter group, 31% were active bisexuals, most having a regular female sexual partner or spouse. Only three of these men used condoms with their female partner (Bennett, Chapman, & Bray, 1989).

Of the bisexual men who died from AIDS, nearly 25% were married at the time of their death. Ethnic and cultural differences may play a role. In a summary of research related to bisexual men, blacks (41%) reported bisexuality more frequently than whites (21%) or Hispanics (31%). Further, older men were more likely to report bisexuality than homosexuality, perhaps reflecting changing societal acceptance. It has also been reported that black and Hispanic women are far less likely to be aware of (or acknowledge awareness of) their partners' bisexuality than white women (Chu, Peterman, Doll, Buehler, & Curran, 1992). Other men may be unfaithful to their steady partner or spouse with a woman who has many sexual contacts or who is or has been an injecting drug user. To begin using protection with the steady partner would be a tacit admission of sexual activity outside the relationship, so most men do not, thereby putting the steady partner at an unknown risk. In still other cases, a woman may not realize that her steady partner either regularly or occasionally is an injecting drug user or has been one in the past.

Even if the woman has knowledge that indicates that her mate is not monogamous or is injecting drugs, to insist upon using protection during mutual sexual encounters is to acknowledge a situation she may be incapable of dealing with and which may destroy their relationship. It may represent the loss of such important things as family life, companionship, protection, financial security, emotional stability, and community standing. Threats to the woman's physical safety or that of her children may be other reasons not to insist on the use of condoms with her male partner.

Cultural beliefs impinge on the use of condoms. For example, Hispanic women who suggest that their partners use condoms may be labeled "bad" (Anastos & Palleja, 1991). Other research found that black and Hispanic women were less likely than white women to have sexual partners who always used condoms (Catania et al., 1992). In many cultures, women learn that they must defer to the wishes of men, and it is men who are empowered as the decision makers. Such values are difficult or impossible for many women to overcome (see Chapters 4 and 13). In other countries, such as many African nations, both custom and law dictate women's deference to men (Ulin, 1992) (see Chapter 15). Furthermore, it is necessary to use latex condoms for protection against HIV, of a quality that will not easily be damaged during use and which may not be affordable. Since women do not have direct control over condom use, it is important that development of new (and evaluation of existing) devices for female-controlled protection be accomplished. This would include devices such as the female condom since the use of a diaphragm or cervical cap alone still permits HIV infection through the vaginal wall (Guinan, 1992; Stein, 1990) (see Chapter 4). While nonoxynol-9 has activity against HIV *in vitro*, use of a contraceptive sponge containing nonoxynol-9 has not been shown to prevent heterosexual acquisition of HIV (Kreiss et al., 1992).

When beginning new sexual relationships, one of the ways persons have been advised to reduce their risk of acquiring HIV through sexual contact is by ascertaining the risk history of their partners. However, partners may not always tell the truth about their history or behavior. In one study, about one-third of college-age males stated that they had told a lie to have sex and were sexually involved with more than one person. Nearly half indicated that they would understate the number of previous partners (Cochran & Mays, 1990). Another study was conducted among 138 HIV seropositive lower-income Hispanic and non-Hispanic white males in Los Angeles. Among the 45% who had been sexually active since learning they were HIV-infected, 52% did not disclose this information to their sexual partners (Marks, Richardson, & Maldonado, 1991). The type of sexual encounter (safe or risky) is even more important than the number or type of partner.

Women prostitutes or sex-industry workers can be considered a high-risk group for contracting AIDS through heterosexual contact. In one study in the Netherlands, prostitutes had unprotected sexual intercourse with an average number of 160 partners in four months (Hooykaas, Pligt, van Doornum, van der Linden, & Coutinho, 1989). There is also variation in the frequency of condom use with customers who are regular versus those that are sporadic (Day, Ward, & Harris, 1988). However, prostitutes may be more likely to use condoms with commercial partners than with their private partners. This behavior may put them at an even greater risk since their private partners are often injecting drug users (Rodrigues, 1991).

Female partners of males with hemophilia are at risk for HIV transmission through sexual contact. The first cases were reported in 1984 (Pitchenik, Shafron, Glasser & Spira, 1984; Ratnoff, Lederman & Jenkins, 1984). As of June 1992, females with AIDS whose infection with HIV was believed to result from heterosexual contact with a partner who had hemophilia represented about 1.2% of the heterosexual exposure category and 0.4% of all females with AIDS (Centers for Disease Control, 1992; see Table 3.4). The average male in the United States with hemophilia had been HIV-infected by 1982–1983 (Alexander, Gabelnick, & Spieler, 1990).

Many HIV seroprevalence studies have been conducted among the sexual partners of hemophiliac males. In the United States, transmission of HIV has ranged from 0% to 21.4%, depending upon the sample size, use of condoms between the couple, and other factors. In Italy, one study revealed HIV seroprevalence of 23%. Many of these studies were conducted in the mid-1980s, may have been with a small number of subjects, or have been biased in some way. Many partners had not been tested. Despite much publicity and education aimed at this group, one study estimated that 75% of sexual encounters by the women in their study with their hemophiliac partner did not involve condoms (Alexander et al., 1990).

Women who have had heterosexual contact with males who have received transfusions of blood or blood products have also contracted AIDS. In one study, 18% of 55 wives of men with transfusion-acquired AIDS had themselves become HIV-infected (Peterman, Stoneburner, Allen, Jaffe, & Curran, 1988).

Recipient of Transfusion of Blood, Blood Components, or Tissue

In this category are more than 7% of female AIDS cases, compared with 1.5% of the cases in adult males. Of all adult cases of AIDS in the United States, less than 1% were both female and classified into this category, compared with about 1.4% who were both male and transfusion recipients (see Table 3-3; Centers for Disease Control, 1992). No evidence in the literature suggests any gender distinctions for this exposure category.

Other/Undetermined

"Undetermined" cases refer to persons with no reported history of exposure to HIV that allows them to be placed in any of the established exposure categories, as explained in Chapter 1. "Other" refers to persons developing AIDS after exposure to HIV-infected blood in the health-care setting. For adult females, this represents about 7% of the total AIDS cases, in adult women in contrast to more than 3% of the total AIDS cases in adult men, as shown in Table 3.3 (Centers for Disease Control, 1992).

SUMMARY

Both the number and proportion of AIDS cases among women in the United States are increasing, rising from 3.2% of the reported cases in 1981 to more than 12% in 1991. In women, the majority of cases occurs in those who are 25–44 years of age, black or Hispanic, urban residents, and fall into the lower socioeconomic range. The most important transmission mechanisms for women are exposure to blood while injecting illicit drugs or heterosexual contact with an HIV-infected partner, who is often using drugs.

REFERENCES

ACT UP/New York Women and AIDS Book Group. (1990). *Women, AIDS and activism.* Boston, MA: South End Press.
AIDS in women. (1991). *Weekly Epidemiological Record, 11,* 75.
Alexander, N. J., Gabelnick, H. L., & Spieler, J. M. (Eds.). (1990). *Heterosexual transmission of AIDS.* New York: Wiley-Liss.
Allen, S., Lindan, C., Serufilira, A., Van de Perre, P., Rundle, A., Nsengumuremyi, F., Carael, M., Schwalbe, J., & Hulley, S. (1991). Human immunodeficiency virus infection in urban Rwanda. *Journal of the American Medical Association, 266,* 1657 1663.
Anastos, K., & Palleja, S. M. (1991). Caring for women at risk of HIV infection. *Journal of General Internal Medicine, 6*(Supp), S40–S46.
Bennett, G., Chapman, S., & Bray, F. (1989). A potential source for the transmission of the human immunodeficiency virus into the heterosexual population: bisexual men who frequent "beats". *Medical Journal of Australia, 151,* 314–318.

Brownworth, V. (1990). HIV testing of rapists raises new ethical questions. *Advocate, 565,* 48.

Catania, J. A., Coates, T. J., Kegeles, S., Fullilove, M. T., Peterson, J., Marin, B., Siegel, D., & Hulley, S. (1992). Condom use in multi-ethnic neighborhoods of San Francisco: The population-based AMEN (AIDS in multi-ethnic neighborhoods) study. *American Journal of Public Health, 82,* 284–287.

Centers for Disease Control (1981). Follow-up on Kaposi's sarcoma and *Pneumocystis* pneumonia. *Morbidity and Mortality Weekly Report, 30,* 409–410.

Centers for Disease Control (1983). Immunodeficiency among female sexual partners of males with acquired immune deficiency syndrome (AIDS)—New York. *Morbidity and Mortality Weekly Report, 31,* 697–698.

Centers for Disease Control (1985). Recommendations for assisting in the prevention of perinatal transmission of human T-lymphotropic virus type III/lymphadenopathy-associated virus and acquired immunodeficiency syndrome. *Morbidity and Mortality Weekly Report, 34,* 721–732.

Centers for Disease Control (1990). AIDS in women—United States. *Morbidity and Mortality Weekly Report, 39,* 845–846.

Centers for Disease Control (1991). *HIV/AIDS prevention, 2*(2), 1–8.

Centers for Disease Control (1992, July). *HIV/AIDS surveillance,* 1–18.

Chin, J. (1990). Current and future dimensions of the HIV/AIDS pandemic in women and children. *Lancet, 336,* 221–224.

Chu, S. Y., Buehler, J. W., & Berkelman, R. L. (1990). Impact of the human immuno-deficiency virus epidemic on mortality in women of reproductive age, United States. *Journal of the American Medical Association, 264,* 225–229.

Chu, S. Y., Buehler, J. W., Fleming, P. L., & Berkelman, R. L. (1990). Epidemiology of reported cases of AIDS in lesbians, United States 1980–89. *American Journal of Public Health, 80,* 1380–1381.

Chu, S. Y., Peterman, T. A., Doll, L. S., Buehler, J. W., & Curran, J. W. (1992). AIDS in bisexual men in the United States: Epidemiology and transmission to women. *American Journal of Public Health, 82,* 220–224.

Cochran, S. D., & Mays, V. M. (1990). Sex, lies and HIV. *New England Journal of Medicine, 322,* 774–775.

Cohen, F. L. (1991). Etiology and epidemiology of HIV infection. In J. D. Durham & F. L. Cohen, *The Person with AIDS: Nursing Perspectives* (pp. 1–59). New York: Springer.

Cohen, F. L. (1984). Clinical genetics in nursing practice. Philadelphia: J. B. Lippincott.

Day, S., Ward, H., & Harris, J. R. W. (1988). Prostitute women and public health. *British Medical Journal, 297,* 1585.

Dicker, B. (1989). Risk of AIDS among lesbians. *American Journal of Public Health, 79,* 1569.

Drug use and sexual behaviors among sex partners of injecting-drug users—United States, 1988–1990. *Morbidity and Mortality Weekly Report, 40,* 855–860.

Ellerbrock, T. V., Bush, T. J., Chamberland, M. E., & Oxtoby, M. J. (1991). Epidemiology of women with AIDS in the United States, 1981 through 1990. *Journal of the American Medical Association, 265,* 2971–2975.

Ellerbrock, T., & Rogers, M. (1990). Epidemiology of human immunodeficiency virus infection in women in the United States. *Obstetrics and Gynecology Clinics of North America, 17*(3), 523–544.

Friedland, G., & Selwyn, P. (1990). Intravenous drug use and HIV infection. *AIDS Clinical Care, 2*(4), 29–32.

Fullilove, R. E., Fullilove, M. T., Bowser, B. P., & Gross, S. A. (1990). Risk of sexually transmitted disease among black adolescent crack users in Oakland and San Francisco, Calif. *Journal of the American Medical Association, 263,* 851–855.

Greenhouse, P. (1987). Female-to-female transmission of HIV. *Lancet, 2,* 401–402.

Guinan, M. E. (1992). HIV, heterosexual transmission, and women. *Journal of the American Medical Association, 268,* 520–521.

Guinan, M. E., & Hardy, A. (1987). Epidemiology of AIDS in women in the United States, 1981 through 1986. *Journal of the American Medical Association, 257,* 2039–2042.

Gwinn, M., Pappaioanou, M., George, J. R., Hannon, W. H., Wasser, S. C., Redus, M. A., Hoff, R., Grady, G. F., Willoughby, A., Novello, A. C., Petersen, L. R., Dondero, Jr., T. J., & Curran, J. W. (1991). Prevalence of HIV infection in child-bearing women in the United States. *Journal of the American Medical Association, 265,* 1704–1708.

Handsfield, H. H. (1988). Heterosexual transmission of human immunodeficiency virus. *Journal of the American Medical Association, 260,* 1943–1944.

Hirsch, J., & Hincks, J. (1990). Young women and AIDS: A worldwide perspective. *Center for Population Options,* 1–2.

Hooykaas, C., van der Pligt, J., van Doornum, van der Linden, & Coutinho (1989). Heterosexuals at risk for HIV: Differences between private and commercial partners in sexual behaviour and condom use. *AIDS, 3,* 525–532.

Kent, M. R. (1991). Women and AIDS. *New England Journal of Medicine, 324,* 1442.

Kreiss, J., Ngugi, E., Holmes, K., Ndinya-Achola, J., Waiyaki, P., & Roberts, P. L., et al. (1992). Efficacy of nonoxynol 9 contraceptive sponge use in preventing heterosexual acquisition of HIV in Nairobi prostitutes. *Journal of the American Medical Association, 268,* 477–482.

Lacey, H., Roberts, R., Wooley, P. D., & Chandiok, S. (1991). Male rape. *British Medical Journal, 302,* 179.

Lyons, C., & Fahrner, R. (1990). HIV in women in the sex industry and/or injection drug users. *NAACOG's Clinical Issues in Perinatal and Women's Health Nursing, 1*(1), 33–40.

Marks, G., Richardson, J. L., & Maldonado, N. (1991). Self-disclosure of HIV infection to sexual partners. *American Journal of Public Health, 81,* 1321–1322.

Marmor, M., Weiss, L. R., Lyden, M., Weiss, S. H., Sacinger, W. C., Spira, T. J., & Feorino, P. M. (1986). Possible female-to-female transmission of human immunodeficiency virus. *Annals of Internal Medicine, 105,* 969.

McCoy, C. B., & Khoury, E. (1990). Drug use and the risk of AIDS. *American Behavioral Scientist, 33,* 419–431.

Mitchell, J. L. (1989). Drug abuse and AIDS in women and their affected offspring. *Journal of the National Medical Association, 81,* 841–842.

Monzon, O. T., & Capellan, J. M. B. (1987). Female-to-female transmission of HIV. *Lancet, 2,* 40–41.

Mundy, D. C., Schinazi, D. C., Gerber, A. R., Nahmias, A. J., & Randall, H. W., Jr. (1987). Human immunodeficiency virus isolated from amniotic fluid. *Lancet, 2,* 459–460.

Novick, L. F., Berns, D., Stricof, R., Stevens, R., Pass, K., & Wethers, J. (1989). HIV seroprevalence in newborns in New York State. *Journal of the American Medical Association, 261,* 1745–1750.

Padian, N. S., Shiboski, S. C., & Jewell, N. P. (1991). Female-to-male transmission of human immunodeficiency virus. *Journal of the American Medical Association, 266,* 1664–1667.

Page, J. B. (1990). Shooting scenarios and risk of HIV-1 infection. *American Behavioral Scientist, 33,* 478–490.

Peterman, T. A., Stoneburner, R. L., Allen, J. R., Jaffe, H. W., & Curran, J. W. (1988). Risk of human immunodeficiency virus transmission from heterosexual adults with transfusion-associated infections. *Journal of the American Medical Association, 259,* 55–58.

Petersen, L. R., White, C. R., & Premarital Screening Study Group. (1990). Premarital screening for antibodies to human immunodeficiency virus type 1 in the United States. *American Journal of Public Health, 80,* 1087–1090.

Pitchenik, A. E., Shafron, R. D., Glasser, R. M., & Spira, T. J. (1984). The acquired immunodeficiency syndrome in the wife of a hemophiliac. *Annals of Internal Medicine, 100,* 62–65.

Pizzo, P. A., & Butler, K. M. (1991). In the vertical transmission of HIV, timing may be everything. *New England Journal of Medicine, 325,* 652–654.

Ratnoff, O. D., Lederman, M. M., & Jenkins, J. J. (1984). Lymphadenopathy in a hemophiliac patient and his sexual partner. *Annals of Internal Medicine, 100,* 915.

Rodrigues, L. (1991). HIV transmission to women in stable relationships. *New England Journal of Medicine, 325,* 966.

St. Louis, M. E., Rauch, K. J., Petersen, L. R., Anderson, J. E., Schable, C. A., Dondero, T. J., and the Sentinel Hospital Surveillance Group. (1990). Seroprevalence rates of human immunodeficiency virus infections at sentinel hospitals in the United States. *New England Journal of Medicine, 323,* 213–218.

Schoenbaum, E. (1990). HIV risk factors among IVDUs. *AIDS Clinical Care, 2*(4), 33.

Schwarcz, S. K., & Whittington, W. L. (1990). Sexual assault and sexually transmitted diseases: Detection and management in adults and children. *Reviews of Infectious Diseases, 12*(Suppl. 6), S682–690.

Searching for women: A literature review on women HIV and AIDS in the United States (2nd ed.). (1991). Boston: University of Massachusetts, Boston, Multicultural AIDS Coalition.

Shayne, V. T., & Kaplan, B. J. (1991). Double victims: Poor women and AIDS. *Women & Health, 17*(1), 21–37.

Shih, D., Walter, E. B., Drucker, R. P., Greenwell, T., Wilfert, C., & Weinhold, K. J. (1990). Seroprevalence of human immunodeficiency virus infection at sentinel hospitals. *New England Journal of Medicine, 323,* 1843–1844.

Smith, P. F., Mikl, J., Truman, B. I., Lessner, L., Lehman, J. S., Stevens, R. W., Lord, E. A., Broaddus, R. K., & Morse, D. L. (1991). VI. HIV infection among women entering the New York State correctional system. *American Journal of Public Health, 81*(Suppl.), 35–40.

Stein, Z. A. (1990). HIV prevention: The need for methods women can use. *American Journal of Public Health, 80,* 460–462.

Stricof, R. L., Nattell, T. C., & Novick, L. F. (1991). VII. HIV seroprevalence in clients of sentinel family planning clinics. *American Journal of Public Health, 81*(Suppl.), 41–45.

Thomas, P., O'Donnell, R., Williams, R., & Chiasson, M. A. (1988). HIV infection in heterosexual female intravenous drug users in New York City, 1977–1980. *New England Journal of Medicine, 319,* 374.

Ulin, P. R. (1992). African women and AIDS: Negotiating behavioral change. *Social Science and Medicine, 34*(1), 63–73.

Weinstein, S. P., DeMaria, P. A., Jr., & Rosenthal, M. (1992). AIDS and alcohol. *Hospital Practice, 27*(2), 98–105.

Wiener, L. S. (1991). Women and human immunodeficiency virus: A historical and personal psychosocial perspective. *Social Work, 36,* 375–378.

World Health Organization. (1992). AIDS—over a million new infections in eight months. *WHO Press,* February 12, 1–2.

4

Prevention of HIV Infection in Women and Children

Barbara Berger and Vida Vizgirda

Designing and implementing effective HIV prevention programs for women requires close attention to the special circumstances and issues that women face. Women's lives involve a variety of complex roles with often conflicting expectations. Illness and premature death from HIV infection can prevent women from fulfilling roles as workers, wives, mothers, and caretakers, and adversely affects the families that may depend on their emotional and financial support. Since more than 85% of pediatric AIDS cases result from vertical transmission from an HIV-infected mother (Chapter 7), preventing HIV infection in women will also prevent perinatal HIV transmission. However, our concern in this chapter is not with women as vectors through which HIV is transmitted to others but rather as individuals who deserve the knowledge and opportunity to protect themselves from HIV.

This chapter will discuss the behaviors that place women at risk for HIV infection, methods for reducing and managing the risk from these behaviors, obstacles to consistent use of preventive practices, and educational approaches that can enable women to recognize their personal risk and modify those behaviors that make them vulnerable to HIV infection.

RISK BEHAVIORS RELATED TO HIV ACQUISITION

HIV prevention efforts continue to be hindered by the public's original perception of AIDS as solely a gay white male disease. More than 10 years of experience with AIDS and HIV disease have shown that unsafe behavior, not "risk group" membership, places individuals at risk for HIV infection. HIV prevention for women requires that they recognize the ways they may be at risk. Despite the fact that both heterosexual activity and injecting drug (ID) use are significant routes of exposure to HIV for women (Chapter 3), many women still believe that, unless they personally inject drugs, they need not worry about contracting HIV.

Risk from Sexual Activity

Worldwide, women risk HIV infection primarily through their heterosexual activities. Any sexual activity that involves the exchange of body fluids, including vaginal, oral, and heterosexual anal intercourse, holds the potential to transmit HIV (Johnson et al., 1989; Lifson et al., 1990; Padian, Shiboski, & Jewell, 1990). The vast majority of heterosexuals practice vaginal intercourse and some form of oral sex: fellatio (oral sex on a man), cunnilingus (oral sex on a woman), or both. In addition, many heterosexual couples report engaging in anal intercourse, which has been associated with an increased risk of HIV transmission if one partner is HIV-infected (European Study Group, 1989; Padian et al., 1990). In studies of heterosexual couples with at least one HIV-positive partner, up to 35% reported anal intercourse (European Study Group, 1989; Johnson et al., 1989; Padian, 1990).

HIV transmission to women may be affected by a number of factors. Heterosexual HIV transmission in Pattern I countries such as the United States occurs more commonly from men to women, placing the woman at greater risk in any sexual encounter. Other sexually transmitted diseases (STDs), especially genital ulcer diseases such as syphilis, chancroid, and genital herpes, may also facilitate the sexual transmission of HIV. Transmission of HIV appears to be more likely during periods when the quantity of cell-free virus in the blood is high (European Study Group, 1989; Laurian, Peynet, & Verroust, 1989). Because an infected individual may have a high virus load before becoming HIV-antibody positive, transmission is possible even with a partner who has recently tested negative for the HIV antibody.

HIV is well established among injecting drug users (IDUs) in many cities in the United States. Battjes, Pickens, and Amsel (1991) report HIV seroprevalence among IDUs admitted to methadone treatment programs ranging from 59% in New York City in 1987 to 23% in Baltimore, 15% in Chicago, and 3% in Los Angeles in 1989. Rhodes and associates (1990) found nearly 6% of IDUs in Long Beach, California, HIV seropositive in 1988.

This population of HIV-infected IDU men constitutes a major vector for HIV infection in women. Up to 59% of IDU men report having heterosexual contact with non-IDU women (Abdul-Quader, Tross, Friedman, Kouzi & Des Jarlais, 1990; Booth, Koester, Brewster, Wiebel & Fritz, 1991). Over 41% of the women found to be HIV seropositive at a New York City STD clinic reported heterosexual contact, primarily with a male IDU, as their only known risk behavior (Chiasson et al., 1991). Many non-IDU women find themselves in established relationships before learning of their partner's ID use (Kane, 1991).

To protect themselves women have been advised to limit their number of sex partners. Although limiting the number of partners can decrease the probability of coming in contact with an HIV-infected partner, women still must be aware that a single encounter can result in HIV transmission (Johnson et al., 1989). While decreasing the number of partners offers some protection, there is no guarantee that the one partner selected is, and will remain, free of HIV.

There is also confusion about what "limiting partners" means (Mays & Cochran, 1988). While women may view themselves as monogamous if they have only one partner in a given time period, the risk of HIV results from the number of partners in a lifetime. In a population that is sexually active at younger ages, marrying later, and facing a significant probability of divorce and remarriage, advising women to have only one sexual partner in a lifetime is unrealistic.

Reiss and Leik (1989) found that condom use was more effective in preventing HIV infection than was limiting the number of partners. This was based on mathematical modeling of the risk of HIV infection at various levels of seroprevalence, HIV infectivity, number of partners, and condom use. The estimated risk of infection with only two lifetime partners and no condom use generally exceeded the risk with condom use and 20 partners.

Knowledge that condoms offer some protection against sexual transmission of HIV does not result in consistent condom use, even among individuals at relatively high risk for HIV infection (Dengelegi, Weber & Torquato, 1990; Kane, 1991; Saxon, Calsyn, Whittaker & Freeman, 1991). Recent reports of condom use are summarized in Table 4.1. Even when at least one partner was known to be HIV-infected, 59% of couples never used condoms (Padian, Shiboski & Jewell, 1991). Excluding studies of discordant couples, no more than 11% of respondents, and sometimes fewer than 1%, reported always using condoms.

TABLE 4.1 Condom Use in Various Studies

Sample	Percent Condom Use			First Author, Year
	Never	Sometimes	Always	
IDUs from outreach	66	—	6	Booth, 1991
STD clinic	—	—	<1	Chiasson, 1991
IDUs in detoxification	—	—	6	Dengelegi, 1990
discordants*	—	—	4	Johnson, 1989
sex partners of IDUs	54	37	9	Kane, 1991
discordants*	—	—	45	Laurian, 1989
male IDUs	73	—	—	Lewis, 1990
female IDUs	63	—	—	Lewis, 1989
IDUs, in past month	68	—	11	Magura, 1990
French heterosexuals	53	37	10	Moatti, 1991
discordants*	59	—	—	Padian, 1991
HIV-negative	—	48 in 1984		Samuel, 1991
heterosexual males	—	61 in 1989		
male IDUs	—	37	—	Saxon, 1991
female IDUs	—	32	—	

*Discordants: couples in which one partner is HIV-infected and the other is not.

Moderate numbers of respondents indicated at least some condom use, which raises questions about the personal and/or situational variables affecting that decision (see Table 4.2).

Risk from Injecting Drug Use

Injecting drug use poses a risk of HIV infection to women in two ways: indirectly via its effect on the HIV seroprevalence among potential sex partners, as previously discussed, and directly as a transmission route for those women who inject drugs. HIV transmission is possible whenever needles are reused without adequate cleaning, whether for illicit intravenous injection or skin-popping, vitamin or steroid shots, tattooing or acupuncture, or where limited medical supplies are reused.

The mechanics of ID use include several techniques that can lead to HIV contamination of the needle and syringe and infection of the user. Powdered drug is combined with water in a "cooker," often a bottlecap or spoon, and heat is applied to dissolve the drug for injection. A small piece of cotton or cigarette filter may be placed into the solution to filter the drug as it is drawn into the syringe. Once the needle is in the vein, blood is drawn back into the syringe to dilute the drug, a process known as "booting" (Greenfield, Bigelow, & Brooner, 1992), in the belief that this increases the drug's effects (Inciardi, 1990).

TABLE 4.2 Factors Influencing Decisions about Condom Use

Personal acceptibility of condoms (5, 9, 10, 13)*
Partner receptivity to condoms (6, 9, 13, 14)
Type of partner, "commercial" vs. "private" (2, 4, 8)
Finding condom use disruptive during intercourse (5, 6, 10)
Degree of concern about AIDS (10, 12)
Discussing AIDS before having sex (11, 12)
Number of partners (3, 6)
Type of sexual activity (oral vs. vaginal) (2, 14)
Duration of relationship (7, 11)
Belief in efficacy of condoms in preventing STDs (10) or AIDS (6)
Embarassed to buy condoms (6, 10)
Feeling that condom use creates doubt about the partner (10, 14)
Peer acceptance of condom use (13)
Knowing someone with HIV (10)
Perceived chance of getting AIDS (3)
Where partner was met (through social network vs. "pickup" location) (12)
Feeling the intoxicating effects of alcohol (12)

*Numbers in parentheses indicate first author and year of source: 1 = Abdul-Quader, 1990; 2 = Booth, 1991; 3 = Campbell, A., 1991; 4 = Campbell, C., 1991; 5 = Dengelegi, 1990; 6 = DiClemente, 1992; 7 = Haines, 1991; 8 = Kane, 1991; 9 = Magura, 1990; 10 = Moatti, 1991; 11 = Nelson, 1992; 12 = Trocki, 1991; 13 = Valdiserri, 1989; 14 = Worth, 1989.

"Frontloading" and "backloading" are methods of moving a drug from one syringe into another to mix two types of drugs and/or to divide a drug between two people. To frontload, the needle is removed from one syringe and the needle of the second syringe is placed inside the first barrel to add or aspirate fluid (Grund, Kaplan, Adriaans, Blanken, & Huisman, 1990). When the needle is not removable, as with a diabetic syringe, the same result may be accomplished by "backloading," removing the plunger to fill the receiving syringe from the back (Inciardi & Page, 1991). "Washing" involves drawing fluid into a recently used syringe and injecting the residual drug to tide a user over until more drugs are available (Mays & Cochran, 1988).

Sharing of needles and syringes occurs for several reasons. Where the legal sale of injection equipment is restricted, supplies in the IDU community may be scarce or available only at high prices (Broadhead, 1991; Des Jarlais & Friedman, 1988). Paraphernalia laws may make IDUs reluctant to carry their personal "outfit" in the event they are stopped by police, especially if on parole (Rhodes et al., 1990; Watters, 1989).

But scarcity of sterile equipment due to legal restrictions is only one reason for sharing. Of necessity, IDUs participate in social networks to obtain money, drugs, and equipment, networks that also serve to reinforce group norms and behaviors. These group norms have often involved sharing drugs and "works," as well as food, clothing, and shelter. Grund, Kaplan, and Adriaans (1991) note that "sharing and the reciprocal aid it promotes provide a practical and emotional balance to the daily hardships of addict life . . . , an expression of the almost universal subcultural code of 'share what you have'" (p. 1606). Mays and Cochran (1988) cite friendship and loyalty as motives in allowing another IDU to "wash" residual drug from one's syringe.

Characteristics of these social networks vary among cities and among neighborhoods within cities (Schoenbaum et al., 1989; Watters, 1988). In New York City, for example, in excess of 100 people per day may inject in large "shooting galleries," often using the "house works" or whatever discarded equipment can be found. Syringes and needles may be passed from user to user until the needle is too dull to use, widening the circle of people who may become infected. By contrast, IDUs in San Francisco more often belong to smaller friendship-based networks and gather in a member's apartment to shoot up (Watters, 1989). In Long Beach, California, for example, 72% of IDUs had injected most recently either at home or at a friend's house (Rhodes et al., 1990). Though fewer people may be involved, HIV transmission can still occur if even one participant is infected.

Even where legal penalties are not an issue and sterile supplies are readily accessible, needle sharing may still occur when IDUs experience intense drug craving (Grund et al., 1991; Rhodes et al., 1990). Sharing is also more likely among novice IDUs, since experienced IDUs have a larger repertoire of alternatives with which to protect themselves (Grund et al., 1991). Experienced IDUs have also been reported to be more likely than novices to adopt new behavioral norms against sharing equipment (Des Jarlais & Friedman, 1988). Though easier access to equipment and changing IDU social norms can decrease needle sharing, the behavior is unlikely to be eliminated.

Injection behaviors and the associated risk of HIV transmission are influenced by the choice of drug, which in turn varies across ethnic groups, age, gender, and geographic location (Booth et al., 1991; Rhodes et al., 1990; Singer, 1991). Use of cocaine among IDUs has been associated with increased volume and frequency of booting (Greenfield et al., 1992), intensified craving, and disruption of previously stable patterns of opiate use (Grund, Kaplan & Adriaans, 1991). Although heroin and cocaine, either alone or combined as a "speedball," are the major drugs of choice for injection (Rhodes et al., 1990), polydrug use, the use of multiple mood-altering substances and routes of administration, has become the norm (Singer, 1991).

Interaction between Sex and Drug Use

The impact of drugs on HIV transmission does not depend solely on injection behaviors. Use of any drug, including alcohol (Anastos & Palleja, 1991; Gilliam, Scott, & Troup, 1989; Trocki & Leigh, 1991), can alter one's judgment and motivation to employ appropriate risk-reduction behaviors, primarily in sexual encounters but also in associated ID use. People using illicit drugs may also be drawn into circles where HIV is more prevalent, making any lapses in preventive technique riskier.

The burgeoning use of smokable cocaine, "crack," is of particular concern. Crack is highly addictive, its use characterized by an intense but brief euphoria, followed quickly by extreme depression, anxiety, and craving (Hannan & Adler, 1990). This dysphoria and craving result in a cycle of frequent, repetitive use. Crack's availability, low price, and reputation as a phenomenal sexual stimulant (Anastos & Palleja, 1991; Hannan & Adler, 1990) have contributed to its rapid spread.

Drug addiction, whether to injectable drugs or crack, is in turn tied to prostitution. The exigencies of addiction commonly lead women to exchange sex for drugs or money as a means of supporting their own, and often their partner's, drug habit (Rosenbaum, 1981; Worth, 1989). Studies report up to 36% (Saxon et al., 1991) of female IDUs having engaged in sex for drugs or money. In Chiasson and associates' (1991) study at a New York City STD clinic, 41% of HIV-positive women without other risk had a history of both crack use and prostitution, a finding supported by Chirgwin, DeHovitz, Dillon, and McCormack (1991).

Women who have sex with women are also at risk for HIV infection. Although HIV transmission has been reported from sexual activity between women, the major source of HIV infection in such cases is IDU (Chu, Buehler, Fleming,

& Berkelman, 1990). These women may incur further risk via heterosexual prostitution to support their addiction (Worth, 1989).

Any sex act or drug use poses some risk of HIV transmission. That risk increases in areas of increased HIV seroprevalence, areas that tend to be disproportionately minority and poor. As prevention methods are discussed, some of the social and cultural influences that promote or inhibit the adoption of risk-reduction strategies will be considered.

PREVENTION STRATEGIES

Sexual Behaviors

For many women, the risk of HIV infection arises solely from their sexual activities. Sexual behavior is influenced by complex cultural, economic, and emotional factors that may interfere with women's ability to protect themselves from HIV. The acceptibility of a given risk-reduction method will be affected by the woman's role expectations in a specific relationship, her partner's anticipated reactions, the cultural definitions associated with the method, its expense and availability, its effects on her reproductive options, and the broader economic and physical consequences of its use (Carovano, 1991; Kane, 1990; Worth, 1989).

In many situations, women are relatively powerless in the relationships in which they are sexually active (Anastos & Palleja, 1991; Stuntzner-Gibson, 1991). Attempts to introduce risk-reduction techniques, particularly in an established relationship, may be viewed as expressions of distrust or admissions of one's own illicit behaviors. Refusal to engage in potentially risky activities may disrupt the relationship and can lead to threats of economic abandonment or physical violence, radically reducing the workable options a woman has for protecting herself from HIV. Evaluating the utility of the following risk-reduction strategies requires attention to these possible conflicts.

Abstinence.   Abstinence from all sexual activity offers complete protection from sexually transmitted HIV. For most women, however, lifelong abstinence will not be an option. Particularly in cultures where a woman's identity and value derive primarily from her roles as wife and mother, abstinence will not be an acceptable method of avoiding the often intangible risk of HIV. Individuals for whom fear of HIV is the sole motivation for abstinence remain vulnerable to impulsive sexual behaviors if their inhibitions are lowered by drug or alcohol use.

Partner History.   The injunction to "know your partner," relying on partners' reports of their risk history and/or a healthy physical appearance, offers no guarantee of protection (Nelson, 1992). People in the early stages of HIV disease have no external physical signs, and may themselves be unaware of their

HIV infection. Also, individuals, both male and female, who know themselves to be HIV-infected may conceal this information from potential partners while taking no precautions to prevent HIV transmission (Brown & Rundell, 1990; Marks, Richardson, & Maldonado, 1991). Even in what is believed to be a monogamous relationship, each partner is depending not only on the other's honesty but also on the knowledge and sophistication of the other about which current or past activities, such as bisexuality or drug use, may constitute a risk for HIV. As one nurse put it, "If I have unprotected sex with my husband is that trust, or is that risk?" (Haines, 1991, p. 16). It is both. Even women who initially insist that a new partner use a condom may, after a few weeks or months, become less vigilant about condom use as they become more comfortable in the relationship (Nelson, 1992). But nothing has changed in terms of their risk of HIV infection (Haines, 1991).

Outercourse. Nonpenetrative sexual activities are safe to the extent that exposure to body fluids does not occur. A partial list of these activities appears in Table 4.3. Additional suggestions and variations may be found in *The New Joy of Sex* (Comfort, 1991), which explicitly addresses the risk of HIV transmission in heterosexual activities. Because many of these activities can be preludes to penetrative sex, both participants must be clear about the point beyond which these behaviors become unsafe without further protection.

Latex Condoms. Whenever there is risk of exposure to body fluids during penetrative sex, latex condoms offer a high degree of protection from HIV. Studies of condom use and subsequent seroconversion among HIV-discordant couples (couples in which only one partner was initially HIV-infected) offer persuasive evidence of condoms' protective effect (Feldblum, 1991; Padian et al., 1990). Pooling data from six studies involving 317 HIV-discordant couples, Feldblum found that 2.3% of condom-using couples experienced new HIV seroconversion, compared to 25.5% of couples not regularly using condoms. The seroconversions in condom-using couples may reflect condom failure or inconsistencies in the way "condom use" was evaluated. Unlike use for contraception, where some couples employ condoms primarily during ovulation, condoms must be used in every sexual encounter to prevent HIV transmission.

Only latex condoms should be used, since the hepatitis B virus, which is about one-third the diameter of HIV (Feldblum & Fortney, 1988), can pass through pores in animal-skin condoms. Table 4.4 contains important information on selecting and using condoms. The majority of condom breakages occurs in only 4% to 6% of condom users and has been attributed to very vigorous sex, use of oil-based lubricants, or attempts to test the condom by unrolling, stretching, or blowing it up before using it (Roylance, 1992). Many vaginal medications are oil-based, and if used concurrently, would contribute to condom failure (Stone & Peterson, 1992). Because condoms may be more likely to rupture during anal

TABLE 4.3 Safer Sex Guidelines for Women

Safe: abstinence, fantasizing, erotic conversation, phone sex, self-masturbation, separate
sex toys, voyeurism
Safe if skin is intact: hugging, cuddling, massaging, frottage (body-to-body rubbing), mutual masturbation, body licking (excluding genitals & anus)
Probably safe: wet kissing
If latex barrier protection is used:
heavy petting with latex barrier (if it can get you pregnant, it can give you HIV)
sharing sex toys covered with condoms
fellatio with a condom (no teeth!)
cunnilingus with latex barrier
vaginal intercourse with a latex condom
anal intercourse with a doubled or extra-strong latex condom
* If the condom or barrier fails (breaks, leaks, or falls off), these activities
become unsafe.
* Condom failure is more likely with vaginal and particularly anal intercourse
than with oral sex.
* See Table 4.4 for proper condom use and considerations regarding nonoxynol-9.
Unsafe: heavy petting without a latex condom
sharing sex toys without a latex condom
fellatio without a latex condom
cunnilingus without latex barrier
vaginal intercourse without a latex condom
anal intercourse without a latex condom
The following do NOT reliably protect against HIV infection:
douching, urinating after sex
coitus interruptus (withdrawal before ejaculation)
birth-control pills, diaphragms, intrauterine devices (IUDs), sterilization (vasec-
tomy, tubal ligation, hysterectomy)
implantable contraceptives such as Norplant
contraceptive sponges
pre/postcoital application of nonoxynol-9 alone
having sex with only one person regardless of his/her risk history or healthy
appearance

Adapted from Anastos, K., & Palleja, S. M., (1991). Caring for women at risk for HIV infection, *Journal
of General Internal Medicine, 6*(Suppl), S40-S46; Raisler, J., (1990), Safer sex for women, *Clinical
Issues in Perinatal and Women's Health Nursing, 1*(1), 28–32.

intercourse (Raisler, 1990), use of extra-strong condoms or two condoms together has been suggested. The issue of spermicide use with condoms is discussed below. A new condom must be used with every episode of intercourse
or fellatio.

Barrier protection during cunnilingus can be accomplished by using a *dental
dam* (a thin layer of latex), or a condom split open to lie flat. Any shared sex
toys must also be covered by a condom. Condoms are available from drugstores
or vending machines at prices ranging from approximately 50 cents to $1, and

TABLE 4.4 Proper Condom Use to Prevent HIV Transmission

General information:
- Use latex condoms only, not lambskin or other natural membranes.
- Condoms come in different colors and flavors and are available to fit all sizes. If one type or size is not comfortable, try others.
- Condoms come individually packaged in foil wrappers. Before using, inspect the wrapper for punctures or slits and discard if damaged. Do *not* unroll the condom itself to inspect for defects; unrolling, stretching, or blowing up condoms before using them has been associated with high rates of condom breakage.
- Condoms must be protected from sunlight, heat, and ozone. Do not leave condoms on the dashboard of the car or carry them in pockets for prolonged periods of time.
- Condoms come with and without lubricant. Adequate lubrication with a water-based product such as KY or diaphragm jelly helps prevent breakage. *Never* use oil-based lubricants such as vaseline, vegetable oil, cold cream, or mineral oil, since they hasten deterioration of the latex; this includes oil-based vaginal medications. Latex condoms can lose 90% of their strength within 60 seconds of exposure to oil-based products. Do not use saliva as lubricant because it may contain infectious material.
- Many condoms come with a water-based spermicide containing nonoxynol-9 already in the tip of the condom. Nonoxynol-9 jelly can be put in the tip of unlubricated condoms and on the outside of all condoms and has been recommended because of evidence that it has virucidal activity against HIV.
- If you have experienced genital irritation when using nonoxynol-9, it is probably better to use water-based lubricants without nonoxynol-9.
- If either partner currently has genital irritation or rash, any genital contact, including frottage, will not be safe.
- If you do *not* experience genital irritation with nonoxynol-9, using it may provide extra protection against HIV infection, especially if the condom breaks.

How to apply a condom:
- Adequate lubrication and leaving an empty tip as a reservoir for ejaculate are your best protection against the condom breaking or leaking. Again, never use oil-based lubricants and do not unroll the condom before use to inspect or test it.
- Apply to erect penis before allowing it to make contact with genitals, since an erect penis can ooze fluid containing HIV. If the man is not circumsized, pull the foreskin back before putting on the condom.
- If the condom is not prelubricated, apply a small amount of water-based lubricant to the tip, then pinch approximately half an inch at the tip of the condom to exclude air and leave room for the ejaculate.
- With the tip of the condom pinched, unroll it until it covers the entire penis. If you see any holes or tears, begin again with a new condom.
- Apply water-based lubricant to the outside of the condom and to the entry point.
- If you feel the condom break during sex, immediately stop and put on a new condom and lubricant.
- As soon as your partner ejaculates, have him withdraw while holding the base of the condom firmly in place to avoid spilling any fluid. Wrap the used condom in a tissue and discard it in the trash. Do not flush it down the toilet since it may cause sewer problems.
- After removing the condom, his penis and genital area will still have semen on it. Before cuddling, he should wash himself thoroughly with soap and water. Some people recommend using rubbing alcohol or dilute disinfectants such as Lysol after the soap.
- If you have no condom, stick to "dry sex"—outercourse.
- *Caution*: Use of drugs or alcohol can adversely affect your judgment and motivation to protect yourself during sex.

Adapted from Anastos, K., & Palleja, S. M., (1991), Caring for women at risk of HIV infection, *Journal of General Internal Medicine*, 6(Suppl), S40–S46; Bird, K. D., (1991), The use of spermicide containing nonoxynol-9 in the prevention of HIV infection, *AIDS*, 5, 791–796; Roylance, F. D., (1992, March 23), Condoms: Keeping them safe, *Chicago Sun-Times*, p. 7.

are often distributed free by health departments, STD clinics, and other programs geared toward women, such as Women, Infants and Children (WIC) and prenatal clinics.

However, obstacles to consistent condom use for HIV prevention are many. Having a condom readily available requires that at least one partner anticipated the need. Even among individuals who would otherwise be willing to use this method, the lack of a condom may result in unprotected sex (Kane, 1990).

Many partners are very resistant to using condoms, believing that they negatively affect physical sensation and spontaneity (Suffet & Lifshitz, 1991; Worth, 1989). A woman may feel that even suggesting a condom implies a lack of trust in her partner or will be viewed as an admission of her own infidelity or knowledge of being HIV-infected. For many men and women, condoms have deeply embedded cultural meanings associated with promiscuity and prostitutes. In relationships where these meanings are particularly strong, women may fear that insisting on condom use will result in physical violence or abandonment (Karan, 1989; Mays & Cochran, 1988).

While condoms prevent HIV transmission, their contraceptive action may be undesirable. The ability to bear children is a major aspect of many women's social status and personal identity. Having children enables both partners to fulfill their roles as parents and offers opportunities for emotional expression that may be unattainable in other aspects of their lives. Children may also represent future economic security for the family, and empowerment of the community (Carovano, 1991; Mays & Cochran, 1988). The contraceptive action of condoms deprives people of all these potential rewards.

Many prostitutes routinely require their clients to use condoms and may become skilled at applying condoms during fellatio without the man's knowledge (Campbell, 1991; Mays & Cochran, 1988). However, many women trading sex for drugs or money are not in a position to dictate terms. To insist on condoms may result in having to accept less money or losing the "trick" altogether (Schilling, El-Bassel, Schinke, Gordon, & Nichols, 1991). Prostitutes may also use condoms to distinguish between commercial and more intimate encounters, often choosing to forgo protection with their steady partner as an expression of their emotional bond (Kane, 1991; Suffet & Lifshitz, 1991; Worth, 1989).

The Female Condom. This is a new development in barrier protection. It consists of a polyurethane sheath that lines the vagina and is held in place by two flexible rings. The inner ring fits over the cervix much like a diaphragm; the outer ring remains outside the vagina to cover the labia (Wisconsin Pharmacal Co., 1991). Though some users have found the outer ring cumbersome (Painter, 1992), most report not noticing it after the first few uses (Wisconsin Pharmacal Co., 1991). Some participants in trials have reported that the female condom transmits body heat better than latex condoms, so it feels more natural (Seligman, 1992). Because it is made of polyurethane, the female condom can be an important alternative for couples in which either partner has a latex allergy. The female condom can be inserted before arousal, making it less disruptive than male condoms. Like male condoms, however, the female condom is intended for single use only. While this product gives a woman more control over whether she is protected, it is not a method that can be used without her partner's awareness (Sakondhavat, 1990).

Provisional approval for the female condom was obtained from the Food and Drug Administration in January 1992, contingent on further testing for effectiveness in preventing HIV and STD transmission and pregnancy. General availability in the United States is expected by the end of 1992, at two to three times the price of latex male condoms. With either male or female condoms, price may be a significant issue for frequent condom users with limited incomes.

Spermicides.   Spermicides, specifically nonoxynol-9, have been shown to kill HIV and HIV-infected lymphocytes at *in vitro* concentrations of 0.05% or greater (Feldblum & Fortney, 1988). Nonoxynol-9 is available in various forms: jelly, foam, sponges, and vaginal suppositories, and as a lubricant in many condoms, though the use of spermicides without a condom is not recommended for HIV prevention. Genital irritation has been reported with frequent use of nonoxynol-9 (Bird, 1991). Because irritation may make membranes more permeable to HIV, it is no longer possible to make a blanket recommendation for nonoxynol-9 use, especially in the context of frequent or high-dose usage (see Table 4-4).

Virucides.   Interest in virucides to protect against HIV transmission has arisen in part because all other methods (abstinence, barriers, and spermicides) inextricably link prevention of HIV with contraception. Virucides that would kill HIV without spermicidal effects have been proposed as an option for dealing with the separate goals of HIV prevention and procreation (Carovano, 1991; Stein, 1990). So far, no products that meet these dual requirements are available.

Other Contraceptives.   Finally, many methods that are effective as contraceptives cannot be recommended for protection from HIV because they do not prevent contact between semen and the vagina (see Table 4.3; also see Chapter 6).

Injecting Drug Use Behaviors

Women who inject drugs risk HIV infection from contaminated injection equipment, in addition to their risk from sexual activities. Although male IDUs tend to have non-IDU female partners, female IDUs' partners are predominantly male IDUs (Booth et al., 1991; Saxon et al., 1991). Preventing HIV transmission among IDUs requires teaching techniques for both safer sex and safer ID use.

In the United States, advocating safer drug use is controversial (Anderson, 1991; Broadhead, 1991). Providing information on how to avoid HIV infection when using injectable drugs is viewed by many as an endorsement of an illegal activity. Politicians may be particularly sensitive to the seeming contradiction of publicly funding safer drug use campaigns while simultaneously waging a war on drugs. An opposing perspective sees efforts to promote safer ID use as a way merely to neutralize the threat of HIV for the general public without concern for IDUs' long-term well-being.

Injecting drug use has been labeled by society as a deviant behavior, stigmatizing IDUs as unworthy of any help or support. Already disenfranchised to some extent because of ethnicity and poverty, many IDUs live without a social safety net. Where more socially acceptable individuals who experience a crisis may have a variety of options and resources to draw upon, IDUs' lives are often financially and emotionally precarious.

The life situation of a female IDU may be even more overwhelming. Even within the IDU subculture, women IDUs are viewed more negatively than their male counterparts (Worth, 1990), perhaps because their ID use violates gender stereotypes. Women IDUs may also experience increased stress related to their caretaking responsibilities, the lack of financial and emotional support, and the threat of physical violence in the outside world and at home (Mondanaro, 1987; Suffet & Lifshitz, 1991). Health problems, including poor nutrition, STDs and other infections, and psychomorbidity are also more common among women IDUs than among men IDUs or non-IDU women (Mondanaro, 1987). Nearly half the women IDUs interviewed by Suffet and Lifshitz had considered suicide but rejected the idea because of their responsibilities for others. In the context of the many threats to survival that women IDUs face daily, the risk of HIV infection and AIDS may seem both overwhelmingly inevitable and far less immediate than finding food, drugs, and safe shelter.

Safer injection behavior can be accomplished either by *not sharing equipment* or by disinfecting shared needles and syringes. IDUs may obtain new needles and syringes through illicit markets, needle exchange programs, or pharmacies if purchase without a prescription is legal.

When new needles and syringes are not available, *bleach* is a convenient, effective method of cleaning used "works" (Broadhead, 1991). Bleach use, because it involves modifying current injection behavior rather than extinguishing it, may be more acceptable to the IDU population than exhortations to stop drug use altogether. The basic catechism for safer drug use as presented by Broadhead (1991) is

- Don't use drugs.
- If you use drugs, don't inject.
- If you inject, don't share.
- If you share, clean equipment with bleach between uses.

Presenting this protocol in reverse order, beginning with the use of bleach, offers IDUs small, concrete, immediate steps they can take to protect themselves from HIV. IDUs who may share equipment are instructed to carry a small bottle of full-strength bleach and to flush used needles and syringes twice with bleach, then rinse twice with water. This procedure can be completed in about 15 seconds (Broadhead, 1991). If clean water is not always available, IDUs should carry water with them.

Although cleaning with bleach will disinfect the needle and syringe, IDUs need to be aware of other steps in their injection routine that can reintroduce HIV. If the outfit or the drug comes in contact with infected material before its next use by sharing cookers or "cottons" (Booth et al., 1991; Rhodes et al., 1990) or using contaminated water to rinse equipment or dilute the drug, the possibility of HIV transmission returns. Also, using bleach will not prevent HIV transmission from such practices as frontloading and backloading unless both outfits have been disinfected. IDUs who do not share needles and syringes are as vulnerable to this type of contamination as IDUs sharing works. "Washing" (injecting residual drug from someone else's outfit) cannot be made safe, even with bleach. The injectable drug practices discussed here are unlikely to include the full repertoire of behaviors being used. Techniques of injection need to be explored with each IDU individually to determine which injection practices make that person vulnerable to HIV infection.

There are some disadvantages in using bleach to prevent HIV transmission among IDUs (Broadhead, 1991). The corrosive nature of bleach shortens the useful life of the equipment, especially the rubber plunger. Although bleach works only if it is available when the necessity for sharing equipment arises, being found in possession of a small bottle of bleach when stopped by police may trigger suspicion of current ID use. A leaking bleach container in a pocket can also stain clothing in a characteristic manner, marking the individual with a limited wardrobe as an IDU.

Outreach work may be more effective than mass-media campaigns in reaching IDUs with HIV prevention information. Outreach workers, often former IDUs themselves, gain considerable insight into the problems of life on the street. Through their interactions with individual IDUs, which may include problem-solving and facilitating access to treatment programs and other services, outreach workers develop relationships in which the risk-reduction messages of safer drug use and safer sex become more credible.

Simply improving IDUs' knowledge about HIV prevention does not necessarily affect their practice of risk behaviors. Outreach programs that also provide bleach bottles and condoms have been more effective in promoting behavior change than programs providing information alone (Broadhead, 1991; Des Jarlais & Friedman, 1988; Watters, 1989). Even when the means for safer injection are provided, not all IDUs will change their injection behavior, and even those who do employ safer injection practices may not do so consistently. Safer sex practices have been adopted less readily among IDUs than safer injection behaviors (Booth et al., 1991; Des Jarlais & Friedman, 1988). Achieving a sustained reduction in risk activities will require changing group behavioral norms (Des Jarlais & Friedman, 1988), which may be more difficult with sexual behaviors that are influenced by entrenched cultural patterns that devalue women.

Drug treatment programs contribute to HIV prevention efforts both by targeting HIV/AIDS education to this high-risk population and by decreasing ID use in general. With the advent of HIV disease, the philosophy of drug treatment has undergone some revision. Rather than focusing solely on drug-free outcomes, there is renewed interest in methadone maintenance programs because of their success in decreasing or preventing heroin injection (Brettle, 1991; Des Jarlais, Friedman, & Casriel, 1990). Cocaine dependence has proven more difficult to treat, which is of particular concern, given the association between cocaine use and HIV infection (Brettle, 1991). Recently, acupuncture has shown promise in acute detoxification and drug-free maintenance for individuals with cocaine, alcohol, and polydrug addictions (Bullock, Culliton, & Olander, 1989; Smith, 1989).

Entering a drug treatment program can be more difficult for women than for men. The chaos and instability of female IDUs' lives may be partially counterbalanced by the status and "normalcy" of having a male partner (Suffet & Lifshitz, 1991). When this partner is an IDU, the stress of a treatment program arises not only from giving up drugs but also from the potential emotional and economic consequences of jeopardizing that relationship. Women IDUs may have fewer financial resources to pay for treatment, having to rely instead on free programs with long waiting lists.

Because of the small proportion of women in treatment, few programs are structured to accommodate women's needs. For example, women with children may have great difficulty entering residential treatment programs or meeting the strict attendance requirements of outpatient programs if childcare is not provided (Cohen, Hauer, & Wofsy, 1989). Moreover, many treatment programs have been unwilling to accept pregnant IDUs because of their special medical requirements (Karan, 1989).

The stigmatization that female IDUs experience within the drug subculture may persist in programs where the majority of participants are males, with lesbian IDUs being particularly affected. Given the relatively high HIV seroprevalence in communities where IDUs live explicit safer-sex education must be incorporated into drug treatment programs. In coeducational treatment programs, women IDUs should have their own groups in which to discuss safer sex techniques and to explore ways of incorporating these into their relationships (Cohen et al., 1989).

As hard as it is to access IDUs for HIV education, it is even more difficult to reach their non-IDU sex partners. Because male IDUs comprise the majority of IDUs in treatment and tend to have non-IDU female partners, drug treatment programs may be one way to contact and educate these women about sexual transmission of HIV (Cohen et al., 1989).

EDUCATION STRATEGIES

All women, regardless of ethnicity or socioeconomic status, need basic information on HIV transmission and risk-reduction methods. As with injectable drug practices, merely presenting the facts about HIV transmission is not sufficient to motivate people to change their behavior. The willingness to act on risk-reduction messages arises from a calculation of the individual's perceived HIV risk balanced against the anticipated costs of adopting risk-reduction practices. Somewhat paradoxically, high-fear messages may actually result in denial and increased high-risk behavior rather than risk reduction (Mays & Cochran, 1988; Sherr, 1990; Worth, 1990).

The goal of HIV prevention education is not to extinguish all sexual and injection behaviors but to teach women manageable approaches to making their behaviors safer. There are few sexual or injection practices that cannot be made safer with modifications such as condoms or bleach. Yet the health-care professional needs to be aware of how difficult changing these behaviors can be, especially sexual behaviors that require partner cooperation. Even small steps represent some reduction of risk and should be acknowledged as indications of a woman's willingness to act to protect herself (Raisler, 1990).

The greatest risk of HIV infection lies with those women who have the least control in their sexual relationships (Carovano, 1991). AIDS education programs must be developed with an awareness of the circumstances of these women's lives, which may include poverty, prostitution, ID use, rigid gender stereotypes, and dysfunctional family dynamics. As Worth (1990) states, "AIDS education targeted at minority women, if it is not based on the knowledge of cultural values and gender politics, will further increase high-risk behavior if individual women feel that their economic and social survival mechanisms are threatened by acknowledging risk-related behavior that they feel powerless to alter" (p. 128).

Hearing about HIV risk only from health-care professionals from the majority culture may reinforce feelings of victimization and powerlessness in minority women (Gilliam et al., 1989). The cultural values and obstacles to change, that women at risk for HIV infection experience, may be difficult for such health-care professionals to understand and respond to. Communication, especially about the sensitive subject matter surrounding HIV, may be complicated by misinterpretations of affect and an appearance of insensitivity (Day, 1990). Many people of color distrust health professionals because of previous efforts to control reproduction and disastrous programs such as the Tuskegee syphillis study (Schilling et al., 1989; Thomas & Quinn, 1991).

Given the disproportionate threat that HIV disease poses to people of color, HIV education programs targeted to these groups are critical. Targeting allows prevention messages to speak to the specific needs and realities of the audience. Depending on the homogeneity of the population being served, HIV prevention programs may vary in the degree to which they incorporate culturally specific approaches. Singer (1991) describes four levels of cultural integration for HIV prevention programs. For instance, "culturally sensitive" programs focus on avoiding unintentional offense and establishing an atmosphere of commitment to clients. "Culturally innovative" programs, in addition, attempt to identify and redefine cultural values in ways that are beneficial to the community. An example of cultural innovation would be redefining condom use as a sign of respect for partner and community rather than an occasion for mistrust or promiscuity. Collaboration with formal and informal community leaders can facilitate the development of culturally appropriate programs that present HIV prevention information in accessible language.

Lay leaders trained in HIV education can be valuable additions to prevention efforts by virtue of their credibility and awareness of sociocultural norms. As women coming from the same background as their audience, these "natural helpers" (Mondanaro, 1987) can serve as role models by talking about how they incorporated safer behaviors into their lives. Such demonstrations of successful change in their own community show women that making changes to reduce HIV risk is possible.

Because women at highest risk of HIV infection may be unlikely to come to traditional health-care settings, HIV education programs must seek opportunities in the community for reaching these women. Knowledge of the community and the "daily round" of its women is necessary to select those access points that will be most productive. Community organizations such as churches and tenant groups can be approached to sponsor HIV prevention programs. WIC programs, which require attendance at health education sessions, Head Start programs, jails, social-service agencies, and homeless shelters are other options. Outreach efforts might also recruit participants from settings such as laundromats and beauty shops. In San Francisco, for instance, community-based outreach to prostitutes sends out a mobile unit to provide HIV education and testing, and conducts safer-sex workshops in crack houses (Centers for Disease Control, 1991).

In locations with high volume but rapid turnover, handing out condoms and information written in language accessible to the community may be all that is possible. Even these brief interactions can raise women's awareness of AIDS. Messages that present AIDS as a family and community concern that women can do something about may attract women to local meetings where they can learn more. Neighborhood schools, churches, and libraries are familiar, convenient meeting sites.

HIV prevention education in small group sessions may be less threatening than direct one-to-one discussions of personal risk. Following a brief presentation of the facts about HIV transmission, group members can focus on ways they personally could be at risk for HIV. Distributing checklists of sexual activities and having women identify which ones they practice can help them evaluate which of their behaviors place them at risk and which do not. Some groups may find it useful to consider their reasons for being sexually active. Is it an expression of emotional intimacy? Is it only for having children? Is it a means of financial support or of obtaining drugs? Is it for physical pleasure? Does their primary relationship depend on sexual activity to maintain it? (Haines, 1991). This exercise can help women anticipate the ramifications of initiating sexual risk reduction and allows the group to acknowledge the potential costs of attempting to change their sexual behaviors.

Haines (1991) describes a game in which cards, each naming a different sexual behavior from hugging to unprotected anal intercourse, are dealt out to participants. As the group determines the HIV risk associated with each activity, the women take turns placing the cards along a line representing the continuum from totally safe to totally unsafe practices. This activity both reinforces the basic information on risk reduction and demonstrates the variety of activities that are safe, expanding the women's repertoire of safe behaviors.

A variety of tactics can be employed to overcome resistance to condom use among women. Condom use is a learned skill and will not necessarily go smoothly the first time. Programs educating women about HIV risk reduction should provide condoms and include opportunities for practicing their application (see Table 4.4). Techniques for increasing sensuality, such as incorporating condoms into foreplay or experimenting with the variety of colors and flavors available, can be shared at these sessions. As part of building peer support for condom use, women might go condom shopping together, buying different types of latex condoms and trading among themselves. Women can share ideas for "creative condomization," such as putting a condom on with the mouth or using a blindfold for either or both partners. While these techniques will not be equally acceptable in all cultures or to all women, they may stimulate participants to come up with their own more manageable suggestions.

In cultures where men expect to be the sexually knowledgeable partner, programs that encourage women to invite partners may facilitate discussion and use of condoms at home. Men may be more willing to use condoms when they are presented as a way of protecting their families and being responsible to their community (Mays & Cochran, 1988; Peterson & Marin, 1988). Negotiating safer sex with one's partner may also be easier at times when the couple is not already engaged in a sexual encounter.

Role-plays provide an opportunity to rehearse verbal and behavioral responses to partner resistance. Scenarios that depict obstacles to risk reduction give participants practice in anticipating and countering objections. Drawing on their understanding of one another's life experiences, peers can then validate or challenge these perceptions of barriers to safer behavior.

The importance of having condoms readily available should be emphasized in all role-plays. Just as introducing condom use may be easier in a new relationship, it may also be easier when the usual pattern of sexual activity is changed. Setting the scene for the role-play can begin by having the women consider the situations that usually precede their sexual encounters, how they might vary those routines, and what effect this might have on their partner.

Role-plays need to address explicitly the possibility of failure. Even if their first attempt at persuading their partner to use a condom is not successful, women need to be encouraged to keep trying and perhaps to reevaluate their approach. Also, many of these suggestions assume that women's sexual relationships follow a "friendship" paradigm in which power is at least somewhat equally shared between partners (Mays & Cochran, 1988). Role-plays may reveal different types of sexual relationships for which these suggestions are not realistic. Encouraging participants to be frank about their relationships can help the group generate alternatives that are better suited to their circumstances.

Finally, in developing HIV prevention programs for women, health-care professionals must recognize that the women at highest risk of HIV infection are those with the fewest options and resources. Helping these women implement HIV risk reduction in their lives will require more than education, condoms, and bleach. HIV educators must be prepared to provide concrete information and help in accessing other services such as drug treatment, crisis intervention, vocational training, financial assistance, parenting classes, and battered-women's shelters.

CONCLUSION

Preventing HIV infection and AIDS in women means confronting a host of personal and social issues that arise from deeply held beliefs and values about sexuality and deviance (see Chapter 13). Educating and enabling women to protect themselves from HIV is both simple and complex (Haines, 1991). Condoms and safer injecting drug use are simple, straightforward methods of markedly decreasing risk. The complexity arises from the variety of emotional, cultural, and socioeconomic factors that affect women's motivation and ability to adopt risk-reduction measures. The effectiveness of HIV prevention programs for women depends in large part on how well these issues are addressed.

REFERENCES

Abdul-Quader, A. S., Tross, S., Friedman, S. R., Kouzi, A. C., & Des Jarlais, D. C. (1990). Street-recruited intravenous drug users and sexual risk reduction in New York City. *AIDS, 4,* 1075–1079.

Anastos, K., & Palleja, S. M. (1991). Caring for women at risk of HIV infection. *Journal of General Internal Medicine, 6*(Suppl), S40–S46.

Anderson, W. (1991). The New York needle trial: The politics of public health in the age of AIDS. *American Journal of Public Health, 81,* 1506–1517.

Battjes, R. J., Pickens, R. W., & Amsel, Z. (1991). HIV infection and AIDS risk behaviors among intravenous drug users entering methadone treatment in selected U.S. cities. *Journal of Acquired Immune Deficiency Syndromes, 4,* 1148–1154.

Bird, K. D. (1991). The use of spermicide containing nonoxynol-9 in the prevention of HIV infection. *AIDS, 5,* 791–796.

Booth, R., Koester, S., Brewster, J. T., Weibel, W. W., & Fritz, R. B. (1991). Intravenous drug users and AIDS: Risk behaviors. *American Journal of Drug and Alcohol Abuse, 17*(3), 337–353.

Brettle, R. P. (1991). HIV and harm reduction for injection drug users. *AIDS, 5,* 125–136.

Broadhead, R. S. (1991). Social constructions of bleach in combating AIDS among injection drug users. *Journal of Drug Issues, 21,* 713–737.

Brown, G. R., & Rundell, J. R. (1990). Prospective study of psychiatric morbidity in HIV-seropositive women without AIDS. *General Hospital Psychiatry, 12,* 30–35.

Bullock, M. L., Culliton, P. D., & Olander, R. T. (1989, June 24). Controlled trial of acupuncture for severe recidivist alcoholism. *Lancet,* pp. 1435–1439.

Campbell, A. A., & Baldwin, W. (1991). The response of American women to the threat of AIDS and other sexually transmitted diseases. *Journal of Acquired Immune Deficiency Syndromes, 4,* 1133–1140.

Campbell, C. A. (1991). Prostitution, AIDS, and preventive health behavior. *Social Science and Medicine, 32,* 1367–1378.

Carovano, K. (1991). More than mothers and whores: Redefining the AIDS prevention needs of women. *International Journal of Health Services, 21*(1), 131–142.

Centers for Disease Control. (1991, April). Targeting prevention programs to women via community-based organizations. *CDC HIV/AIDS Prevention Newsletter, 2*(1), 11.

Chiasson, M. A., Stoneburner, R. L., Hildebrandt, D. S., Ewing, W. E., Telzak, E. E., & Jaffe, H. W. (1991). Heterosexual transmission of HIV-1 associated with the use of smokable freebase cocaine (crack). *AIDS, 5,* 1121–1126.

Chirgwin, K., DeHovitz, J. A., Dillon, S., & McCormack, W. M. (1991). HIV infection, genital ulcer disease, and crack cocaine use among patients attending a clinic for sexually transmitted diseases. *American Journal of Public Health, 81,* 1576–1579.

Chu, S. Y., Buehler, J. W., Fleming, P. L., & Berkelman, R. L. (1990). Epidemiology of reported cases of AIDS in lesbians, United States 1980–89. *American Journal of Public Health, 80,* 1380–1381.

Cohen, J. B., Hauer, L. B., & Wofsy, C. B. (1989). Women and IV drugs: Parenteral and heterosexual transmission of human immunodeficiency virus. *Journal of Drug Issues, 19,* 39–56.

Comfort, A. (1991). *The New Joy of Sex.* New York: Crown.

Day, N. A. (1990). Training providers to serve culturally different AIDS patients. *Family and Community Health, 13*(2), 46–53.

Dengelegi, L., Weber, J., & Torquato, S. (1990). Drug users' AIDS-related knowledge, attitudes, and behaviors before and after AIDS education sessions. *Public Health Reports, 105,* 504–510.

Des Jarlais, D. C., & Friedman, S. R. (1988). The psychology of preventing AIDS among intravenous drug users. *American Psychologist, 43,* 865–870.

Des Jarlais, D. C., Friedman, S. R., & Casriel, C. (1990). Target groups for preventing AIDS among intravenous drug users: 2. The "hard" data studies. *Journal of Consulting and Clinical Psychology, 58*(1), 50–56.

DiClemente, R. J., Durbin, M., Siegel, D., Krasnovsky, F., Lazarus, N., & Comacho, T. (1992). Determinants of condom use among junior high school students in a minority, inner-city school district. *Pediatrics, 89*(2), 197–202.

European Study Group. (1989). Risk factors for male to female transmission of HIV. *British Medical Journal, 298,* 411–415.

Feldblum, P. J. (1991). Results from prospective studies of HIV-discordant couples. *AIDS, 5,* 1265–1266.

Feldblum, P. J., & Fortney, J. A. (1988). Condoms, spermicides, and the transmission of human immunodeficiency virus: A review of the literature. *American Journal of Public Health, 78,* 52–54.

Flaskerud, J. H., & Nyamathi, A. M. (1990). Effects of an AIDS education program on the knowledge, attitudes and practices of low income black and Latina women. *Journal of Community Health, 15,* 343–355.

Gilliam, A., Scott, M., & Troup, J. (1989). AIDS education and risk reduction for homeless women and children: Implications for health education. *Health Education, 20*(5), 44–47.

Greenfield, L., Bigelow, G. E., & Brooner, R. K. (1992). HIV risk behavior in drug users: Increased blood "booting" during cocaine injection. *AIDS Education and Prevention, 4,* 95–107.

Grund, J-P C., Kaplan, C. D., & Adriaans, N. F. P. (1991). Needle sharing in The Netherlands: An ethnographic analysis. *American Journal of Public Health, 81,* 1602–1607.

Grund, J-P C., Kaplan, C. D., Adriaans, N. F. P., Blanken, P., & Huisman, J. (1990). The limitations of the concept of needle sharing: The practice of frontloading. *AIDS, 4,* 819–820.

Haines, J. (1991). Women and AIDS. *Canadian Nurse, 87*(2), 15–17.

Hannan, D. J., & Adler, A.G. (1990). Crack abuse: Do you know enough about it? *Postgraduate Medicine, 88*(1), 141–147.

Inciardi, J. A. (1990). HIV, AIDS and intravenous drug use: Some considerations. *Journal of Drug Issues, 20,* 181–194.

Inciardi, J. A., & Page, J. B. (1991). Drug sharing among intravenous drug users. *AIDS, 5,* 772–773.

Johnson, A. M., Petherick, A., Davidson, S. J., Brettle, R., Hooker, M., Howard, L., McLean, K. A., Osborne, L. E. M., Robertson, R., Sonnex, C., Tchamouroff, S., Shergold, C., & Adler, M. W. (1989). Transmission of HIV to heterosexual partners of infected men and women. *AIDS, 3,* 367–372.

Kane, S. (1990). AIDS, addiction and condom use: Sources of sexual risk for heterosexual women. *Journal of Sex Research, 27,* 427–444.

Kane, S. (1991). HIV, heroin and heterosexual relations. *Social Science and Medicine, 32,* 1037–1050.

Karan, L. D. (1989). AIDS prevention and chemical dependence treatment needs of women and their children. *Journal of Psychoactive Drugs, 21,* 395–399.

Laurian, Y., Peynet, J., & Verroust, F. (1989). HIV infection in sexual partners of HIV-seropositive patients with hemophilia. *New England Journal of Medicine, 320,* 183.

Lewis, D. K., & Watters, J. K. (1989). Human immunodeficiency virus seroprevalence in female intravenous drug users: The puzzle of black women's risk. *Social Science and Medicine, 29,* 1071–1076.

Lewis, D. K., Watters, J. K., & Case, P. (1990). The prevalence of high-risk sexual behavior in male intravenous drug users with steady female partners. *American Journal of Public Health, 80,* 465–466.

Lifson, A. R., O'Malley, P. M., Hessol, N. A., Buchbinder, S. P., Cannon, L., & Rutherford, G. W. (1990). HIV seroconversion in two homosexual men after receptive oral intercourse with ejaculation: Implications for counseling concerning safe sexual practices. *American Journal of Public Health, 80,* 1509–1511.

Longoria, J. M., Turner, N. H., & Phillips, B. U. (1991). Community leaders help increase response rates in AIDS survey. *American Journal of Public Health, 81,* 654–655.

Magura, S., Shapiro, J. L., Siddiqi, Q., & Lipton, D. S. (1990). Variables influencing condom use among intravenous drug users. *American Journal of Public Health*, *80*, 82–84.

Marks, G., Richardson, J. L., & Maldonado, N. (1991). Self-disclosure of HIV infection to sexual partners. *American Journal of Public Health*, *81*, 1321–1322.

Mays, V. M., & Cochran, S. D. (1988). Issues in the perception of AIDS risk and risk reduction activities by black and Hispanic/Latina women. *American Psychologist*, *43*, 949–957.

Moatti, J-P, Bajos, N., Durbec, J-P, Menard, C., & Serrand, C. (1991). Determinants of condom use among French heterosexuals with multiple partners. *American Journal of Public Health*, *81*, 106–109.

Mondanaro, J. (1987). Strategies for AIDS prevention: Motivating health behavior in drug dependent women. *Journal of Psychoactive Drugs*, *19*, 143–149.

Nelson, S. (1992, February). Talking smart, acting stupid about AIDS. *Glamour*, pp. 174–175, 190–191.

Padian, N. S. (1990). Sexual histories of heterosexual couples with one HIV-infected partner. *American Journal of Public Health*, *80*, 990–991.

Padian, N. S., Shiboski, S. C., & Jewell, N. P. (1990). The effect of number of exposures on the risk of heterosexual HIV transmission. *Journal of Infectious Diseases*, *161*, 883–887.

Padian, N. S., Shiboski, S. C., & Jewell, N. P. (1991). Female-to-male transmission of human immunodeficiency virus. *Journal of the American Medical Association*, *266*, 1664–1667.

Painter, K. (1992, January 30). FDA to consider "female condom." *USA Today*, p. 6D.

Peterson, J. L., & Marin, G. (1988). Issues in the prevention of AIDS among Black and Hispanic men. *American Psychologist*, *43*, 871–877.

Raisler, J. (1990). Safer sex for women. *Clinical Issues in Perinatal and Women's Health Nursing*, *1*(1), 28–32.

Reiss, I. L., & Leik, R. K. (1989). Evaluating strategies to avoid AIDS: Number of partners vs. use of condoms. *Journal of Sex Research*, *26*, 411–433.

Rhodes, F., Corby, N. H., Wolitski, R. J., Tashima, N., Crain, C., Yankovich, D. R., & Smith, P. K. (1990). Risk behaviors and perceptions of AIDS among street injection drug users. *Journal of Drug Education*, *20*(4), 271–288.

Rosenbaum, M. (1981). When drugs come into the picture, love flies out the window: Women addicts' love relationships. *The International Journal of the Addictions*, *16*, 1197–1206.

Roylance, F. D. (1992, March 23). Condoms: Keeping them safe. *Chicago Sun-Times*, p. 7.

Sakondhavat, C. (1990). The female condom. *American Journal of Public Health*, *80*, 498.

Samuel, M. C., Guydish, J., Ekstrand, M., Coates, T. J., & Winkelstein, W., Jr. (1991). Changes in sexual practices over 5 years of follow-up among heterosexual men in San Francisco. *Journal of Acquired Immune Deficiency Syndromes*, *4*, 896–900.

Saxon, A. J., Calsyn, D. A., Whittaker, S., & Freeman, G., Jr. (1991). Sexual behaviors of intravenous drug users in treatment. *Journal of Acquired Immune Deficiency Svn-dromes*, *4*, 938–944.

Schilling, R. F., El-Bassel, N., Schinke, S. P., Gordon, K., & Nichols, S. (1991). Building skills of recovering women drug users to reduce heterosexual AIDS transmission. *Public Health Reports*, *106*, 297–304.

Schilling, R. F., Schinke, S. P., Nichols, S. E., Zayas, L. H., Miller, S. O., Orlandi, M. A., & Botvin, G. J. (1989). Developing strategies for AIDS prevention research with black and Hispanic drug users. *Public Health Reports*, *104*, 2–11.

Schoenbaum, E. E., Hartel, D., Selwyn, P. A., Klein, R. S., Davenny, K., Rogers, M., Feiner, C., & Friedland, G. (1989). Risk factors for human immunodeficiency virus infection in intravenous drug users. *New England Journal of Medicine, 321*, 874–879.

Seligman, J., (1992, February 10). A condom for women moves one step closer to reality. *Newsweek*, p. 45.

Sherr, L. (1990). Fear arousal and AIDS: Do shock tactics work? *AIDS, 4*, 361–364.

Singer, M. (1991). Confronting the AIDS epidemic among IV drug users: Does ethnic culture matter? *AIDS Education and Prevention, 3*, 258–283.

Smith, M. O. (1989, July 25). *The Lincoln Hospital Acupuncture Drug Abuse Program.* Testimony presented to the Select Committee on Narcotics of the House of Representatives.

Stein, Z. A. (1990). HIV prevention: The need for methods women can use. *American Journal of Public Health, 80*, 460–462.

Stone, K. M., & Peterson, H. B. (1992). Spermicides, HIV, and the vaginal sponge. *Journal of the American Medical Association, 268*, 521–523.

Stuntzner-Gibson, D. (1991). Women and HIV disease: An emerging social crisis. *Social Work, 36*(1), 22–28.

Suffet, F., & Lifshitz, M. (1991). Women addicts and the threat of AIDS. *Qualitative Health Research, 1*(1), 51–79.

Thomas, S. B., & Quinn, S. C. (1991). Public health then and now: The Tuskegee syphilis study, 1932 to 1972: Implications for HIV education and AIDS risk education programs in the black community. *American Journal of Public Health, 81*, 1498–1505.

Trocki, K. F., & Leigh, B. C. (1991). Alcohol consumption and unsafe sex: A comparison of heterosexuals and homosexual men. *Journal of Acquired Immune Deficiency Syndromes, 4*, 981–986.

Valdiserri, R. O., Arena, V. C., Proctor, D., & Bonati, F. A. (1989). The relationship between women's attitudes about condoms and their use: Implications for condom promotion programs. *American Journal of Public Health, 79*, 499–501.

Waring, N. (1990, June 17). Needle exchange. *Boston Globe Magazine.*

Watters, J. K. (1988). Meaning and context: The social facts of intravenous drug use and HIV transmission in the inner city. *Journal of Psychoactive Drugs, 20*, 173–177.

Watters, J. K. (1989). Observations on the importance of social context in HIV transmission among intravenous drug users. *Journal of Drug Issues, 19*, 9–26.

Wisconsin Pharmacal Co. (1991). *Reality intravaginal pouch: Instructions for use.* Jackson, WI: Author.

Worth, D. (1989). Sexual decision-making and AIDS: Why condom promotion among vulnerable women is likely to fail. *Studies in Family Planning, 20*(6), 297–307.

Worth, D. (1990). Minority women and AIDS: Culture, race, and gender. In D. A. Feldman (Ed.), *Culture and AIDS* (pp. 111–135). New York: Praeger.

5

Clinical Manifestations and Treatment of HIV Infection and AIDS in Women

Felissa L. Cohen

This chapter will discuss the clinical spectrum of HIV infection as it relates to HIV-infected women. This chapter will not attempt to review all of the signs and symptoms seen in HIV infection or the conditions defining full-blown AIDS. For such a review, see Chapter 1 or Cohen (1991).

Little information regarding clinical manifestations of HIV infection and AIDS specific to women has appeared in the scientific literature, and that information is relatively recent. Women have also been notoriously underrepresented in the federally sponsored AIDS clinical treatment trials. The CDC definition of AIDS, based on observations in males (mostly homosexual males), excluded many of the conditions now believed by many researchers to define AIDS in women. Thus, female-specific symptoms associated with HIV infection, such as chronic vaginitis, often go unrecognized.

There are few data available on the presentation of HIV infection or AIDS in women. In addition, symptoms of HIV infection and AIDS that would be recognized as such if they occurred in a male may go unrecognized in relation to their true significance in females. For example, one author reports on the case of a 55-year-old white woman with fever, diarrhea, weight loss, and night sweats for two months. During chart review, it was noticed that she had received multiple transfusions during surgery in 1982, and it was that information that led to the discovery that she was HIV-infected (Gravell, 1990). However, many health professionals still do not maintain a high index of suspicion regarding HIV infection when the client is female. Consequently, women may be diagnosed later in their disease than men, may not be diagnosed with HIV infection, or may be misdiagnosed. Awareness of what to look for can allow health caregivers to conduct a thorough and knowledgeable assessment of their female clients, including referral for testing when indicated to avoid overlooking HIV infection.

Both biological and social conditions may influence the response of females to HIV infection and AIDS (Minkoff & DeHovitz, 1991). For example, sexual dimorphism in both the humoral and cell-mediated immune response has been described with more immune activity in females than males. This might explain the increased autoimmune reactions reported in females. It is postulated that one reason for increased immune activity might be to compensate for the physiological stress accompanying reproduction, thus ensuring survival of the species (Grossman, 1989). The interaction between sex hormones and the components, function, and activity of the immune system has not been well studied in females. Gender-specific differences also exist in the rate and qualitative metabolism of various drugs and chemicals. Thus it would not be unexpected to see a gender effect of some type in the acquisition and course of HIV infection and response to its therapy. The social conditions affecting HIV-infected women may include poverty, stress, cultural boundaries, health-services access, and caretaking responsibilities. These are discussed in more detail in Chapters 3, 4, 10, and 14.

CLINICAL CONDITIONS ACCOMPANYING HIV INFECTION IN WOMEN

As discussed in Chapter 1, the CDC has determined conditions that are AIDS-defining diagnoses both in the presence of a positive HIV test and in its absence, and in relation to the CD4+ lymphocyte count (Centers for Disease Control, 1987, 1991). These definitions were developed largely on information determined from the study of homosexual males, who comprised the majority of known early cases of AIDS. Many clinicians are concerned that the AIDS indicator conditions do not include enough female-specific conditions and thus exclude a proportion of women from the AIDS definition. Vaginal candidiasis and other gynecological conditions have been observed by clinicians to be related to HIV infection in women. Further, there are real questions as to (1) whether initial clinical manifestations of HIV infection are similar in men and women, (2) whether the AIDS-defining diagnostic events are similar, (3) what the similarities and differences are between males and females in the opportunistic infections, neoplasms, and nervous-system dysfunctions observed, and (4) what similarities and differences exist in the natural history of HIV infection. Relatively few studies have addressed these issues.

In an attempt to describe the spectrum of HIV infection among women, a CDC project reviewed the medical records of 465 women with HIV infection, of whom 23% had AIDS and 17% had potentially severe opportunistic infections. Genital infections were found in 31%, including vaginal yeast infections, genital herpes, trichomonas, and PID. Six women had cancers not included in the AIDS definition (Buehler, Farizo, Berkelman et al., 1991).

In a study of AIDS among 24 women in Rhode Island, major AIDS-defining diagnostic events were identified. The four most frequent were *Candida albicans* esophagitis (38%), HIV-related constitutional wasting syndrome (25%), *Pneumocystis carinii* pneumonia (13%), and *Toxoplasma gondii* encephalitis (8%). Opportunistic infections had occurred in all of the women. Fungal infections were most common (about 95%), followed by viral infections (about 83%), and protozoal infections (about 51%). In this study only 2 (about 8%) developed neoplasms, neither of which was Kaposi's sarcoma. The most frequent of the fungal infections was vaginitis due to *Candida albicans* (Carpenter, Mayer, Fisher, Desai, & Durand, 1989). The findings of this study must be considered in light of the very small sample size studied.

In another comparative study reported from Atlanta, 204 women and 2,435 men were studied. Women were more likely than men to have *Candida* esophagitis, *Mycobacterium avium* complex, or atypical myobacterial infections. By organ system, women were more likely than men to have genitourinary infections, psychological and neurologic conditions, while men were more likely to have skin diseases (Thompson, Whyte, Morris, Rimland, & Thompson, 1991). When men and women were compared as to their AIDS-defining illness in New York City, no statistically significant differences were observed except for Kaposi's sarcoma which was more frequently observed in men (Grant, Anastos, & Ernst, 1991). In examining the prevalence of AIDS-indicative diagnoses for cases diagnosed in 1988 and 1989, CDC found that esophageal candidiasis and herpes simplex infections were statistically more frequent in women (Fleming, Cleslelski, & Berkelman, 1991).

A 1991 report described experiences of Carpenter and coworkers with 200 HIV-infected women in Rhode Island, one of the most comprehensive studies available. The length of the study was not longer than four years for any woman, and shorter for most. At the time of the report, 117 of these 200 women were symptomatic, and 83 remained asymptomatic. Forty-four women were diagnosed with AIDS during the course of the study. The *first* recognized documented HIV-related clinical manifestation in the group of symptomatic women in descending order of frequency were

Recurrent vaginal candidiasis (36.7%)
Lymphadenopathy (14.5%)
Bacterial pneumonia (12.8%)
Acute retroviral syndrome (6.8%)
Constitutional symptoms (6.8%)
Oropharyngeal candidiasis (thrush) (5.1%)
Thrombocytopenic purpura (5.1%)
Oral hairy leukoplakia (3.4%)
Herpes zoster (1.7%)
Pneumocystis carinii pneumonia (1.7%)

AIDS encephalopathy (0.85%)
Cytomegalovirus (0.85%)

Because many of the women who entered this study had presumably been HIV-infected for many years, milder initial clinical manifestations such as the flulike symptoms often associated with primary infection might have been overlooked (Carpenter et al., 1991).

Among the 44 women actually diagnosed with AIDS, the major *AIDS-defining diagnoses* were

Esophageal candidiasis (34%)
Pneumocystis carinii pneumonia (20.5%)
Chronic herpes simplex infections (18.2%)
Cryptococcus neoformans meningitis (4.5%)
Toxoplasma gondii encephalitis (4.5%)

Other diagnoses present in single patients (2.2%) were AIDS-wasting syndrome, progressive multifocal leukoencephalopathy, extrapulmonary tuberculosis, *Mycobacterium avium* complex, HIV encephalopathy, *Cryptosporidium* enteritis, *Isospora belli* enteritis, and central nervous system lymphoma (Carpenter et al., 1991).

The number of women of the 117 with specific opportunistic infections and neoplasms occurring at *any time* during the study period was also determined. The major ones are shown in descending order of frequency:[*]

Recurrent vaginal candidiasis (76.1%)
Oropharyngeal candidiasis (30.8%)
Viral genital warts (27.3%)
Bacterial pneumonia (22.2%)
Esophageal candidiasis (20.5%)
Pneumocystis carinii pneumonia (12.8%)
Chronic mucocutaneous herpes simplex (8.5%)
Recurrent genital herpes simplex (8.5%)
Oral hairy leukoplakia (7.7%)
Herpes zoster (6.8%)
Recurrent oral herpes simplex (6%)
Cutaneous candidiasis (6%)

Cervico-vaginal squamous intraepithelial lesions were present in 25% of 65 women examined from the group of 117 described above (Carpenter et al., 1991).

---

[*]Multiple disorders could be present in one individual.

The above information indicates that the major types of infections most frequently seen in HIV-infected women to date, particularly early in their clinical course, are fungal (predominately *Candida*), mucocutaneous and genital herpes simplex infections, *Pneumocystis carinii* pneumonia, and acute bacterial pneumonias. Protozoal infections seen commonly in males, such as *Toxoplasma gondii* encephalitis and enteritis due to *Cryptosporidium* or *Isospora belli*, are described far less frequently in females, as are nongynecological neoplasms. However, various studies report some differing information. These differences might be a reflection of small sample size or length of time of observation, or may represent real nonuniformity.

INFECTIONS

Like infections in males, infections in HIV-infected females may be more aggressive, are more likely to be caused by unusual organisms, and are generally less responsive to standard treatment regimens than in those who are not HIV-infected (Anastos, & Palleja, 1991). Those infections most commonly observed in females will be discussed below. The reader is referred elsewhere for in-depth discussions of the clinical spectrum of HIV-related illness (Chapter 1; Cohen, 1991).

Fungal Infections

In HIV-positive women, the most prevalent type of fungal infection is caused by members of the genus *Candida*, usually *Candida albicans*. Predisposition to fungal infections may occur secondary to chemotherapy, irradiation, antibacterial treatment, corticosteroid use, and indwelling venous catheters as well as primary immune suppression due to HIV (Saral, 1991). *Candida* has been associated for a long time with immune defects, especially those affecting T-cells, and otherwise unexplained oral candidiasis (thrush) has been recognized as both a presenting sign of AIDS and a prognostic indicator of progressive disease (Rhoads, Wright, Redfield, & Burke, 1987; Selwyn, 1986).

Localized *Candida* infections occur frequently in patients with AIDS, and oral candidiasis may at some time affect more than 90%. Disseminated candidiasis is less usual, particularly early in AIDS (Diamond, 1991). Imam and colleagues (1990) observed that in their cohort of HIV-infected women, vaginal candidiasis occurred first, followed by oropharyngeal candidiasis and then by esophageal candidiasis in a hierarchical manner relating to the degree of declining immune function.

Several researchers have observed that vaginal candidiasis occurred as a new infection or recurred with increased frequency, severity, or duration in women who were later determined to be HIV-infected. Usually it was refractory to standard treatment (Imam et al., 1990; Rhoads et al., 1987). Symptoms of vaginal candidiasis typically include severe vaginal itching that may be associated with a thick, white or yellow clumped discharge that is usually without a prominent odor (Handsfield, 1992). Most frequently, clinicians do not associate vaginal candidiasis with HIV infection, although it occurs more often in women who are HIV-infected than in those who are not. In many of the studies it was the presenting complaint and the *only* clinical indication of underlying immunodeficiency but was not recognized as such at the time of presentation (Imam et al., 1990; Rhoads et al., 1987). While vaginal candidiasis also occurs among women without HIV infection, women who present with it should be carefully questioned for a history that might put them at risk for HIV infection and should be carefully examined for other signs and symptoms such as lymphadenopathy or patterns of genital-tract infections or irregularities. HIV testing and counseling should be encouraged when appropriate (Carpenter et al., 1991; "Me first!" 1990). Vaginal candidiasis in women without HIV infection is generally responsive to imidazole antifungal creams or suppositories such as clotrimazole or to oral fluconazole (Handsfield, 1992; Saral, 1991; Sobel, 1992). Sobel defines recurrent vaginal candidiasis as "the occurrence of at least four mycologically proven symptomatic episodes within 12 months, with the exclusion of other common vaginal pathogens" (p. S148). However, others counsel that one should be suspicious of HIV infection in women who have more than two episodes within six months or persistence of candidiasis after two treatment courses (Allen & Marte, 1991).

Oropharyngeal candidiasis may coexist on a clinical or subclinical level in HIV-infected women with vaginal candidiasis or may develop later (Diamond, 1991). The incidence of oropharyngeal candidiasis in HIV-infected women appears similar to that seen in men. The most common type is synonymous with thrush and is known as pseudomembranous. In this type, white removable plaques can be seen on the oral mucosa, which can be removed, leaving behind an erythematous or bleeding surface (Greenspan, Greenspan, & Winkler, 1990). Treatment can vary. Topical therapy includes nystatin suspension, oral pastilles, or clotrimazole troches. Oral ketoconazole or fluconazole may also be used (Galgiani, 1990; Greenspan, Greenspan & Winkler, 1990).

Esophageal candidiasis is usually accompanied by dysphagia, odynophagia (painful swallowing), and retrosternal pain without swallowing (Cello, 1988). Some observations suggest that in the United States esophageal candidiasis is more common as an AIDS-defining event in women than in men (Carpenter et al., 1991), but in Haiti, it is a common presenting event for both men and women (Pape et al., 1983). Treatment usually consists of fluconazole and may require amphotericin B in refractory cases (Galgiani, 1990). Despite therapy, painful esophageal lesions may persist, resulting in inadequate nutrition and weight loss (Cohen, 1991). Since esophageal candidiasis is usually preceded by oropharyngeal candidiasis, thrush should be adequately treated early, particularly in immunocompromised patients (Imam et al., 1990).

Bacterial Infections

In one of the largest reported studies of women with HIV infection, bacterial pneumonias were the third most frequent initial clinical manifestation of HIV infection and occurred during the study period in nearly one-quarter of these patients. In most of these cases, the etiology was undetermined, but in about a third, the pneumonia was caused by *Streptococcus pneumoniae* (Carpenter et al., 1991). Bacterial pneumonias are seen in persons with HIV infection more commonly than in the general population, especially pneumococcal pneumonia. The incidence of bacterial pneumonias appears higher among injecting drug users (IDUs) and heterosexual persons with AIDS than in homosexual men with AIDS (Cohn, 1991).

The organisms involved in bacterial pneumonias in HIV-infected patients are numerous. Recurrent pneumonias are more common in HIV-infected persons than those who are uninfected. Symptoms may include fever, chills, productive cough, dyspnea, and pleuritic chest pain. The majority of patients respond well to specific antimicrobial therapy despite the frequent occurrence of bacteremia (Cohn, 1991). Only one of the women in one study who presented with bacterial pneumonia was tested for HIV infection (Carpenter et al., 1991); however, HIV testing should be considered in such situations, particularly if the woman is known to be an IDU.

HIV-infected women are also subject to tuberculosis and to disease resulting from infection with *Mycobacterium avium* complex (MAC), but the prevalence has not been generally described as varying significantly from that described in HIV-infected males except in a few reports (Thompson et al., 1991). Mycobacterial infections are discussed in Chapter 1.

Viral Infections

Mucocutaneous herpes simplex infections may be caused by herpes simplex viruses (HSV) types 1 and 2. Although overlap exists, HSV-1 is generally responsible for oral-facial lesions, visceral infections, and encephalitis, while HSV-2 is associated with genital-tract infections and neonatal disease (Still, 1992). After early initial infection, HSV can lie dormant until it is reactivated following stressful events that include decreased cellular immunity ("Herpes simplex virus," 1989). HSV-2 antibodies (representing previous infection) are more common in blacks than whites, and black women are more likely to have HSV-2 antibodies than black men. HSV-2 antibodies are more common in inner-city residents of lower socioeconomic class (Aral & Holmes, 1991). Less than one-third of persons with HSV-2 antibody were aware of having symptoms associated with genital herpes, and new cases often occur after exposure to a sex partner with an asymptomatic infection (Aral & Holmes, 1991).

There are three categories of genital herpes disease:

1. Primary disease. Signs and symptoms can last three or more weeks and range from barely noticeable to severe. Symptoms can include mucosal lesions, cervicitis, fever, lymphadenopathy, headache, and neurologic symptoms resulting from sacral nerve involvement such as urinary retention. Neither HSV-1 or HSV-2 antibody is present.

2. Nonprimary initial disease. This is the first recognized outbreak of genital herpes in a person who had HSV before, either because of HSV-1 infection or previous HSV-2 infection that was not recognized. The person may have HSV-1 antibody. Systemic symptoms are mild or absent.

3. Recurrent disease. The person has mild manifestations lasting a short period. Overt lesions appear as vesicle clusters or ulcers in the genital area, followed by crusting and healing. Many persons experience a prodrome consisting of tingling or numbness a few days before lesions occur (Handsfield, 1992; Still, 1992).

Infection with HSV-1 and HSV-2 is common in persons who are HIV-infected. Lesions may be oral, genital, or anorectal. Treatment is most commonly with acyclovir and with foscarnet for lesions resistant to acyclovir (Cotton, 1991). Nearly 20% of the women in one study had herpes simplex lesions as their AIDS-defining diagnosis, and such lesions were commonly seen as opportunistic infections in women (Carpenter et al., 1991).

Persons who are HSV-infected but who are asymptomatic can still transmit HSV to their sexual partners. Condoms are useful in preventing transmission but offer only partial protection because of the location of the lesions (Mertz, Benedetti, Ashley, Selke, & Corey, 1992). While herpes ulcers normally heal within one to three weeks, in persons with HIV infection, they may persist for months (Aral & Holmes, 1991).

Genital herpes may act in women to increase their chances of acquiring HIV infection, and in women with HIV infection genital herpes infections may be more severe, have a longer duration, and be more resistant to the usual acyclovir therapy (Allen, 1990). In fact, a recent study found that persons with genital herpes had double the risk for acquiring HIV infection than those who did not, after controlling for other factors (Quinn, Groseclose, Spence, Provost, & Hook, 1992).

Other viral infections specific to gynecological disorders in HIV-positive women are discussed under gynecological manifestations, below.

Parasitic Infections

Pneumocystis carinii is an organism frequently causing pneumonia in persons with AIDS. While it typically is classified as a parasite, there is some evidence that it might actually be a fungus (Edman et al., 1988).

As an AIDS-defining event, the frequency of *Pneumocystis carinii* pneumonia has been similar for males and females and in most studies has been the most common AIDS-defining event for both (Grant et al., 1991; Spence & Reboli, 1991). Most of the other studies examining clinical manifestations in women do not find an increased rate of parasitic infections in HIV-infected women compared with HIV-infected men. PCP and other parasitic infections commonly found in AIDS are discussed in detail in Chapter 1 and elsewhere (Cohen, 1991). Gynecological infections such as *Trichomonas* vaginitis are discussed below.

NEOPLASMS

The most frequently observed neoplasms in persons with AIDS have been Kaposi's sarcoma (KS) and malignant lymphomas, particularly of the central nervous system. KS is most frequently observed in homosexual and bisexual males, affecting 15–20% of that group in contrast to its lower prevalence in injecting drug users (IDUs) where the prevalence is estimated at about 3% (Brettle & Leen, 1991; Lassoued et al., 1991). Currently it is postulated that KS might result from an infectious sexually transmitted agent, inhalation of nitrites, or other factors since KS has been observed in HIV-seronegative homosexual males (Beral, Peterman, Berkelman, & Jaffe, 1990; Root-Bernstein, 1990). Among IDUs, the most common HIV-associated malignancy is lymphoma, occurring in about 8% (Brettle & Leen, 1991).

KS is relatively rare among women. It is estimated that between 1% and 3% of HIV-infected women have developed KS in the United States or Europe (Johnson & Webster, 1989; Lassoued et al., 1991). Relatively few studies of KS in women with AIDS have been conducted. In one series of 12 women with AIDS conducted in France, it was the first manifestation of AIDS in 10 of them (Lassoued et al., 1991). Nine had acquired HIV through sexual contact and 3 after blood transfusion. KS was associated with a more aggressive presentation than had been observed in men, and the affected women had severe immunodeficiency. While many of the lesions (described in Chapter 1) occurred in similar sites as those observed in men, some patients had lesions in pubic, perianal, anal, and vaginal areas before being observed elsewhere (Lassoued et al., 1991). These findings, plus the observation in other studies that KS is four times more likely to be present in female partners of bisexual men than other risk groups, and because it is more common in Africa, appear to support KS as a sexually transmitted disease (Beral et al., 1990). However, the numbers of affected persons in these studies is small, and another study failed to confirm this observation (Benedetti, Greco, Figoli, & Tirelli, 1991).

The disease course observed for women with KS has been severe and progressive, and the reported prognosis is correspondingly poor. This is in contrast to what has been reported in males with AIDS who have KS and no opportunistic infections (Brettle & Leen, 1991; Rothenberg et al., 1987).

Except for gynecological malignancies, there is little information in the literature regarding the prevalence of other malignancies among women. In males, lymphomas occurring subsequent to long-term antiviral therapy for AIDS have been described (Raub, 1990). Since women were not included in many of the clinical trials of early zidovudine therapy, it is too early to predict whether the same observations will be made in women. There is a need for more systematic definitive information regarding all types of malignancies, including KS, in females. Gynecological malignancies are discussed in the section on gynecological manifestations of HIV infection, below.

GYNECOLOGICAL MANIFESTATIONS

Gynecologic conditions appearing in HIV-infected women most frequently include but are not limited to

Pelvic inflammatory disease
Cervical dysplasia and neoplasia
Vaginal fungal infections, especially candidiasis

Vaginal candidiasis has been discussed in detail earlier; other vaginal infections are considered below, as are sample protocols for gynecological manifestations in HIV-infected women.

Pelvic Inflammatory Disease

About 1 million women per year are treated for acute pelvic inflammatory disease (PID), and one in seven American women of reproductive age have had PID (Aral, Mosher, & Cates, 1991; Peterson et al., 1991). PID refers to infection of the upper genital tract, often resulting from complications of sexually transmitted diseases (STDs), especially those caused by *Chlamydia trachomatis* and *Neisseria gonorrhoeae* as well as secondary to intrauterine devices (Aral et al., 1991; Handsfield, 1992; Rice & Schachter, 1992). A classically thought-of presentation includes severe lower abdominal pain, tenderness, and fever, often accompanied by vaginal discharge or bleeding. Vomiting and an elevated leukocyte count and sedimentation rate may be seen. However, a vast majority of patients have mild or no symptoms (Handsfield, 1992). The minimum diagnostic criteria as established by the CDC are shown in Table 5.1 (Centers for Disease Control, 1991). PID can result in acute or more chronic conditions that include ectopic pregnancy, infertility, tubo-ovarian abscesses, salpingitis, endometritis, and pelvic peritonitis, among others. Between 10% and 20% of women experience scarring and

TABLE 5.1 Diagnostic Criteria for Pelvic Inflammatory Disease

Minimal Criterial for Clinical Diagnosis of PID

Lower abdominal tenderness
Bilateral adnexal tenderness
Cervical motion tenderness

Additional Criteria Useful in Diagnosing PID

Routine	*Elaborate*
Oral temperature > 38.3 C	Histopathologic evidence on endometrial biopsy
Abnormal cervical or vaginal discharge	
Elevated erythrocyte sedimentation and/or C-reactive protein	Tubo-ovarian abscess on sonography
Culture or non-culture evidence of cervical infection with *N. gonorrhoeae* or *C. trachomatis*	Laparoscopy

Tests Recommended for All Suspected Cases of PID

Cervical cultures for *N. gonorrhoeae*
Cervical culture or non-culture test for *C. trachomatis*

Source: Centers for Disease Control. (1991). Pelvic inflammatory disease: Guidelines for prevention and management. *Morbidity and Mortality Weekly Report, 40*(RR-5), 1–25, p. 16.

obstruction of the Fallopian tubes, leading to infertility as a result of their first episode of PID. Medical opinion is divided on the desirability of hospitalization for women with PID, usually for intravenous antibiotic therapy, and many women are treated as outpatients or at home (Handsfield, 1992).

Given the association between PID and STDs and many epidemiological similarities with women who are HIV-infected, it is not surprising to find an association between PID and HIV; however, little definitive information is available. Among women admitted to San Francisco General Hospital during a four-year period with acute PID, the proportion of women with HIV infection rose from 0% in 1985 to 6.7% in 1988 (Safrin, Dattel, Hauer, & Sweet, 1990). Does the presence of PID confer susceptibility to becoming infected with HIV? Does the presence of HIV result in an increased susceptibility to PID? Or is there some more complex interaction between the two conditions?

Hoegsberg and colleagues (1990) studied HIV infection among women with PID in New York City. They found that those women hospitalized with PID who were also HIV-infected had more tubo-ovarian abscesses and more operative intervention than those who were HIV-negative and suggested that the PID might be more refractory in the HIV-positive women (Hoegsberg et al., 1990).

PID is actually very nonspecific. It is interesting that little effort has been made by the majority of the medical establishment to more stringently describe the actual conditions rather than lumping many conditions together under one broad umbrella. So doing might shed more light on the relationship between PID and HIV infection in women.

Cervical Abnormalities

In 1986, the first reports detailing the presence of HIV in both cervical and vaginal secretions appeared (Vogt et al., 1986; Wofsy et al., 1986). Subsequently it was found that monocyte-macrophages, endothelial cells, and other cells in the cervix can harbor HIV (Pomerantz et al., 1988).

Bradbeer (1987) proposed that HIV infection might be a risk factor for cervical intraepithelial neoplasia. Cervical neoplasia has been said to have many characteristics of sexually transmitted diseases, and the papillomaviruses have been associated with its development.

The human papillomaviruses (HPVs) belong to the papovavirus family, and more than 60 types are known. HPVs can cause (1) benign lesions such as genital warts; (2) cervical intraepithelial neoplasias (CIN) or invasive carcinomas; and (3) latent or asymptomatic infections (Allen, 1990; Aral & Holmes, 1991). A few types of HPV (e.g., types 16, 18, and 31) have been strongly associated with malignant cervical and vulvar cancer in women (Handsfield, 1992). HPV-induced cervical infections have been shown to be increased in severity in women with low CD4 lymphocyte counts (Johnson, Burnett, Willet, Young, & Doniger, 1992).

It is possible that the immunosuppression resulting from HIV infection might be a cofactor in the development of cervical dysplasia and/or neoplasia. The observation that women who are HIV-infected but still immunocompetent had a prevalence of cervical dysplasia-neoplasia that was comparable to the prevalence seen in HIV-negative women with a comparable risk for HPV infection supports this theory. Studies have also found that the frequency and severity of cervical dysplasia in HIV-infected women appeared to increase with diminishing numbers of CD4 lymphocytes (Schafer, Friedmann, Mielke, Schwartlander, & Koch, 1991). In women who were immunosuppressed for reasons other than HIV infection (Hodgkin's disease and renal transplant recipients), an increased prevalence of cervical cancer has been observed (Schneider, Kay, & Lee, 1983; Shakri-Tabizzadeh, Koss, Molnar, & Ramney, 1981). It has been proposed that for those with HIV infection, the subsequent immunosuppression results in active HPV infection leading to cervical dysplasia and neoplasia. There may be a dose-response relationship between increased immunosuppression and the severity of HPV-induced disease. Thus it may be that human papillomavirus-induced cervical dysplasia and/or neoplasia may actually be an opportunistic disease (Schafer et al., 1991; Vermund et al., 1991). HIV-infected women may not respond well to conventional therapy for HPV lesions, and therefore these lesions may continue to progress (Vermund et al., 1991).

Researchers in London reported that 95% of the HIV-infected women in their clinic showed clinical or subclinical evidence of HPV infection. Half of the women had multicentric disease involving both the cervix and lower genital tract, especially the vulva and perianal regions. Routine cervical cytology screening revealed dyskaryotic cells that suggested cervical intraepithelial neoplasia in 47% of HIV-infected women, compared with a 12% prevalence in the routine clinic population. Colposcopy was necessary to ascertain the subclinical HPV lesions (Byrne, Taylor-Robinson, Munday, & Harris, 1989). Other investigators have noted that Pap smear results may not correlate well with findings from colposcopy and biopsy (Allen, 1990; Centers for Disease Control, 1990).

In New York City, women attending two ambulatory care clinics were tested for cervical dysplasia by use of the Papanicolaou (Pap) smear. Dysplasia was found in 32% and 33% of the HIV-positive women, compared to 4% and 3% of HIV-negative women in the community (Centers for Disease Control, 1990). Further evidence suggests that cervical intraepithelial neoplasia appears more severe and extensive in HIV-positive women compared with HIV-negative women (Maiman et al., 1990).

Vermund and coworkers (1991) found that HIV-infected women who were symptomatic were more likely (70%) to have HPV infection than those who were asymptomatic (22%) or HIV negative (22%). The symptomatic HIV-infected women with HPV infection were at higher risk for genital squamous intraepithelial lesions than those who had either HIV or HPV alone. The prognostic importance of severe squamous intraepithelial lesions in women has not yet been assessed, and it is possible that they are similar in implication to other opportunistic infections already included in the AIDS surveillance definition (Vermund et al., 1991).

Although the CDC has identified methodological shortcomings in studies examining the relationship between HIV infection in women and cervical disease, clinical observations have supported such an association. Identified risk factors for cervical cancer may include number of sexual partners; age at first intercourse; infectious agents such as HPV, smoking, diet, and immunosuppression; it has been suggested that cervical cancer may be an STD (Centers for Disease Control, 1990). In any case, the findings from the studies discussed above and others suggest guidelines that might decrease the risk of cervical cancer in HIV-infected women. These include at least a yearly Pap smear and gynecologic examination for sexually active women and those after age 18 (Centers for Disease Control, 1990). For women at high risk for HIV infection or those who are already HIV-infected, it might be desirable to decrease the time interval to four to six months with liberal use of colposcopy. More aggressive treatment protocols may be necessary in HIV-positive women for many of the conditions discussed above such as HPV, HSV, PID, and cervical dysplasia or neoplasia (Allen, 1990). Further, practitioners working with women should be alert for genital infections that are resistant to the usual therapies and discuss the possibility of HIV testing and counseling with the client. Finally, prospective, well-designed studies with state-of-the-art protocols and treatment are necessary to determine the most optimum therapies for HIV-infected women with gynecologic disorders. The CDC has proposed adding invasive cervical cancer to the AIDS surveillance case definition (CDC, 1992).

Other Gynecologic Infections

Since HIV infection for many women is a sexually transmitted disease (STD), there may be a relationship between other STDs and AIDS. It has been postulated that certain STDs, especially those causing genital ulcers, may increase the risk of acquiring HIV infection. Genital ulcers alone due to syphilis, herpes simplex, and chancroid have been shown to be bidirectional risk factors for HIV transmission, increasing the susceptibility of the HIV-negative person and increasing the infectivity of the HIV-positive person (Allen, 1990; Johnson & Webster, 1989). In African women, gonorrheal or chlamydial cervical infections or *Trichomonas* vaginal infections have been associated with a higher risk of HIV acquisition (Aral & Holmes, 1991). Hepatitis B (and to a lesser extent C) infections have shown a decrease among homosexual men but are increasing in poor minority populations in the United States (Handsfield, 1992). Because of the close relationships among behaviors associated with the acquisition of STDs and the acquisition of HIV, persons with STDs should be educated, counseled, and offered HIV testing. More than ever it is important to ensure adequate treatment and follow-up.

Vaginal infections may also be observed in women with HIV infection. Most commonly seen in addition to *Candida*, as discussed above, are bacterial infections, other yeast infections such as *Monilia*, and *Trichomonas vaginalis* infections.

Gynecological Protocols

A suggested gynecology protocol for HIV-infected women in medical clinics has been developed by Allen and Marte and is shown in Table 5.2.

HIV INFECTION AND PREGNANCY

The reciprocal questions of how HIV infection affects pregnancy and how pregnancy affects the course of HIV infection are important ones. If a woman infected with HIV has decided to become pregnant, are pregnancy outcomes related to the stage of her HIV infection? At this time, many of these issues are still not well understood (Brettle & Leen, 1991). The European Collaborative Study (1992) reports an increased risk of vertical transmission when the HIV-infected woman has p24-antigenemia or a low CD4+ count. These issues are discussed further in Chapter 6.

TABLE 5.2 Suggested Gynecology Protocol for HIV-infected Women in Medical Clinics

I. *Routine gynecologic care* for the HIV-infected woman requires a pelvic exam every 6 months.

II. *Routine pelvic exam should include*:
   - Pap test
   - Chlamydia and gonorrhea assay
   - Wet mount and KOH prep of any cervical or vaginal discharge
   - Serum RPR

III. *Counselling* at time of initial pelvic exam on: candidiasis, STDs, cervical cancer and HPV, contraception and pregnancy, safe sex.

IV. *Management*:

Recurrent Candidiasis

Vaginal anti-fungal cream or suppository as needed (patient should have medication available for self-administration).

If candidiasis is *non*-responsive to topical therapy (and unless contraindicated by known liver disease):
   - Confirm *Candida* by fungal culture or wet mount.
   - Initiate therapy with ketoconazole 200 mg po qd or bid or with fluconazole 200 po followed by 100 mg po qd or bid until the woman is asymptomatic for two weeks (avoid the use of concomitant antacids if possible).
   - Maintain ketoconazole therapy indefinitely with ketoconazole 200mg or fluconazole 100 mg po qd for 5 days/month at the onset of each menses, or ketoconazole 100 mg or fluconazole 50 mg po qd.
   - Liver function tests must be monitored closely; transaminase three times normal requires evaluation for discontinuation of ketoconazole or fluconazole.
   - Ulcerative candidiasis may require higher doses, up to 800 mg daily of ketoconazole or 400 mg daily of fluconazole.

Recurrent Herpes Simplex
   - Confirm herpes simplex by viral culture.
   - Initiate therapy during the acute phase with acyclovir 400 mg po q 4 h, with or without acyclovir ointment 5% q 3 h.
   - Maintain acyclovir therapy indefinitely with 200 mg po bid or tid.
   - Renal function must be monitored closely and dosing interval extended for renal insufficiency.

Abnormal Pap (Papanicolaou) *Test*

If atypia: repeat Pap test 90 days after treatment. (Treat an identified infection with the appropriate agent; treat nonspecific vaginosis with metronidazole 500 mg po bid for 7 days.)

If atypia on repeat Pap test: refer to colposcopy clinic for endocervical curettage and biopsy of any visible lesions.

If dysplasia and/or evidence of (HPV) human papillomavirus: refer to colposcopy clinic. Endocervical curettage in addition to biopsy of any visible lesions must be performed in every HIV infected woman.

Severe dysplasia, CIN III or CIS should be colposcoped immediately.

If biopsy is negative, recolposcope in 3 months.

Condyloma Acuminata

Refer to a gynecologist or gynecology clinic for topical treatment. Persistent or recurrent lesions should be brought to the attention of a gynecologist or clinic familiar with management of HIV-infected women.

(continued)

Table 5.2 (*continued*)

(Topical therapies include trichloroacetic acid (TCA), cryosurgery, surgical excision, CO_2 laser. Podophyllin is less effective in this population.)

Women should be advised that there may be a risk of increased HIV transmission after biopsy or treatment procedures which result in open wounds.

Persistent Ulcerative Lesions

RPR and dark field exam (even if patient has nonreactive RPR); bacterial culture and sensitivity; viral and fungal cultures. Treat for identified infection with appropriate agent.

Persistent Inguinal Adenopathy

Aspirate and send contents for culture and sensitivity. Treat for identified infection with appropriate agent.

Syphilis

• *Primary, secondary, early latent* (less than one year) should be treated with Penicillin G benzathine 2.4 million units IM weekly × 3 weeks.
• *Late* (*more than one year*): Lumber puncture and/or treatment as for neurosyphilis.
• Any potential *neurosyphilis or recurrent syphilis*:
  • Penicillin G 2 to 4 million units IV q 4 hours × 10 days; or
  • Penicillin G procaine 2.4 million units IM daily plus probenecid 500 mg qid orally, both for 10 days; and
  • Either one followed by penicillin G benzathine 2.4 million units weekly × 3 weeks.
• Serial RPR's should be drawn at 1, 2, 3, 6, 9, 12 months and every 6 months thereafter.
• Whenever possible, penicillin allergic patients should be referred to an infectious disease specialist for desensitization because of reports that tetracycline and erythromycin may be inadequate for HIV-infected patients.

Adapted from Allen, M. H. & Marte, G. Gynecology protocol for HIV-infected women (mimeographed). Used with permission.

NATURAL HISTORY AND SURVIVAL
OF WOMEN WITH AIDS

Many of the natural occurrences in women, such as the menstrual cycle and its hormonal changes, pregnancy, and the onset of menopause, and basic biologic differences between males and females (pharmacokinetics, for example) have not been systematically evaluated in regard to HIV infection, AIDS, or therapeutic approaches for women. Of interest are the questions of the time (1) from initial HIV infection to the development of symptoms (2) until the development of full-blown AIDS and (3) between infection and death. The majority of studies attempting to address these questions have been conducted in homosexual males and males with hemophilia; few have examined progression in women (Brettle & Leen, 1991).

In one study examining survival of adult women with AIDS in San Francisco, 125 women were followed. The survival range was 0.1 to 61.8 months with a median survival of 11.1 months for women. Survival was significantly shorter in women than in men and did not differ by initial diagnosis or race.

Independent predictors of improved survival were younger age (below 39 years) and use of zido-vudine or ddI (Araneta et al., 1991). Another study with similar findings observed that survival times did not differ by gender if both males and females were receiving antiretroviral therapy. However, among those not receiving such therapy, survival times were significantly shorter for females (Lemp et al., 1992). Royce, Tu, and Papano (1991) found an increased mortality risk after diagnosis in women when compared with men, with increased mortality for blacks and Hispanics as well as adults over 50 years of age. In another study, when extraneous variables including IDU and age were controlled for, females did not have decreased predicted survival (Horsburgh, Hanson, Fann, Havlik, & Thompson, 1991).

Still others demonstrate that prognosis is worse for women who are IDUs. In New York, the cumulative probability of survival at one year for white males with KS was 75.4%, compared with 37% for black female IDUs with PCP (Rothenberg et al., 1987).

In regard to both progression and survival, many factors play a role, including genetic susceptibility, age, smoking, cofactors, risk activities, viral strain, and so forth. It would not be unreasonable to expect that the natural history of HIV infection and AIDS in women would be somewhat different than in men. What might partially explain the studies that do find decreased survival in women is that HIV-infected women tend to be minorities, of lower socioeconomic status, may be IDUs, have been diagnosed later, not have received early zidovudine treatment, and have impaired access to quality care due to their social situations (for example, child-care responsibilities and financial status). Women who receive episodic health services may not have any continuity of health-care providers, further lessening the chance of appropriate diagnosis and treatment. It is important to maximize a favorable course for women by being alert to the possibility of HIV infection and offering HIV testing and counseling, conducting appropriate education, recognizing gender specific symptoms and issues, initiating prompt and optimal treatment, and facilitating access to treatment, care, and supportive services.

SUMMARY

HIV infection in women may still be overlooked. Nonspecific symptoms found in both men and women with HIV infection may be overlooked in women unless health-care providers develop a high index of suspicion regarding HIV. Evidence from various research studies is beginning to accumulate, indicating that certain gynecological conditions such as vaginal candidiasis occur early in HIV-infected women and that others, such as cervical disturbances, are also associated with HIV infection. In women who are IDUs, either HIV-related symptoms may mimic other infections seen in IDUs or the health-care provider may (because of their own values) not spend the necessary time to assess properly the HIV risk and recommend testing and counseling. In women who are neither prostitutes nor IDUs, the health-care provider may neglect to consider HIV infection as a cause of the presenting problems, falsely assuming that the client is not at risk for HIV infection.

Important to optimal care for HIV-infected women are the issues of access to, and facilitation of, optimal services and care. Nursing has an important role to play in providing these.

REFERENCES

Allen, M. H. (1990). Primary care of women infected with the human immunodeficiency virus. *Obstetrics and Gynecology Clinics of North America, 17*(3), 557–569.

Allen, M. H., & Marte, C. (1991). Gynecology protocol for HIV-infected women.

Anastos, K., & Palleja, S. M. (1991). Caring for women at risk of HIV infection. *Journal of General Internal Medicine, 6*(Suppl), S40–S46.

Araneta, M. R., Lemp, G. F., Cohen, J. B., Derish, P. A., Carmona, I., & Clevenger, A. C. (1991). Survival trends among women with AIDS in San Francisco. In *Abstracts of the VII International Conference on AIDS* (Vol. 1, p. 328) (abstract M.C. 3122). Florence, Italy.

Aral, S. O., & Holmes, K. K. (1991). Sexually transmitted diseases in the AIDS era. *Scientific American, 264*(2), 62–69.

Aral, S. O., Mosher, W. D., & Cates, W., Jr. (1991). Self-reported pelvic inflammatory disease in the United States, 1988. *Journal of the American Medical Association, 266,* 2570–2573.

Benedetti, P., Greco, D., Figoli, F., & Tirelli, U. (1991). Epidemic Kaposi's sarcoma in female AIDS patients. *AIDS, 5,* 466–467.

Beral, V., Peterman, T. A., Berkelman, R. L., & Jaffe, H. W. (1990). Kaposi's sarcoma among persons with AIDS: A sexually transmitted infection? *Lancet, 335,* 123–128.

Bradbeer, C. (1987). Is infection with HIV a risk factor for cervical intraepithelial neoplasia? *Lancet, 2,* 1277–1278.

Brettle, R. P., & Leen, C. L. S. (1991). The natural history of HIV and AIDS in women. *AIDS, 5,* 1283–1292.

Buehler, J., Farizo, K., Berkelman, R., & Adult/Adolescent Spectrum of Disease Project Group. (1991). The spectrum of HIV disease in women. In *Abstracts of the VII International Conference on AIDS* (Vol 1, p. 453) (M. D. 4253) Florence, Italy.

Byrne, M. A., Taylor-Robinson, D., Munday, P. E., & Harris, J. W. (1989). The common occurrence of human papillomavirus infection and intraepithelial neoplasia in women infected by HIV. *AIDS, 3,* 379–382.

Carpenter, C. C. J., Mayer, K. H., Fisher, A., Desai, M. B., & Durand, L. (1989). Natural history of acquired immunodeficiency syndrome in women in Rhode Island. *American Journal of Medicine, 86,* 771–775.

Carpenter, C. C. J., Mayer, K. H., Stein, M. D., Leibman, B. D., Fisher, A., & Fiore, T. C. (1991). Human immunodeficiency virus infection in North American women: Experience with 200 cases and a review of the literature. *Medicine, 70,* 307–325.

Centers for Disease Control. (1987). Revision of the CDC surveillance case definition for acquired immunodeficiency syndrome. *Morbidity and Mortality Weekly Report, 36*(1), 1S–15S.

Centers for Disease Control. (1990). Risk for cervical disease in HIV-infected women— New York City. *Morbidity and Mortality Weekly Report, 39,* 846–849.

Centers for Disease Control. (1991). Pelvic inflammatory disease: Guidelines for prevention and management. *Morbidity and Mortality Weekly Report, 40* (RR-5), 1–25.

Centers for Disease Control. (15 November 1991). 1992 revised classification system for HIV infection and expanded AIDS surveillance case definition for adolescents and adults. Draft (unpaginated).

Centers for Disease Control. (July, 1992). *HIV/AIDS Surveillance* (pp. 1–18).

Centers for Disease Control. (1992). Addendum to the proposed expansion of the AIDS surveillance case definition, October 22, 1992.

Cohen, F. L. (1991). The clinical spectrum of HIV infection and its treatment. In J. D. Durham & F. L. Cohen (Eds.), *The person with AIDS: Nursing perspectives* (2nd ed., pp. 135–205). New York: Springer.

Cohn, D. L. (1991) Bacterial pneumonia in the HIV-infected patient. *Infectious Disease Clinics of North America, 5*(3), 485–507.

Cotton, P. (1991). Medicine's arsenal in battling 'dominant dozen,' other AIDS-associated opportunistic infections. *Journal of the American Medical Association, 266,* 1476–1481.

Diamond, R. D. (1991). The growing problem of mycoses in patients infected with the human immunodeficiency virus. *Reviews of Infectious Diseases, 13,* 480–486.

Edman, J. C., Kovacs, J. A., Masur, H., Santi, D. V., Elwood, H. J., & Sogin, M. L. (1988). Ribosomal RNA sequence shows *Pneumocystis carinii* to be a member of the fungi. *Nature, 334,* 519–522.

European Collaborative Study. (1992). Risk factors for mother-to-child transmission of HIV-1. *Lancet, 339,* 1007–1012.

Fleming, P., Cleslelski, C. A., & Berkelman, R. L. (1991). Sex-specific differences in the prevalence of reported AIDS-indicative diagnoses, United States, 1988–1989. In *Abstracts of the VII International Conference on AIDS* (Vol. 1, p. 350) (abstract M.C. 3210). Florence, Italy.

Galgiani, J. N. (1990). Fluconazole, a new antifungal agent. *Annals of Internal Medicine, 113,* 177–179.

Grant, I. H., Anastos, K., & Ernst, J. (1991). Gender differences in AIDS-defining illnesses. In *Abstracts of the VII International Conference on AIDS* (Vol. 1, p. 346) (abstract M.C. 3192). Florence, Italy.

Gravell, C. (1990) Progression of HIV infection in women: Asymptomatic state to frank AIDS. *NAACOG's Clinical Issues in Perinatal and Women's Health Nursing, 1*(1), 20–27.

Greenspan, J. S., Greenspan, D., & Winkler, J. R. (1990). Diagnosis and management of the oral manifestations of HIV infection and AIDS. In M. A. Sande & P. A. Volberding (Eds.), *The medical management of AIDS* (2nd ed., pp. 131–144). Philadelphia: Saunders.

Grossman, C. (1989). Possible underlying mechanisms of sexual dimorphism in the immune response, fact and hypothesis. *Journal of Steroid Biochemistry, 34,* 241–251.

Handsfield, H. H. (1992). Recent developments in STDs: II. Viral and other syndromes. *Hospital Practice, 27*(1), 175–200.

Herpes simplex virus latency. (1989). *Lancet, 1,* 194–195.

Hoegsberg, B., Abulafia, O., Sedlis, A., Feldman, J., Des Jarlais, D., Landesman, S., & . Minkoff, H. (1990). Sexually transmitted diseases and human immunodeficiency virus infection among women with pelvic inflammatory disease. *American Journal of Obstetrics and Gynecology, 163,* 1135–1139.

Horsburgh, C. R., Hanson, D., Fann, S. A., Havlik, J. A., & Thompson, S. E. (1991). Predictors of survival in HIV infection include CD4+ cell count, AIDS defining condition and therapy but not sex, age, race or risk activity. In *Abstracts of the VII International Conference on AIDS* (Vol 1, p. 341) (M.C. 3175). Florence, Italy.

Imam, N., Carpenter, C. C. J., Mayer, K., H., Fisher, A., Stein, M., & Danforth, S. B.

(1990). Hierarchical pattern of mucosal Candida infections in HIV-seropositive women. *American Journal of Medicine, 89,* 142–146.

Johnson, J. C., Burnett, A. F., Willet, G. D., Young, M. A., & Doniger, J. (1992). High frequency of latent and clinical human papillomavirus cervical infections in immunocompromised human immunodeficiency virus-infected women. *Obstetrics and Gynecology, 79,* 321–327.

Johnson, M. A., & Webster, A. (1989). Human immunodeficiency virus infection in women. *British Journal of Obstetrics and Gynaecology, 96,* 129–134.

Lassoued, K., Clauvel, J-P, Fegueux, S., Matheron, S., Gorin, I., & Oksenhendler, E. (1991). AIDS-associated Kaposi's sarcoma in female patients. *AIDS, 5,* 877–880.

Lemp, G. F., Hirozawa, A. M., Cohen, J. B., Derish, P. A., McKinney, K. C., & Hernandez, S. R. (1992). Survival for women and men with AIDS. *Journal of Infectious Diseases, 166,* 74–79.

Maiman, M., Fruchter, R. G., Serur, E., Remy, J. C., Feuer, G., & Boyce, J. (1990). Human immunodeficiency virus infection and cervical neoplasia. *Gynecologic Oncology, 38,* 377–382.

Me first! Medical manifestations of HIV in women. (1990). New Brunswick, NJ: New Jersey Women and AIDS Network.

Mertz, G. J., Benedetti, J., Ashley, R., Selke, S. A., & Corey, L. (1992). Risk factors for the sexual transmission of genital herpes. *Annals of Internal Medicine, 116,* 197–202.

Minkoff, H. L., & DeHovitz, J. A. (1991). Care of women infected with the human immunodeficiency virus. *Journal of the American Medical Association, 266,* 2253–2258.

Pape, J. W., Liautaud, B., Thomas, F., Mathurin, J. R., St. Amand, M-M. A., Boney, M., Pean, V., Pamphile, M., Laroche, A. C., & Johnson, W. D., Jr. (1986). Risk factors associated with AIDS in Haiti. *American Journal of Medical Science, 29,* 4–7.

Peterson, H. B., Walker, C. K., Kahn, J. G., Washington, A. E., Eschenbach, D. A., & Faro, S. (1991). Pelvic inflammatory disease. *Journal of the American Medical Association, 266,* 2605–2611.

Pomerantz, R. J., de la Monte, S. M., Donegan, S. P., Rota, T. R., Vogt, M. W., Craven, D. E., & Hirsch, M. S. (1988). Human immunodeficiency virus (HIV) infection of the uterine cervix. *Annals of Internal Medicine, 108,* 321–327.

Quinn, T. C., Groseclose, S. L., Spence, M., Provost, V., & Hook, E. W., III. (1992). Evolution of the human immunodeficiency virus epidemic among patients attending sexually transmitted disease clinics: A decade of experience. *Journal of Infectious Diseases, 165,* 541–544.

Raub, W. (1990). High probability of lymphoma found after long-term, anti-HIV therapy. *Journal of the American Medical Association, 264,* 2191.

Rhoads, J. L., Wright, D. C., Redfield, R. R., & Burke, D. S. (1987). Chronic vaginal candidiasis in women with human immunodeficiency virus infection. *Journal of the American Medical Association, 257,* 3105–3107.

Rice, P. A., & Schachter, J. (1991). Pathogenesis of pelvic inflammatory disease. *Journal of the American Medical Association, 266,* 2587–2593.

Root-Bernstein, R. S. (1990). AIDS and Kaposi's sarcoma pre-1979. *Lancet, 335,* 969.

Rothenberg, R., Woelfel, M., Stoneburner, R., Milberg, J., Parker, R., & Truman, B. (1987). Survival with the acquired immunodeficiency syndrome. *New England Journal of Medicine, 317,* 1297–1302.

Royce, R. A., Tu, X., & Pagano, M. (1991). Gender differences in survival after AIDS diagnosis: U.S. surveillance data. In *Abstracts of the VII International Conference on AIDS* (Vol 1, p. 331) (M.C. 3135). Florence, Italy.

Safrin, S., Dattel, B. J., Hauer, L., & Sweet, R. L. (1990). Seroprevalence and epidemiologic correlates of human immunodeficiency virus infection in women with acute pelvic inflammatory disease. *Obstetrics & Gynecology, 75*, 666–670.

Saral, R. (1991). Candida and Aspergillus infections in immunocompromised patients: An overview. *Reviews of Infectious Diseases, 13*, 487–492.

Schafer, A., Friedmann, W., Mielke, M., Schwartlander, B., & Koch, M. A. (1991). The increased frequency of cervical dysplasia-neoplasia in women infected with the human immunodeficiency virus is related to the degree of immunosuppression. *American Journal of Obstetrics and Gynecology, 164*, 593–599.

Schneider, V., Kay, S., & Lee, H. M. (1983). Immunosuppression: high risk factor for the development of condyloma acuminatum and squamous neoplasia of the cervix. *Acta Cytologica, 27*, 220–224.

Selwyn, P. A. (1986). AIDS: What is now known. Clinical aspects. *Hospital Practice, 21*(9), 119–153.

Shakri-Tabibzadeh, S., Koss, L. G., Molnar, J., & Ramney, S. (1981). Association of human papillomavirus with neoplastic processes in genital tract of four women with impaired immunity. *Gynecologic Oncology, 12*, 129–140.

Sobel, J. D. (1992). Pathogenesis and treatment of recurrent vulvovaginal candidiasis. *Clinical Infectious Diseases, 14* (Suppl. 1), S148–S153.

Spence, M. R. & Reboli, R. C. (1991). Human immunodeficiency virus infection in women. *Annals of Internal Medicine, 115*, 827–829.

Still, J. M.(1992). Helping patients cope with genital herpes infections. *OB/GYN Nursing & Patient Counseling, 4*(1), 4–6.

Thompson, M., Whyte, B., Morris, A., Rimland, D., & Thompson, S. (1991). Gender differences in the spectrum of HIV disease in Atlanta. In *Abstracts of the VII International Conference on AIDS* (p. 32) (M. C. 3115). Florence, Italy.

Vermund, S. H., Kelley, K. F., Klein, R. S., Feingold, A. R., Schreiber, K., Munk, G., & Burk, R. D. (1991). High risk of human papillomavirus infection and cervical squamous intraepithelial lesions among women with symptomatic human immunodeficiency virus infection. *American Journal of Obstetrics and Gynecology, 165*, 392–400.

Vogt, M. W., Witt, D. J., Craven, D. E., Byington, R., Crawford, D. F., Schooley, R. T., & Hirsch, M. S. (1986). Isolation of HTLV-III/LAV from cervical secretions of women at risk for AIDS. *Lancet, 1*, 525–527.

Wofsy, C. B., Cohen, J. B., Hauer, L. B., Padian, N. S., Michaelis, B. A., Evans, L. A., & Levy, J. A. (1986). Isolation of AIDS-associated retrovirus from genital secretions of women with antibodies to the virus. *Lancet, 1*, 527–529.

6

Reproductive Issues, Pregnancy, and Childbearing in HIV-Infected Women

Ann Kurth

Terminal illness is not generally within the province of reproductive health professionals. The appearance of HIV infection, however, broadens that purview while at the same time forcing a reexamination of many personal assumptions about sexual and substance-use behaviors and reproductive choices. As discussed in Chapter 3, the vast majority of the women with AIDS in the United States are in the reproductive potential years: 15–44. In the coming decade, nurses will see an increasing number of women who are affected by HIV.

UNIQUE CONCERNS

At the national level, HIV is predominantly a diagnosis of socially and economically disenfranchised women; moreover, AIDS has appeared in this country at a time when the reproductive rights of women are being challenged on a variety of fronts. Low-socioeconomic nonwhite women have historically been most vulnerable to the erosion of reproductive autonomy (Gertner, 1990). This and other realities compound the story of women and HIV. Some of these factors are briefly reviewed below.

Reproductive Roles and Self-Care Issues

Many women still have traditional roles that can have an adverse influence on an HIV diagnosis. Women often see themselves as care providers, as the ones who must take care of everyone else's needs, thus affecting their experiences with HIV disease from testing to clinical care. The experience of one HIV counseling center, for example, has been that women "to an incomparably larger extent than men [feel] responsible for the life, the well-being and the distress of their partners, friends and relatives" (Hutterer, Blaas, Oberauer, Ogris, & Zupan, 1991); thus some women take excellent care of their children but neglect to take care of themselves. Part of the nurse's role may be to help such women learn the difference between "healthy nurturance—something they may never have experienced themselves—and codependent caretaking, that is, pathologically putting the needs of others before their own" (Benson & Maier, 1990, p. 1).

Motherhood is very important to many women and for some constitutes the primary source of self-expression and self-esteem. The power of the parenting role should never be underestimated. Because children are central to the lives of many women, pregnancy can be a time when chemically dependent women are motivated to stop their substance use entirely (Williams, 1990). The implications of HIV infection for these women's reproductive capacities can pose an enormous threat to their sense of self.

Chemical Dependence

Many women with HIV and/or their sexual partners are chemically dependent. Women have traditionally had trouble accessing drug treatment, a situation particularly acute for the pregnant woman. Only a few addiction treatment centers in the country will accept a pregnant substance user into a program (see Chapter 14).

HIV TESTING AND COUNSELING FOR WOMEN OF REPRODUCTIVE AGE

The American Nurses Association has endorsed the availability of voluntary, anonymous HIV testing with informed consent and appropriate counseling by qualified health-care professionals (Barrick, 1989). Excellent protocols for HIV counseling in pregnancy and in general populations have been published elsewhere (Carr & Gee, 1986; Holman et al., 1989; McMahon, 1988; Moroso & Holman, 1990; Tuomala, 1990; WHO, 1990). General information about HIV testing is discussed in Chapter 1. Because most HIV tests detect antibodies to HIV, false positive results can occur in multiparous women (due to cross-reactivity with HLA-DR5 antibody) and in pregnant women (McMahon, 1988). Several factors that the nurse must consider before beginning HIV testing and counseling of pregnant and nonpregnant women are briefly reviewed below.

Consent and Documentation

The nurse-counselor should be familiar with state and local laws regarding patient consent and documentation of HIV testing. It is highly advisable that health-care workers obtain verbal or written consent before testing. If the test site is not run on an anonymous basis (i.e., using a numerical assignment rather than patient name and demographic identifiers) the patient should be informed that the results are kept confidential. It is important for the counselor to explain the limits of confidentiality. If the test result goes into the patient's medical record, insurance companies may see the result if they request access to the chart. It is generally agreed that those staff with a "medical need to know" of the patient's blood-borne pathogen status will have access to that information on the chart. The institution of universal precautions in most settings precludes the need to "label" these patients for the information of health-care workers with whom they may come in contact. Each institution should devise its own system of documentation on the medical chart (coded "body fluids precautions," etc.) to ensure patient confidentiality and the staff's desire to be informed.

The health professional should know that there are several important reasons why women of reproductive (or any) age can benefit from HIV testing. Women should be informed of these. These include empowerment to make lifestyle and health changes; to seek needed clinical, pharmacological, and psychosocial care; and to make informed life decisions for oneself and one's children (see Tuomala, 1990). Mounting evidence of the benefits of early clinical intervention lend an effective counterweight to the stigma and discrimination that can result from being known to be HIV-positive. Williams (1990) has warned, however, that clinicians should not slip into treating the HIV test as "routine" as these indications for testing accumulate.

Knowledge of HIV status can assist the health-care worker in tailoring prenatal (Minkoff et al., 1990a) and pediatric care (Nolan, 1990), and in reinforcing safe behaviors with women who test negative (Tuomala, 1990). Discovery of a patient's HIV serostatus for health-care workers' purposes, on the other hand, may not be ethically justifiable. As with any information gathered by health-care workers, the old adage applies: "Don't ask the question unless you are prepared to deal with the result." It is crucial to ensure that there are adequate clinical and psychosocial (not just testing) services in place for those women who find out that the result of their HIV test is positive. An intrinsic part of the nursing process is an ongoing assessment of the patient's referral needs. In the case of women with HIV infection, specific services may not exist (e.g., child care and transportation to a clinic site), and even accessibility to clinical care may be limited. In these situations nurses may need to interpret their role as that of an advocate for improving or increasing the availability of needed services.

It is important to reinforce with patients as well as with colleagues that it is risk behaviors, not membership in risk groups, that increase the likelihood of HIV acquisition. If women and men are having unprotected sex or sharing used or nondisinfected needles with anyone who is HIV-positive or whose HIV status is unknown, they are engaging in risky behavior that can result in HIV infection (see Chapter 4).

Who, then, should be tested? Several schools of thought about prenatal testing have evolved and can be summed up as the "routine" versus "targeted" testing approaches. Those who advocate routine prenatal testing point to data showing that health-care workers' assessments of patient risk are accurate only in identifying a portion of women who actually are HIV-positive (Barbacci, Repke, & Chaisson, 1991; Landesman, Minkoff, Holman, McCalla, & Sijin, 1987). Furthermore, requiring women to self-identify their previous risk history and risk behaviors may well make these women feel singled out or "branded." Being asked to label oneself as "promiscuous," a drug user, or prostitute may seem punitive. Advocates of targeted testing, on the other hand, say that such risk assessment is generally adequate, likely to reduce costs associated with testing and improve the positive predictive value of the HIV antibody test in those populations that are low seroprevalence/low risk (Carlson et al., 1985). The American Academy of Pediatrics has recommended that HIV testing be routinely offered to all pregnant and childbearing women and encouraged for those at increased risk of HIV infection because of behaviors or residence in a place "with an HIV seroprevalence rate among pregnant women and newborns of 1:1000 or more" (Task Force on Pediatric AIDS, 1992, p. 792).

Still another approach, as Moroso and Holman outline (1990), is to provide information to clients about risk behaviors and the HIV antibody test and then to ask women to request the test if they desire without having to state their reasons for doing so. HIV testing on a routine basis, without having to "confess" risk behaviors, should always be done with written consent, confidentiality provisions, and pre- and posttest counseling (Minkoff & Landesman, 1988; Working Group on HIV Testing of Pregnant Women and Newborns, 1990).

Counseling Models

Nurses play vital roles in counseling, testing, and patient teaching regarding HIV disease (Barrick, 1989). Whether the nurse is functioning in a clinical-nurse-specialist role in doing all the pre- and posttest HIV counseling (McMahon, 1988) or is complementing the work of other clinicians, in most settings the nurse has primary responsibility for education and provision of emotional support for patients (Moroso & Holman, 1990). Reproductive counseling is discussed below.

HIV AND REPRODUCTIVE CHOICES

Although women have experienced HIV disease since the beginning of the epidemic, only recently were women discussed in terms other than as "vectors" of transmission to potential children and to clients (in roles as sex workers or prostitutes). At one end of the extreme, some have proposed that all HIV-positive women be forced to undergo abortion and/or sterilization (Newman, 1987). Others have suggested mandatory HIV-antibody testing of all pregnant women and all women of reproductive age, with an assumption that knowledge of HIV serostatus will lead to a significant reduction in the incidence of perinatal AIDS. Still others recommend, like the U.S. Public Health Service, that prenatal HIV testing be made routinely available to women of reproductive potential (Centers for Disease Control, 1985; Centers for Disease Control, 1987a). The CDC and others recommend that women with HIV postpone childbearing "until more is known" (Rogers, 1987, p. 109) about HIV vertical transmission. However, since the risk of perinatal transmission may increase with advancing maternal HIV disease and decreasing CD4+ cell counts (Landers & Sweet, 1990), other authors have pointed out that a woman may have a better chance of an HIV seronegative pregnancy earlier in the disease process.

Nurses and other health-care workers who discuss HIV with clients should have a thorough knowledge of HIV disease and its physical and psychosocial implications. They should assess their own biases and values regarding sexuality, substance use, and reproductive decisions, and should be aware of any other issues that may affect their provision of appropriate education and care (Moroso & Holman, 1990). There is no question that HIV infection, particularly in the emotional context of female and pediatric AIDS, can stir up a number of issues for the health-care worker. As Middleton (1990) advises, "Professional crisis resolution is essential before effective patient care can begin" (p. 349). Strong administrative support, opportunities for peer feedback and continuing education, and clear protocols with guidelines and confidentiality provisions should also be in place for the nurse who functions in a primary counselor role (McMahon, 1988).

Most reproductive health workers recommend that reproductive counseling be based on the genetic counseling model, that is, the presentation of factual information in a nondirective manner. The role of the counselor is to present the most recent information available and encourage the patient to assume a decision-making role (Francis & Chin, 1987). Olds, London, and Ladewig (1984) have defined seven major principles that govern genetic counseling: accurate diagnosis, confidentiality, truthfulness, nondirective counseling, timing, team approach, and follow-up counseling. HIV infection raises concerns in several of these areas, leading to difficulties for the nurse who is counseling the affected patient or family.

At the present time, there is no accurate prenatal method of diagnosing which women will definitively transmit HIV or which fetus will become HIV-infected. Moreover, maintaining the confidentiality of HIV test results is expected of professional nurses, but they cannot guarantee that the woman who tests positive will not lose her family, job, insurance, or housing if test results are inappropriately revealed or insurance companies gain access to the medical record. Truthfulness in discussing the possible outcomes of HIV infection for the woman or her fetus can involve a certain degree of subjectivity that may be a direct outgrowth of unconscious or conscious personal biases in the nurse. An example of this unintentional bias is illustrated by the counselor who decides to stress a

"50% or more" transmission figure to the injecting drug-using woman with four children but a "30% or so" figure to the wife of a hemophiliac couple who desperately want children. The rule of nondirectiveness in the counselor's approach to fact giving is obviously contravened by such an inconsistent approach. Discussion of reproduction and HIV issues optimally takes place prior to conception. However, this timing is not always possible. Many women still find out about their HIV status only after they or their child become ill (Centers for Disease Control, 1990). A multidisciplinary team approach is best suited to meet the needs of women with HIV infection. These clients need not only excellent nursing care but access to clinical research protocols for experimental therapies, medical services, social services, financial and legal counseling, and psychological support. The nurse will ideally function as an integral part of a team that may include physicians (adult and pediatric), social workers, mental health workers, and community-based organizations. However, this well-integrated multidisciplinary team that follows the woman and her children is not the norm for every health-care setting or community (see Chapter 11).

Finally, follow-up counseling is perhaps the most important element of the genetic counseling model. Yet it is the piece most often missing in the systems that serve women with HIV. Much of the discussion about HIV testing and modes of counseling conducted prenatally focus on fetal implications. What is obvious but often ignored is the fact that HIV infection is nearly unique among illnesses that can be screened for during pregnancy because the results of maternal testing holds implications for both the woman and the fetus. The woman who is told that she is HIV positive will require ongoing support beyond the pregnancy interval.

Emotional and Psychological Concerns

The genetic counseling paradigm is a necessary but insufficient approach to the woman with HIV infection considering reproduction. Identifying HIV infection in a woman puts that woman on notice that she now faces a life-threatening illness. This illness is one that might be passed on to any potential children, but it is one from which she already may be suffering consequences. Adapting to this news necessarily involves a grief process. Anyone suffering from grief has "work to do" (Kubler-Ross, 1969). This work has implications for reproductive decision making and women's lives and should not be ignored by nurses as they counsel the whole person. Little has been written about the interaction between grief and pregnancy, yet grief may have important implications for women with HIV infection. One non-AIDS-related study, for example, showed how a loss event (death of a parent) precipitated unplanned pregnancy in seven women (Swigar, Bowers, & Fleck, 1976). For these women, sexual intimacy and pregnancy fulfilled their loss-related needs. Whether similar processes occur with HIV disease is not known.

Women with HIV infection are living not only with the implications of this diagnosis for their own lives but with its potential impact on a child. HIV infection without clinical symptoms carries tremendous ambiguity that may be even more difficult to resolve than an AIDS diagnosis. The difficulties inherent in adaptation to ambiguity have been described in the context of emotional resolution of an abnormal pregnancy or a pregnancy in which there is an indication of a poor fetal outcome (i.e., congenital anomaly). Penticuff (1982) suggests that a diagnosis of a high-risk pregnancy may be met with denial until symptoms of the problem are physically apparent and thus indisputable.

The classic Kubler-Ross (1969) stages of adaptation to terminal illness may have limited applicability with respect to adaptation to a diagnosis of asymptomatic HIV infection. Important, however, is her identification of denial as a necessary grief stage, one that most often occurs as the initial response to a diagnosis but that in some cases may continue until shortly before death. In this model, a fixation on the stage of denial is not viewed pejoratively but as a reflection of how an individual has historically responded to stress. Denial "is a common coping mechanism and when patients begin to break through this, it is important that supportive counseling be available" (VanDevanter et al., 1987). The nurse must be prepared to assess for suicidal ideation, depression, and other adverse responses in the client coping with HIV infection and be able to intervene or make appropriate referrals in a timely manner.

Since the ability to process grief may be compromised by the emotionally intense, time-limited concurrent psychological processes of pregnancy, counseling should ideally be continued through the nonpregnant intervals of women's lives. Such caregiving acknowledges that a woman's needs extend beyond her capacity as a maternal-fetal unit. Studies suggest that for some, pregnancy is a time of emotional crisis and that many women become more introverted and have lower levels of self-acceptance and independence (Bailey & Hailey, 1986; Leifer, 1977). Counselors should also be aware that women who choose to abort may be at risk for grief reactions (McAll & Wilson, 1987). This reaction may be compounded by HIV infection and if unresolved may have implications for future reproduction.

Nurses and other counselors must bear in mind that a reproductive decision takes place along a spectrum of life events. Though it occurs at a distinct point in time, the confluence of factors that come to bear will be unique with each pregnancy decision. Prior reproductive decisions are not necessarily repeated or predictors of behavior. Counselors must strive, therefore, to eradicate assumptions about how a woman will think or act on the basis of her history (e.g., previous therapeutic abortion). Unfounded assumptions about the existence of familial and community support systems must also be avoided; careful estimation of the woman's perceptions of her support networks will best enable the counselor to address deficiencies in those systems. Assessment should also be made of her sense of access to health-care systems since this may influence how one chooses to assist the woman in negotiation of resources and referrals.

Research Regarding HIV and Reproductive Decision Making

Studies from around the world find that often a majority of HIV-positive women choose not to abort their pregnancies (Rudin, Lauper, Biedermann et al., 1991; Sunderland, 1990). These and other studies show that HIV-positive women make reproductive choices similar to those of HIV-negative women (Johnstone et al, 1990). This reality is uncomfortable for some people in the nursing and medical community because of *health-care worker* perception of the risks involved. In this context, a 1987 study is instructive. A group of pregnant women were asked for their attitude toward abortion of fetuses with neural tube defects. More women stated that they would continue pregnancy if there was only a 5% chance of having a normal child than if there was no such likelihood (32% vs. 4%; Faden et al., 1987). Vertical HIV transmission rates average about 30%, with the chance of having a HIV-negative child from an HIV-positive mother as high as 70%, depending on a variety of factors that are not entirely understood. It has been pointed out that these risk levels may not be seen by many woman as an overriding factor in pregnancy decision making (Selwyn et al., 1989a).

Only a few studies have looked at HIV infection and reproductive decision making. For example, one recent study found that HIV-positive women who had a child living at home were more likely to terminate pregnancy than women who had lost children to child welfare bureaus (Pivnick et al., 1991). I conclude that policies should try to encourage mother-child residence so that women will not be influenced in their current reproductive decisions by unnecessary separations from existing children. Another study conducted with eleven HIV-positive women who had faced pregnancy decisions within the previous 24 months found that the decision to abort or take a pregnancy to term involves a multitude of factors, HIV infection being one among several (Hutchison & Kurth, 1991). Moral thought systems employed by these women are varied, complex, and often child-centered, although the same fundamental concern may translate into different decisions—therapeutic abortion to prevent the potential suffering of a child versus taking the pregnancy to term because of the belief that even a life shortened by HIV infection is of value.

These preliminary findings underscore the possibility that pregnancy decision making is not necessarily only a cognitive process. Many cultural and affective, emotion-based elements may come into play. Women will respond to the crisis of HIV infection in ways that reflect their life history. Nurses and other health-care workers must learn to recognize this likelihood and adapt their approaches accordingly.

Referrals

A list of available clinical and psychosocial service providers should be developed so that the nurse can make necessary referrals (Moroso & Holman, 1990). Figure 6.1 presents an algorithm that may be useful when testing and counseling pregnant and nonpregnant women.

Clients are routinely provided with information
re: risk behaviors, antibody test; client can
request test without identifying "risk history"

PRE-TEST COUNSELING
- Continuum of HIV disease
- HIV transmission routes
- HIV antibody test, waiting period for & meaning of result
- Usefulness of knowing HIV serostatus for own health/
  pregnancy/pediatric care
- Risk reduction: safer sex, needle avoidance or cleansing
  with bleach if shared

BLOOD TEST (with informed consent)
- ELISA x 2 If either or both are positive or indecisive
- Do confirmatory western blot

-RESULT
- Review "window period" of antibody production
- If recent exposure, avoid risk behavior &
  repeat test in 3 - 6 months
- Reinforce need to practice risk reduction behaviors
- Negative result does *not* imply "immunity"

+ RESULT
- Review client's support network & have follow-up
  referral plan before meeting
- Consider having two staff in client meeting
- Discuss meaning of HIV positive antibody result by
  reviewing spectrum of disease; HIV ≠ AIDS
- Review how HIV is *not* transmitted
- Reinforce need to practice risk reduction behaviors
  (provide couples counseling with sex or needle
  partner if client requests)
- Instruct re: benefits and importance of clinical early
  intervention (antiviral and/or opportunistic infection
  prevention)
Before leaving initial session:
- Have client identify a support person who will
  respect the client's confidentiality
- Schedule follow-up session to assess coping and
  review above information
- Assess needed clinical & psychosocial referrals &
  client's ability to access them (money, car, etc.)

REPRODUCTIVE HEALTH

Maternal Assessment
* T-cell panel
* p24 antigen
* Physical Examination
* CDC disease stage
* Need for anti-HIV
  and/or anti-opportunistic
  infection therapies

If Pregnant/Considering Pregnancy:
- Review vertical transmission
  (≈ 30% but may be related to
  maternal disease status)
- Options include therapeutic abortion
  if < 24 wks; or taking pregnancy to
  term
- Need for thorough HIV disease
  monitoring and/or treatment as part of
  prenatal care

Reproductive Options:
- Barrier birth control methods/
  condoms (LATEX &
  SPERMICIDE)
- Alternative, non-penetrative
  sexual expression
  techniques
- Sterilization *at client request*
  (continued need for barriers)

FIGURE 6.1 HIV testing and counseling.

EFFECT OF PREGNANCY
ON WOMEN'S HEALTH STATUS

Pregnancy and HIV disease involve changes in cellular immunity, with a specific focus on T-helper (T4) cells. In particular, the T4:T8 ratio becomes inverted in both pregnancy and HIV disease (Minkoff, deRegt, Landesman, & Schwarz, 1986). Pregnancy therefore mimics a state of immunosuppression, but it is not necessarily the case that overall clinical immunocompetence in the normal pregnancy is impaired (Coyne & Landers, 1990). Because of alterations in immune levels of normal pregnancy, it was hypothesized that pregnancy might accelerate disease progression in HIV-positive women. Findings from early studies seemed to demonstrate that the mother of an infant diagnosed with AIDS was at increased risk for development of AIDS, especially in a second or subsequent pregnancy (Minkoff, Nanda, Menez, & Fikrig, 1987a; Scott et al., 1985). Confounding factors that made the specific impact difficult to assess included subjects' low socioeconomic status, limited access to timely health care, drug addiction, and concurrent illness (Koonin et al., 1989). It is also true that many symptoms of HIV infection—fatigue, weight loss, anorexia, nausea, vomiting, shortness of breath—may be mistakenly attributed to normal symptoms of pregnancy (Coyne & Landers, 1990; Poole, 1989). Additional case-control prospective studies are needed to definitively determine the effects of pregnancy during different stages of HIV disease.

Studies that have been able to control for confounding factors have concluded that there is no marked effect of pregnancy on disease progression when women are still asymptomatic (Johnstone, MacCallum, Brettle, Inglis, & Peutherer, 1988). Selwyn and colleagues (1989b) found that only 1 out of 39 asymptomatic HIV-positive women developed symptomatic HIV disease during pregnancy. While these women were slightly more likely than the control group to be hospitalized for bacterial pneumonia, the authors concluded that "an acceleration in HIV-disease status during pregnancy is uncommon" with asymptomatic HIV infection. The Project AWARE women's study at San Francisco General Hospital also found no evidence that HIV disease progressed more rapidly in pregnant and postpartum subjects. The author concluded that there is a theoretical risk that pregnancy can accelerate HIV disease progression but found no firm evidence of it (Poole, 1989). Ellerbrock and Rogers (1990) pointed out that while pregnancy may not significantly exacerbate disease progression in symptomatic women in the short term, the long-term effects are not known. These authors compare survival intervals of pregnant and nonpregnant HIV-positive women from one study (mean of 59 versus 187 days) (Koonin et al., 1989) and conclude that these differences "support the notion that pregnancy aggravates the course of HIV infection in women who are in advanced stages of disease" (Ellerbrock & Rogers, 1990, p. 541).

There does appear, moreover, to be a correlation between low T-cell counts and disease progression in women. Minkoff and coworkers (1990a) found that serious infections during pregnancy were experienced only by those women with CD4+ counts of less than 300 cells/mm^3. Opportunistic infections (OIs) experienced by these women can be especially fulminant in pregnancy and carry an inherent risk to both the woman and the fetus (Poole, 1989). *Pneumocystis carinii* pneumonia, for example, which affects up to 80% of all persons with HIV disease, may result in severe maternal and fetal hypoxia and can cause mortality in both (Minkoff et al., 1990a). Studies have reported the rapidly progressive and fatal course of some pregnant women with OIs (Jensen et al., 1984; Minkoff et al., 1986; Wetli, Roldan, & Fojaco, 1983).

EFFECT OF HIV INFECTION ON OBSTETRICAL AND NEONATAL OUTCOME

A prospective cohort study conducted in Kenya matched HIV-positive with HIV-negative women and found that women infected with HIV were at greater risk for premature delivery and stillbirth and that four of the HIV-positive women died within one month after delivery (Temmerman, Hawala, Ndinya-Achola, Plummer, & Piot, 1991). Controlled studies in the United States, however, show no higher incidence of obstetrical complication, low birth weight, or prematurity in HIV-positive women. Minkoff and colleagues (1990b) controlled for a number of possible variables in comparing 101 HIV-positive and 129 HIV-negative women. The HIV-positive women experienced statistically significantly more sexually transmitted diseases (STDs, 18% vs. 7%) and medical complications (43% vs. 25%) during pregnancy. No other obstetrical complications (e.g., chorioamnionitis, endometritis, toxemia, or placental problems) or differences in neonatal outcomes (birth weight, gestational age, head circumference or Apgar scores) were associated with the woman's serological status. In keeping with results from several multicenter studies, the Hemophilia-AIDS Collaborative Study Group found that "maternal HIV infection does not necessarily lead to clinically significant intrauterine growth retardation or prematurity" (Jason & Evatt, 1989, p. 489). Selwyn and associates (1989b) found no increase in the frequency of spontaneous abortion, ectopic pregnancy, preterm delivery, stillbirth or low-birth-weight infants of relatively asymptomatic HIV-positive women compared to seronegative controls.

VERTICAL TRANSMISSION

HIV can be transmitted from an infected mother to the infant in the antepartum, intrapartum, or postpartum periods, as discussed in Chapter 7. Why HIV is transmitted in some cases and not in others is not well understood. Women have given birth to an HIV-infected infant and then, in another pregnancy, to an uninfected infant; there have also been several occurrences of HIV-discordant monozygotic twins (Viscarello, 1990a), as has also been documented with rubella. Like hepatitis B (HBV), vertical transmission of HIV may increase if the woman develops a primary infection in the third trimester and when advanced HIV disease is present (Hague, Mok, MacCallum, Burns, & Yap, 1991). Risk factors for vertical transmission of HIV may include advanced maternal age and advanced maternal disease (Zylke, 1991). It is now believed that the risk of vertical transmission is higher in advanced maternal disease and when there is positivity for the HIV p24 antigen (European Collaborative Study, 1992; Muggiasca et al., 1991). In fact, one study found that women who had low CD4 counts and CDC disease stage IV with HIV p24 antigen positive levels transmitted HIV to their offspring in 92% of cases versus 11% transmission in women who were less clinically advanced (D'Arminio Monforte, et al., 1991). If this finding is supported by future research, it may be possible to predict more accurately which women are likely to transmit HIV and thus to tailor counseling individually.

Conversely, the possibility exists that certain maternal antibodies to HIV (notably to gp120, an envelope glycoprotein) may have a "protective" or neutralizing effect preventing vertical transmission. Goedert and colleagues (1989) reported that preterm infants were at greater risk of acquiring HIV infection than term infants and that those women with high reactivity to gp120 were less likely to transmit HIV to their term infants. Other studies, however, have found no relationship between levels of maternal HIV antibody and rates of transmission (Shaffer et al., 1991). No clear evidence from large-scale studies yet exists to answer conclusively the "protective antibody" theory. Other researchers are investigating the role of the placenta as a modulator of vertical transmission (Valente & Main, 1990).

Future Diagnostic Trends

Researchers have pointed out that truly informed reproductive decision making would include determining if and when the fetus is infected (Viscarello, 1990a). Potential methods of fetal diagnosis include looking directly for evidence of fetal infection (via percutaneous umbilical blood sampling [PUBS] and chorionic villus sampling), looking for indirect markers (detecting if there are any protective antibodies in maternal serum), and conducting diagnostic screening to distinguish maternal from fetal HIV antibodies. While some of these techniques, such as PUBS, run the risk of introducing HIV into the fetal bloodstream, the possible benefits may warrant further investigation under controlled conditions (Nolan, 1990).

Future research is exploring potential ways to interrupt vertical transmission, as by the administration of anti-HIV therapies (e.g. zidovudine) and immune strategies (hyperimmune antibody infusions, vaccines) (Heagarty & Abrams, 1992). These strategies are controversial, however, since at present the majority of infants in the United States will turn out not to be truly HIV-infected (Zylke, 1991). Women's health activists have also raised objections to these proposals because, as with the AIDS Clinical Trials Group's (ACTGs) study investigating the administration of zidovudine in the third trimester, a main goal is to prevent possible transmission to the fetus (rather than primarily to maintain the health of the mother). This approach could appear to treat the woman as a carrier or vessel for the fetus and not as a person in her own right. Researchers have also encountered difficulties with federal regulations that require the permission of the fetus's father before any treatment can be given to a pregnant woman. Many women, and some researchers, find these regulations paternalistic, insulting to women, and outmoded (Kolata, 1991).

CLINICAL ISSUES OF HIV-SEROPOSITIVITY IN PREGNANCY

Antepartum Management

Perhaps the most important services that the nurse and other women's health providers can give during the antepartum period are counseling and psychosocial support. This counseling should be both religiously and culturally sensitive and should be provided whether the woman chooses to continue or to terminate her pregnancy (Schwarz, 1989). Evidence suggests that a higher rate of genitourinary tract infections and an increased incidence of sexually transmitted diseases occur in HIV-positive women during pregnancy. Gloeb, O'Sullivan, and Efantis (1988) found that over one-third of the 50 HIV-positive women they followed through pregnancy suffered infections, including urinary tract infections, syphilis and/or gonorrhea, or herpes simplex; only 15 women (28.8%) had uncomplicated antenatal courses.

It is necessary that women with HIV infection have baseline cytomegalovirus (CMV) and toxoplasmosis titres drawn since these infections can have implications for the fetus. HIV-positive women should continue receiving careful monitoring of gynecological manifestations during the pregnancy. Monitoring during pregnancy should include Pap tests, examination for primary HSV or recurrences, syphilis and HBsAG titres, cultures for gonorrhea, and chlamydial infection and other pertinent cultures in the first and third trimesters, more often if exposure warrants. *Mycobacterium tuberculosis* should also be ruled out.

HIV-infected pregnant women should be encouraged to report all symptoms as some HIV-related effects may otherwise be attributed to the pregnancy (Feinkind & Minkoff, 1988). Health-care workers should advise patients to see their health provider for an evaluation immediately if they develop fever, sweats, cough, or diarrhea (Minkoff, 1988). These women should also receive nutritional counseling and be encouraged to gain weight appropriately (Schwarz, 1989).

As Minkoff and coworkers point out, if an HIV-positive woman's T4 cells drop below 300 mm^3, she may well need prophylaxis for opportunistic infections, especially PCP. A baseline T-cell panel should be drawn, and CD4 counts should be taken at least every trimester, with careful monitoring in the third trimester when T-cells reach their nadir and risk of infection appears most prevalent (Minkoff et al., 1990a). Other laboratory tests pertinent to pregnant women with HIV include a complete blood count (CBC) with differential/platelet count to rule out thrombocytopenia and anemia, both of which can have implications at delivery (Feinkind & Minkoff, 1988; Viscarello, 1990b.) The risks of possible fetal side effects from aerosolized pentamidine, sulfa drugs, and/or folic acid antagonists must be weighed against the very real risks of fetal impact from maternal disease to which women with T4 cells less than 300 mm^3 are predisposed. While research is under way to test formally the use of zidovudine in the third trimester, some physicians around the country have already been giving zidovudine to pregnant women on a compassionate-use basis. More data on the natural history of HIV infection in women are needed to determine whether different therapeutic strategies may be required.

It is important to point out that women who test as HIV negative at the beginning of pregnancy may seroconvert during gestation, especially if risk behavior has occurred. HIV can be acquired during pregnancy. If the woman has been placed at risk of HIV acquisition during pregnancy, HIV antibody testing can be repeated around the time of delivery (Rudin, Lauper, & Biedermann, 1991).

Intrapartum Management

HIV has been cultured from cervical secretions and can directly infect cells that line the vagina and other mucosal regions (Langhoff et al., 1991; Vogt et al., 1986; Wofsy et al., 1986). Thus it was conjectured that operative delivery (cesarean) might reduce HIV transmission to the fetus. For operative delivery to make an impact, however, one must assume that intrauterine HIV transmission has not yet occurred. To date, there are no definitive clinical data to indicate any pronounced protective effect from operative versus vaginal delivery. Recently a possible protective effect of cesarean section delivery on vertical transmission has been suggested (European Collaborative Study, 1992). However, the effects of the anesthesia and surgery on the mother must also be considered (Fuith, Czarnecki, Wachter, & Fuchs, 1992). Data from twin studies suggest a higher risk of infection in firstborn as opposed to second born twins (Goedert et al., 1991). These data suggest that transmission during the intrapartum period may be highly likely from passage through the birth canal for some infants. Some researchers have suggested "cleansing the birth canal with a non-traumatic antiviral solution" at delivery (Duliege et al., 1992). It has been pointed out that cesarean sections do carry maternal risk that may be enhanced in a potentially immunocompromised individual and do not guarantee neonatal well-being (Minkoff et al., 1987b; Peckham, Senturia, & Ades, 1987). When possible, practitioners should avoid certain invasive procedures that could expose the fetus to maternal blood. These include internal fetal scalp electrodes, scalp pHs, artificial rupture of membranes or multiple vaginal exams following rupture of membranes, amniocentesis, chorionic villus sampling, cordocentesis/percutaneous blood sampling, internal uterine pressure monitoring, and episiotomies (Feinkind & Minkoff, 1988; Mendez & Jule, 1990; Shannon & Coats, 1990). For similar reasons, practitioners have also advised that vacuum extraction should be avoided (Swift, 1988; Viscarello, 1990b). If these procedures are needed, they should be performed after a careful analysis and discussion of risks, alternatives, and benefits.

Postpartum Management

Although there is no clear evidence to suggest that HIV-positive women experience increased rates of postpartum or postoperative morbidity, the HIV-positive woman should be monitored for the development of any signs and symptoms of infectious morbidity (Minkoff, 1988; Shannon & Coats, 1990).

A SAFE WORKING ENVIRONMENT FOR NURSING CARE

Universal Precautions for Staff

Universal precautions can be summed up as "clinical common sense." Because HIV antibodies can take several months to reach detectable levels, the HIV or other blood-borne pathogen status of patients (or staff) cannot always be known, even if testing is done routinely. It is therefore prudent not to treat patients on the basis of their presumed blood-borne pathogen status but to treat all patients' blood and body fluids as potentially infectious. Management of the HIV-positive parturient and infant should proceed in a way that maximizes prevention of nosocomial HIV acquisition by obstetric and neonatal personnel (Minkoff, 1988). This means adhering to universal precautions guidelines promulgated by the CDC and found in the policies and procedures of institutions.

Obstetric, gynecologic, and neonatal nurses; nurse-midwives; nurse-practitioners; and other women's health workers are exposed to many body fluids on the job. These include blood, cervical and vaginal secretions, semen, urine, stool, amniotic fluid, vernix, meconium, lochia, breast milk, tears, saliva, and endotracheal and gastric secretions. The CDC (1988) has emphasized that blood remains the single most important source of occupational exposure for health workers but also recommends that universal precautions apply to cerebrospinal fluid, synovial fluid, pleural fluid, peritoneal fluid, pericardial fluid, and amniotic fluid. An infection-control nurse and coworkers (Jackson, Lynch, McPherson, Cummings, & Greenwalt, 1987) have taken the universal precaution approach one step further by advocating that all patient fluids, not just blood or visibly blood-contaminated fluids, be treated as infectious.

For prenatal and gynecologic visits, gloves should be worn on both hands for pelvic examinations and collection of cervical, vaginal, and rectal cultures. The practitioner should use instruments and specula that are disposable or auto-clavable. Glutaraldehyde should be used to disinfect cryocautery probe tips and vaginal ultrasound tips (soak 10 to 45 minutes and rinse with tap water after-ward). Diaphragm-fitting rings should be washed with soap and water, then immersed in 70% alcohol for 15 minutes (Mead, 1988). Sharps should be dis-posed of in puncture-resistant containers and placed out of reach of children in the examination area. Venipuncture and vascular access procedures—blood draws, IV starts and discontinuations—should be performed wearing gloves. It is useful to prepare strips of adhesive tape for anchoring before putting on gloves: tear strips, folding down a quarter inch of one end of each (providing a stick-free surface to handle once gloves are on). Once the site is stabilized with an initial butterfly fold of tape and blood wiped off, gloves can be removed to apply extra tape (Wiley & Grohar, 1988). Gloves are not needed for physical exami-nation of intact skin or assessing a patient's vital signs. Nurses should wash hands thoroughly following glove removal and keep fingernails trimmed and smooth. Unfortunately compliance with hand-washing among health profession-als still remains less than what is necessary for control of infection (Goldmann & Larson, 1992). Institutional policies and CDC recommendations should be followed for those situations involving glove allergy/contact dermatitis or if exudative lesions are present on hands (Centers for Disease Control, 1988). All health workers should be knowledgeable about the standards regarding blood-borne pathogens in the workplace, such as the December 1, 1991, standard on bloodborne pathogens enforced by the Occupational Safety and Health Admin-istration.

Above and beyond universal precaution techniques and technologies, it is important to analyze obstetrical and gynecological procedures. In one study, the two factors found to be significantly related to intraoperative exposure to blood were operative procedures lasting more than three hours and an associated blood loss in excess of 300 ml (Gerberding, Littell, Tarkington, Brown, & Schecter, 1991). Where patient safety is not compromised, making certain procedural changes may have widespread benefit. It may, for example, be sensible to elimi-nate passing sharp instruments from hand to hand, instead using trays or emesis basins to hand off instruments (Mead, 1989). Sharp instruments should not be placed on surgical drapes, and health workers may consider using staples and electrocautery rather than sharp tools if merited (Mead, 1988).

Labor and Delivery

The above precautions are needed during labor and delivery, with the use of masks, protective eyewear or face shields, and gowns or aprons to avoid possible mucous membrane exposure to potentially infectious blood or blood-contaminated body fluids. Some practitioners complain that goggles make seeing difficult. It is im-portant to try different brands of protective eyewear to find an optimal product that will be routinely used by labor and delivery personnel. At a minimum, staff can wear eyeglasses (clear glass lenses if they have normal vision) with side shields to protect from lateral splashes. Staff wearing prescriptive eyeglasses who wish additional protection can wear face shields (Crombleholme, 1990). Practitioners in high HIV, HBV, hepatitis C, STD and other blood-borne pathogen prevalence areas will often double-glove during procedures. One study looking at double-gloving found a perforation rate of 17.7% in the outer and 5.5% in the inner glove. The first (inner) glove should be one half-size larger than usually worn, with the second (outer) glove used being one's usual size. This will allow for tactile flexibility without risking tears and air pockets (Crombleholme, 1990).

In the labor and delivery-operating room, as everywhere else, care must be taken with needles, scalpels, and other sharp instruments. The vast majority of occupationally acquired HIV (and HBV) cases have involved parenteral exposures, usually with hollow needles. It is important not to recap needles, though many health workers seem to find this habit hard to break. Many workplaces are now moving to "needleless" systems that may help minimize exposure to unsheathed needles.

Staff in the delivery room should wear long-sleeved gloves, preferably with impervious material covering the arms. These gowns should be used for all operative deliveries and procedures where prolonged exposure to copious amounts of blood are likely. Elbow-length gloves should be worn if placental removal is necessary (Bailey, 1991). Fingers should never be used as retractors during operative procedures. Impermeable paper or rubber boots are also useful for avoiding prolonged skin exposure to the puddles of blood and fluids that tend to accumulate in cesarean and vaginal deliveries (Crombleholme, 1990). The nurse should exercise caution when removing sheets and wastes following delivery, as large amounts of fluid generally pool in these materials (avoid slinging or dragging soiled materials across the room). Some drape packs for cesarean sections now come with plasticized folds/pockets in the laparotomy sheet surrounding the incision aperture to collect fluid and minimize leakage to the floor (Crombleholme, 1990).

Gloves should be worn for all cord care and handling of the placenta. Practitioners should get in the habit of "stripping" the cord of blood before cutting to avoid splattering of attendant staff. (Place the first clamp; squeeze cord downward several centimeters; then place second clamp and cut.) Practitioners should avoid using syringes and needles to draw cord samples or arterial and venous blood gases. Sterile tubes for cord-blood specimen collection should be a standard part of the delivery supply kit; the nurse can unclamp the cord and let the specimen flow into the tube. Gloves should also be worn when handling blood-contaminated materials such as blood tubes, alcohol wipes, gauze squares (Crombleholme, 1990).

Health workers should always use pick-ups (instruments), not fingers, when suturing. For additional protection, some have recommended that thimbles be used as well (Bailey, 1991). The person doing the suturing should count and place all used needles in one spot, such as the emesis basin or lidocaine cup, to avoid accidental sticks to nursing staff during cleanup. When placing deep interrupted stitches during vaginal laceration/episiotomy repair, health workers should not palpate for the needle tip with fingers. Because administration of paracervical blocks and pudendal anesthesia involves similar palpation of the needle tip in a blind body cavity for correct placement, the use of pudendals should be restricted and alternative methods of pain relief used where possible (Swift, 1988; Viscarello, 1990b).

Neonate, Nursery

Mouth-operated DeeLee mucous suction traps should never be used to clear blood and fluids from the neonatal airway (Mendez & Jule; 1990; Viscarello, 1990b). Wall-operated or hand-powered suction at 80–100mm Hg negative pressure or bulb suction should be used instead (Mead, 1988). Resuscitation bags, mouthpieces, and endotracheal tubes should be available in all areas where a delivery may occur (including precipitous births) to avoid the need for mouth-to-mouth or mouth-to-endotracheal-tube patient resuscitation (Mendez & Jule, 1990).

Because HIV-exposed neonates do not differ from their seronegative controls in maternal history, mode of delivery, rate of obstetric complications, Apgar score, and initial physical examination, recommendations for their management are those that usually apply to all neonates (Mendez & Jule, 1990). Gloves should be worn by all persons handling the infant until blood and body fluids are removed. The infant's skin should be cleansed thoroughly using alcohol swabs prior to administration of vitamin K, heel sticks, and any other procedure that breaks the skin (including administration of resuscitation medications through the umbilical cord). The infant warming area should be cleansed between deliveries and all wastes disposed of or towels laundered according to institutional infection control procedures (Mendez & Jule, 1990).

Figure 6.2 summarizes universal precautions for staff working in gynecological, obstetrical, and neonatal healthcare settings.

Maternal Care

Women should be allowed to spend ample time to bond with their baby following delivery. The use of private rooms for inpatients with HIV is not necessary unless there is a documented contagious respiratory infection present and if other patients in the room are also immunocompromised (Ungvarski, 1990). It is recommended that nurses wear gloves while giving perineal care and changing dressings, chuxs, and peripads (Wiley & Grohar, 1988). Nurses can continue the important role of assisting in development of self- and infant-care skills that they perform with all patients. Patient education is a premier function of the nurse, and postpartum is a good time to review universal precautions with the

Procedures	Precautions
Gynecological	
Pelvic Exams	Wear gloves
Pelvic Surgery	Gloves; impervious gowns & leg cover; masks; eye/face shield
Labor & Delivery	
Venipuncture/access	Gloves; be cautious with needles
Vaginal delivery	Cover skin wounds & wear gloves; masks; impervious gown & foot cover; eye cover
Operative delivery	Gloves; impervious gowns & legcover; masks; eye/face shield; pass sharps on tray; use retractors; double glove p.r.n.
Placental removal	Wear elbow-length gloves
Suturing	Use pick-ups; avoid blind needletip palpation; count & dispose of used needles carefully
Cord samples/handling	Wear gloves; "strip" cord before cutting; avoid needles in obtaining blood samples
Injections	Don't re-cap; dispose of needles properly
Anesthesia	Avoid paracervicals, pudendals unless necessary
Clean-up/disinfection	Wear gloves while handling bloody materials; beware of sharps; dispose of or sterilize equipment according to protocols
Neonatal	
Suctioning	Never use DeeLee/mouth operated suction; use wall suction @ 80mm Hg or bulb
Injections/heel sticks	Wipe fluids off infant skin before using needle
Resuscitation	Use mechanical suction; + - pressure bags & masks; wipe umbilical stump before administering medications/volume expanders
Postpartum	
Maternal care	Wear gloves to change blood-soaked materials; gloves not needed for examining intact skin & for other nursing care (no body fluid contact)
Breastfeeding	Review recommendations; wear gloves if handling milk in milk banks
Infant care	Gloves not needed for routine bath, feeding, diaper change unless blood present or caretaker's skin non-intact

FIGURE 6.2 Universal precautions in reproductive health settings.

HIV-infected mother as it pertains to her and her baby's care. There is no evidence of horizontal HIV transmission to household contacts, so the mother should be reassured that she can handle her infant, simply taking care to prevent exposure to her blood or body fluids (Nanda, 1990).

This review of universal precautions for the home should include discussion of breast-feeding (see next section), the use of gloves when the baby's stools contain blood or when the mother's hands have lacerations or irritation, and the fact that normal soap and water and the hot cycle of laundry machines are sufficient to kill HIV if present on dishes and clothes. Articles soiled with large amounts of blood should be double-bagged and spills cleaned up with a solution of one part bleach to nine parts water. While saliva is not known to transmit HIV, toys should be washed in hot soap and water if excessive drooling occurs and the toys are shared with others. The nurse should advise the infected woman to hug and kiss her child as much as she wants, as can her friends and family. Before discharge from the hospital, the nurse should answer any questions the woman may have to reinforce the teaching already done. With the help of a multidisciplinary team (if in place), the nurse should ensure that contraceptive plans have been discussed and that the woman is scheduled not only for her six-week postpartum and pediatric appointments but her HIV surveillance visits every three to six months (Shannon & Coats, 1990).

Infant Care

Nursing staff should wear sterile gloves during the initial infant bath and for administration of antimicrobial cord care. Prophylaxis against ophthalmia neonatorium should be administered according to usual guidelines. After skin, cord, and eye care and the administration of vitamin K are completed, the use of gloves is no longer required for practices such as weighing, bathing, and feeding the newborn. Gloves are not required while changing diapers because of the doubtful importance of urine and stool in transmitting HIV (though if the nurse's hands are chapped, abraded, or cut, it may be advisable to wear gloves when changing diapers or giving baths) (Wiley & Grohar, 1988). Hands should be washed after diaper changes to reduce nosocomial transmission of pathogens (American Academy of Pediatrics, 1988). Barrier precautions (e.g., gloves) should be used to prevent exposure to the infant's blood or bloody secretions (Mendez & Jule, 1990).

Recommendations Regarding Breastfeeding

HIV can be cultivated from both the cellular and liquid portion of breastmilk (Ellerbrock & Rogers, 1990). Breastfeeding has been implicated in several documented cases of HIV transmission (Ellerbrock & Rogers, 1990; European Collaborative Study, 1992). For women who have access to safe, alternative infant nourishment, the CDC states that HIV-infected women should be advised against breastfeeding (Centers for Disease Control, 1985). Further evidence for transmission of HIV through breastfeeding was presented at the VIII International Conference on AIDS held in July 1992 in Amsterdam. Nonetheless, the WHO/UNICEF Consultation on HIV Transmission and Breastfeeding has concluded that the risks of HIV transmission through breastfeeding are outweighed by the benefits wherever the primary causes of infant deaths are infectious disease and malnutrition ("Breastfeeding benefits usually . . .", 1992). This issue is more fully discussed in Chapter 7.

For those women who are chemically dependent, particularly on cocaine, refraining from breastfeeding is recommended because cocaine and other lipid-soluble drugs can concentrate in breast milk. For the chemically dependent woman whose HIV status is unknown, the breastfeeding issue becomes difficult. Breastfeeding can enhance bonding and parenting skills, both of which tend to be poor in chemically dependent women. Harlem Hospital's approach is not to recommend breastfeeding in those chemically dependent women who do not wish to find out their HIV status (Mitchell, Brown, Lofman, & Williams, 1990).

REPRODUCTIVE HEALTH FOR WOMEN WITH HIV INFECTION

Reproductive choice must be determined by the patient, and nurses must assist her in obtaining those services required by her informed choice. Women with HIV infection need the same access to therapeutic abortion, prenatal care, birth control, or sterilization as their HIV-negative peers. Women with HIV infection have been denied access to needed reproductive services such as pregnancy termination, have faced discrimination in gynecological offices, and have been pressured into sterilization procedures (American Public Health Association, 1988; Nolan, 1990). The nurse should be able to make referrals to providers who do not (illegally) discriminate on the basis of HIV status.

Birth Control, Safer Sex Methods and Techniques

Pregnancy is frequently an unplanned event in women's lives regardless of HIV status. The few studies that have looked at the use of birth-control methods in HIV-positive and HIV-negative women have not found significant differences in the rates of birth-control use (Casolati et al., 1991), although one study did find that HIV-positive women had significantly higher rates of sterilization following delivery (Dattel et al., 1991).

Deciding if and when to get pregnant is an issue for many people, not just those with HIV infection. HIV infection has not been shown to be the major factor in many women's reproductive decision making (Williams, 1990). It may not be a predominant factor in decision making of men either (Williams, 1990). Jason and Evatt (1990) found that in 280 couples in an HIV-AIDS hemophiliac study group, the female partner became pregnant despite recommendations against unprotected intercourse with HIV-positive men. This study group's pregnancy rate was comparable to the U.S. fertility rate for that period. For both HIV-positive and HIV-negative women, the nurse-counselor should review the benefits and risks of available birth-control methods and safer sex techniques. Barrier and spermicidal methods of contraception, including the female condom, are discussed in Chapter 4.

Oral contraceptives.   Oral contraceptives prevent pregnancy by interfering with ovulation, implantation, and gamete transport, among other mechanisms. While some have postulated a theoretical advantage for oral contraceptives in terms of HIV transmission (due to decreased number of "bleeding" days and the development of thick cervical mucous), those same authors have stated that hormonal contraceptives may have systemic effects that impact upon the likelihood of transmission and/or course of disease due to alterations in liver metabolism and increased susceptibility to some common viral pathogens (Hatcher et al., 1988). An early study of sex workers in Nairobi seemed to suggest a link between oral contraceptives and an increased risk of HIV infection; at least two subsequent studies, however, have found no such relationship (WHO, 1990). Other recent studies have found an association between HIV-1 infection and the use of oral contraceptives (Plourde et al., 1992). What is known is that oral contraceptives, because they offer no physical barrier, are not inherently protective against HIV; other infections such as syphilis, gonorrhea, chlamydia; and other viruses such as herpes simplex and the human papilloma virus.

Oral contraceptives became a mainstay of the family-planning system in the 1960s. It is critical to stress that today pregnancy prevention should not be the woman's only concern. Birth-control methods should ideally protect against the panoply of epidemic STDs, HIV infection foremost among them. The nurse should discuss the benefits of barrier protection in this regard. However, only latex condoms, along with spermicides, have been demonstrated to be protective against sexual transmission of HIV. Women's health providers often recommend use of both condoms and oral contraceptives for extra protection.

For those women who are HIV-positive, it should be stressed that not much is known about the interaction of oral contraceptives (most of which contain varying levels of estrogen and progesterone) with the immune system in the context of HIV disease. While estrogen and progesterone do have complex effects on target cells in the immune system, it is not known if this is detrimental or contributory to HIV disease progression (Peterman, Cates, & Curran, 1988). The interaction of HIV with injectable (Depo-Provera) and/or implantable (Norplant) hormonal contraceptives is also not known.

Intrauterine Devices (IUDs).   IUDs function by creating an inflammatory response in the uterus, thus preventing implantation. Because a correlation has been found between a history of other STDS and an increased risk of pelvic inflammatory disease (PID), the IUD is contraindicated in women with HIV infection and women at risk of acquiring HIV (WHO, 1990). Some researchers have documented an increased risk of HIV acquisition through sexual contact in women who use IUDs (Gervasoni, Lazzarin, Musicco, Saracco, & Nicolosi, 1992).

Sterilization

HIV can be transmitted by the pre-ejaculate fluid and by ejaculate of men who have undergone vasectomies (WHO, 1990). For this reason, couples at risk should use condoms and spermicide even if one or both have undergone a sterilization procedure.

Artificial Insemination

It is not uncommon to encounter HIV-discordant couples (where one partner is HIV-positive and the other negative) and lesbian and other women who wish to become pregnant by artificial insemination. HIV is found as an extracellular virus in seminal fluid and in the white cells of the ejaculate (WHO, 1990). HIV transmission has resulted from artificial insemination with both cryopreserved and fresh semen in cases where the donor was HIV-positive (Ellerbrock & Rogers, 1990). Media reports of the theoretical ability to separate HIV seminal fluid from the sperm itself prior to artificial insemination have received wide coverage (Kolata, 1988). More recently, however, evidence has accumulated that the virus may be incorporated into the surface of the sperm itself (Scofield, Rao, & Clisham, 1991). It is important that the nurse discuss current information with patients to ensure that they are aware of the risks inherent to artificial insemination procedures. Guidelines for HIV testing of semen donors have been published and should be followed by all institutions involved in artificial insemination procedures.

SUMMARY

The nursing care of women with HIV infection can be complex. For female nurses in particular, there can sometimes be conscious or unconscious emotions engendered by these patients, a phenomenon known as countertransference (Macks, 1988). These patients often have many of the same concerns (family, loved ones, holding a household together) as the nurse. It can be helpful, and indeed appropriate, for nurses to develop a forum to discuss the fears, joys, sadness, and small triumphs that can arise from caring for these often involved patients.

REFERENCES

Allen, M. H. (1990). Primary care of women infected with the human immunodeficiency virus. *Obstetrics and Gynecology Clinics of North America, 17*(3), 557–569.

American Academy of Pediatrics. (1988). Pediatric guidelines for infection control of human immunodeficiency virus (acquired immunodeficiency virus) in hospitals, medical offices, schools, and other settings. *Pediatrics, 82,* 801–807.

American Public Health Association. (1988, September). Counseling and testing for peri-natal transmission of AIDS. *The Nation's Health*, 17–18.

Bailey, L. A., & Hailey, B. J. (1986). The psychological experience of pregnancy. *International Journal of Psychiatry in Medicine*, *16*(3), 263–274.

Bailey, M. (1991). What is the risk of AIDS to health workers? Save the Children Fund.

Barbacci, M., Repke, J. T., & Chaisson, R. (1991). Routine prenatal screening for HIV infection. *Lancet*, *337*, 709–711.

Barrick, B. (February/March, 1989). Teaching safer sex: a nursing intervention in the AIDS epidemic. *Imprint*, *36*, 47–53.

Benson, D. J. D., & Maier, C. (1990). Challenges facing women with HIV. *Focus, A Guide to AIDS Research and Counseling*, *6*(1), 1–2.

Breast-feeding benefits usually outweigh HIV risk. (1992). *Global AIDS News*, *2*, 4, 19.

Burrow, G. N., & Ferris, T. F. (Eds.). (1988). *Medical complications during pregnancy* (3rd ed). Philadelphia: W. B. Saunders.

Carlson, J. R., Bryant, M. L., Hinrichs, S. H. Yamamoto, J. K., Yee, J., Higgins, J. Levine, A. M., Holland, P., Gardner, M. B., & Pederson, N. C. (1985). AIDS serology testing in low- and high-risk groups. *Journal of the American Medical Association*, *253*, 3405–3408.

Carr, G. S., & Gee, G. (1986). AIDS and AIDS-related conditions: Screening for populations at risk. *Nurse Practitioner*, *11*(10), 25–48.

Casolati, E., Agarossi, A., Muggiasca, M. L., Ravasi, L., Brambilla, T., Conti, M., & Zampini, L. (1991, June). Sexual behavior in HIV positive past intravenous drug abuser women. (abstract M.D. 4089). In *VII International Conference on AIDS Abstract Book, 1* (p. 412). Florence, Italy.

Centers for Disease Control. (1985). Recommendations for assisting in the prevention of perinatal transmission of human T-lymphotropic virus type III/lymphadenopathy-associated virus and acquired immunodeficiency syndrome. *Morbidity and Mortality Weekly Report*, *34*, 721–726, 731–732.

Centers for Disease Control. (1987a). Public health service guidelines for counseling and antibody testing to prevent HIV infection and AIDS. *Morbidity and Mortality Weekly Report*, *36*(31), 509–515.

Centers for Disease Control. (1987b). Recommendations for prevention of HIV trans-mission in health-care settings. *Morbidity and Mortality Weekly Report*, *36* (Suppl. 2S, 35–185).

Centers for Disease Control. (1988). Update: Universal precautions for prevention of transmission of human immunodeficiency virus, hepatitis B virus, and other blood-borne pathogens in health-care settings. *Morbidity and Mortality Weekly Report*, *37*(24), 337–382, 387–388.

Centers for Disease Control. (1990). AIDS in women—United States. *Morbidity and Mortality Weekly Report*, *39*, 845–846.

Centers for Disease Control. (1991a). Recommendations for preventing transmission of human immunodeficiency virus and hepatitis B virus to patients during exposure-prone invasive procedures. *Morbidity and Mortality Weekly Report*, *40* (Suppl. RR-8), 1–9.

Centers for Disease Control. (1991b). Purified protein derivative (PPD)-tuberculin anergy and HIV infection. Guidelines for anergy testing and management of anergic persons at risk of tuberculosis. *Morbidity and Mortality Weekly Report*, *40* (Suppl. RR-5), 27–33.

Coyne, B. A., & Landers, D. V. (1990). The immunology of HIV disease and pregnancy and possible interactions. *Obstetrics and Gynecology Clinics of North America*, *17*(3), 595–606.

Crombleholme, W. R. (1990). HIV infection, managing exposure risks for the obstetrician/gynecologist. *Obstetrics and Gynecology Clinics of North America*, *17*(3), 627–636.

D'Arminio Monforte, A., Ravizza, M., Muggiasca, M. L., Novati, R., Bini, T., Tornaghi, R., Zuccotti, G. V., Cavalli, G., Musicco, M., Giovanni, M., Principi, N., Conti, M., Pardi, G., & Lazzarin, A. (1991). HIV infected pregnant women: possible predictors of vertical transmission (abstract W.C. 49). In *VII International Conference on AIDS Abstract Book, 2* (p. 35). Florence, Italy.

Dattel, B. J., Padian, N., Shannon, M., Miller, J., Crombleholme, W. R., & Sweet, R. L. (1991, June). HIV serostatus and risk unrelated to pregnancy planning or contraceptive use (Abstract M.D.4233). In *VII International Conference on AIDS Abstract Book, 1* (p. 448). Florence, Italy.

Duliege, A., Felton, S., & Goedert, J. J., & the International Registry of HIV-exposed Twins (1992, July). High risk of HIV-1 infection for first-born twins: The role of intrapartum transmission. (WeC1062.1,We56) VIII International Conference on AIDS Abstracts, Amsterdam, the Netherlands.

Ellerbrock, T. V., Bush, T. J., Chamberland, M. E., & Oxtoby, M. J. (1991). Epidemiology of women with AIDS in the United States, 1981 through 1990. *Journal of the American Medical Association, 265*, 2971–2981.

Ellerbrock, T. V., & Rogers, M. (1990). Epidemiology of human immunodeficiency virus infection in women in the United States. *Obstetrics and Gynecology Clinics of North America, 17*(3), 523–544.

European Collaborative Study. (1992). Risk factors for mother-to-child transmission of HIV infection. *Lancet, 339*, 1007–1012.

Faden, R. R., Chwalow, A. J., Quaid, K., Chase, G. A., Lopes, C., Leonard, C. O., & Holtzman, N. A. (1987). Prenatal screening and pregnant women's attitudes toward the abortion of defective fetuses. *American Journal of Public Health, 77*, 288–290.

Feinkind, L., & Minkoff, H. L. (1988). HIV in pregnancy. *Clinics in Perinatology, 15*(2), 189–202.

Fenyo, E. M., Keys, B., Fredriksson, R., & Chiodi, F. (1992, July). Mother-to-child transmission. State of the Art Discussion. VIII International Conference on AIDS, July, 1992, Amsterdam, the Netherlands, *1*, 199.

Francis, D. P., & Chin, J. (1987). Counseling the HIV-positive woman regarding pregnancy. *Journal of the American Medical Association, 257*, 3361.

Fuith, L. C., Czarnecki, M., Wachter, H., & Fuchs, D. (1992). Mode of delivery in HIV-1 infected women. *Lancet, 339*, 1603.

Gerberding, J. L., Littell, C., Tarkington, A., Brown, A., & Schecter, W. R. (1991). Risk of exposure of surgical personnel to patients' blood during surgery at San Francisco General Hospital. *New England Journal of Medicine, 322*, 1788–1793.

Gertner, N. (1990, October). Interference with reproductive rights summary. Paper presented at Forum for Reproductive Laws for the 1990s, Newark, New Jersey.

Gervasoni, C., Lazzarin, A., Musicco, M., Saracco, A., & Nicolosi, A. (1992). Contraceptive practices and man-to-woman HIV sexual transmission. (PoC4651) VIII International Conference on AIDS Abstracts, Amsterdam, the Netherlands, *2*, C351.

Giovannini, M., Tagger, A., Ribero, M. L., Zuccotti, G., Pogliani, L., Grossi, A., Ferroni, P., & Fiocchi, A. (1990). Maternal-infant transmission of hepatitis C virus and HIV infections: a possible interaction. *Lancet, 335*, 1166.

Gloeb, D. J., O'Sullivan, M. J., & Efantis, J. (1988). Human immunodeficiency virus infection in women. I. The effects of human immunodeficiency virus on pregnancy. *American Journal of Obstetrics and Gynecology, 159*, 756–761.

Goedert, J. J., Duliege, A-M, Amos, C. I., Felton, S., Biggar, R. J., & the International Registry of HIV-exposed Twins. (1991). High risk of HIV-1 infection for first-born twins. *Lancet, 338*, 1471–1475.

Goedert, J. J., Mendez, H., Drummond, J. E., Robert-Guroff, M., Minkoff, H., Holman, S., Stevens, R., Rubenstein, A., Blattner, W. A., Willoughby, A., & Landesman, S.

(1989). Mother-to-infant transmission of HIV type 1: association with prematurity or low anti-gp 120. *Lancet, 2*, 1351–1354.

Goldmann, D., & Larson, E. (1992). Hand-washing and nosocomial infections. *New England Journal of Medicine, 327*, 120–122.

Hague, R. A., Mok, J. Y. Q., MacCallum, L., Burns, S., & Yap, P. L. (1991). Do maternal factors influence the risk of vertical transmission HIV? (Abstract W.C. 3237). In *VII International Conference on AIDS Abstract Book, 2* (p. 355). Florence, Italy.

Hatcher, R. A., Guest, F., Stewart, F., Stewart, G. K., Trussell, J., Bowen, S. C., & Cates, W. (1988). *Contraceptive Technology* (14th ed). New York: Irvington.

Heagarty, M. C., & Abrams, E. J. (1992). Caring for HIV-infected women and children. *New England Journal of Medicine, 326*, 642–643.

Holman, S., Berthaud, M., Sunderland, A., Moroso, G., Cancellieri, F., Mendez, H., Beller, E., & Marcel, A. (1989). Women infected with human immunodeficiency virus: counseling and testing during pregnancy. *Seminars in Perinatology, 13*(1), 7–15.

Hutchison, M., & Kurth, A. (1991). "I need to know that I have a choice": A study of women, HIV, and reproductive decision-making. *AIDS Patient Care, 5*(1), 17–25.

Hutterer, J., Blaas, P., Oberauer, C., Ogris, M., & Zupan, B. (1991, June). Differences in HIV/AIDS counselling for women and for men. Poster presented at the VII International Conference on AIDS, Florence, Italy.

Jackson, M. M., Lynch, P., McPherson, D. C., Cummings, M. J., & Greenwalt, N. C. (1987). Why not treat all body substances as infectious? *American Journal of Nursing, 87*, 1137–1139.

James, M. E. (1988). HIV seropositivity diagnosed during pregnancy: Psychosocial characterization of patients and their adaptation. *General Hospital Psychiatry, 10*, 309–316.

Jason, J., & Evatt, B. L. (1990). Pregnancies in human immunodeficiency virus infected sex partners of hemophilac men. *American Journal of Diseases of Children, 144*, 485–490.

Jensen, L. P., O'Sullivan, M. J., Gomez-del-Rio, M., Setzer, E. S., Gaskin, C., & Penso, C. (1984). Acquired immunodeficiency (AIDS) in pregnancy. *American Journal of Obstetrics and Gynecology, 148*, 1145–1146.

Johnstone, F. D., Brettle, R., MacCallum, L., Mok, J., Peutherer, J. F., & Burns, S. (1990). Women's knowledge of their HIV antibody status: Its effect on their decision whether to continue the pregnancy. *British Medical Journal, 300*, 23–24.

Johnstone, F. D., MacCallum, L., Brettle, R., Inglis, J. M., & Peutherer, J. F. (1988). Does infection with HIV affect the outcome of pregnancy? *British Medical Journal, 296*, 467.

Kolata, G. (1988, October 17). Discovery on AIDS virus raises a possibility of safe fatherhood. *The New York Times.*

Kolata, G. (1991, August 25). U.S. rule on fetal studies hampers research on AZT. *The New York Times.*

Koonin, L. M., Ellerbrock, T. V., Atrash, H. K., Rogers, M. F., Smith, J. L., Hogue, C. J. R., Harris, M. A., Chavkin, W., Parker, A. L., & Halpin, G. J. (1989). Pregnancy-associated deaths due to AIDS in the United States. *Journal of the American Medical Association, 261*, 1306–1307.

Kubler-Ross, E. (1969). *On death and dying.* New York: MacMillan.

Landers, D. V., & Sweet, R. L. (1990). Perinatal infections. In *Danforth's Obstetrics and Gynecology* (6th ed., p. 535). Philadelphia: Harper & Row.

Landesman, S., Minkoff, H., Holman, S., McCalla, S., & Sijin, O. (1987). Serosurvey of human immunodeficiency virus infection in patients. *Journal of the American Medical Association, 258*, 2701–2703.

Langhoff, E., Terwilliger, E. F., Poznansky, M. C., Bos, H., Kalland, K. H., & Haseltine, W. A. (1991, June). Prolific HIV-1 growth in human dendritic cells. Paper presented at the VII International Conference on AIDS, Florence, Italy.

Laurence, J. (1987). Diagnostic tests for HIV infection. *PA/The AIDS Report, 87*, 159–163, 170.

Leifer, M. (1977). Psychological changes accompanying pregnancy and motherhood. *Genetic Psychology Monographs, 95*, 55–96.

Macks, J. (1988). Women and AIDS: Countertransference issues. *Social Casework: The Journal of Contemporary Social Work, 69*, 340–347.

McAll, K., & Wilson, W. P. (1987). Ritual mourning for unresolved grief after abortion. *Southern Medical Journal, 80*, 817–821.

McMahon, K. M. (1988). The integration of HIV testing and counseling into nursing practice. *Nursing Clinics of North America, 23*(4), 803–821.

Mead, P. B. (1988). Infection control in the era of AIDS. *Contemporary OB/GYN, 32*(3), 116–119.

Mead, P. B. (1989). AIDS: risk to the health profession. *Clinical Obstetrics and Gynecology, 32*(3), 485–496.

Mendez, H., & Jule, J. E. (1990). Care of the infant born exposed to human immunodeficiency virus. *Obstetrics and Gynecology Clinics of North America, 17*(3), 637–649.

Middleton, J. (1990). Voluntary screening at the first prenatal visit. *Journal of Nurse-Midwifery, 34*(6), 349–351.

Minkoff, H., (1988). Managing AIDS in pregnant patients. *Contemporary OB/GYN, 32*(3), 106–114.

Minkoff, H., deRegt, R. H., Landesman, S., & Schwarz, R. (1986). *Pneumocystis carinii* pneumonia associated with acquired immunodeficiency syndrome in pregnancy: A report of three maternal deaths. *Obstetrics and Gynecology, 67*, 284–287.

Minkoff, H. L., Henderson, C., Mendez, H., Gail, M. H., Holman, S., Willoughby, A., Goedert, J. J., Rubinstein, A., Stratton, P., Walsh, J. H., & Landesman, S. H. (1990b). Pregnancy outcomes among mothers infected with human immunodeficiency virus and uninfected controls. *American Journal of Obstetrics and Gynecology, 163*, 1598–1604.

Minkoff, H., & Landesman, S. H. (1988). The case for routinely offering prenatal testing for human immunodeficiency virus. *American Journal of Obstetrics and Gynecology, 159*(4), 793–796.

Minkoff, H., Nanda, D., Menez, R., & Fikrig, S. (1987a). Pregnancies resulting in infants with acquired immunodeficiency syndrome or AIDS-related complex: Follow-up of mothers, children, and subsequently born siblings. *Obstetrics and Gynecology, 69*, 288–291.

Minkoff, H., Nanda, D., Menez, R., & Fikrig, S. (1987b). Pregnancies resulting in infants with acquired immunodeficiency syndrome or AIDS-related complex. *Obstetrics and Gynecology, 69*, 285–287.

Minkoff, H. L., Willoughby, A., Mendez, H., Moroso, G., Holman, S., Goedert, J. J., & Landesman, S. H. (1990a). Serious infections during pregnancy among women with advanced human immunodeficiency virus infection. *American Journal of Obstetrics and Gynecology, 162*, 30–34.

Mitchell, J. (1988). What about the mothers of HIV infected babies? NAN *Multi-Cultural Notes on AIDS Education and Service, 10*, 1–2.

Mitchell, J., Brown, G., Loftman, P., & Williams, S. (1990). HIV infection in pregnancy: detection, counseling, and care. *Pediatric AIDS and HIV Infection, 1*(5), 78–82.

Moroso, G., & Holman, S. (1990). Counseling and testing women for HIV. *NAACOG's Clinical Issues in Perinatal and Womens Health Nursing, 1*(1), 10–19.

Muggiasca, L., Agarossie, A., Casolati, E., Brambilla, T., Imperiale, D., Scopacasa, P., & Conti, M. (1991). Pregnancy, maternal stage and vertical transmission of HIV infection (Abstract W.B. 2000). In *VII International Conference on AIDS Abstract Book, 2* (p. 182). Florence, Italy.

Muska, S., Schilling, R., Hadden, B., El-Bassel, N., Icard, L., Freeman, L., & Leeper, M. (1991). The WPC-333 female condom: perceptions of male and female drug users (Abstract M.D. 4257). In *VII International Conference on AIDS Abstract Book, 1* (p. 454). Florence, Italy.

Nanda, D. (1990). Human immunodeficiency virus in pregnancy. *Obstetrics and Gynecology Clinics of North America, 17*(3), 617–626.

Newman, A. (1987). Patterns of AIDS spread elicit proposals to tighten precautions. Involuntary sterilization? *Obstetrics and Gynecology News, 22*, 36–37.

Nolan, K. (1990). Human immunodeficiency virus infection, women, and pregnancy. *Obstetrics and Gynecology Clinics of North America, 17*(3), 651–668.

Olds, S. B., London, M. L., & Ladewig, P. A. (Eds.). (1984). Maternal-newborn nursing: A family-centered approach (2nd ed., pp. 152–155). Menlo Park, CA: Addison-Wesley.

Oxtoby, M. J. (1988). Human immunodeficiency virus and other viruses in human milk: placing the issue in broader perspective. *Pediatric Infectious Disease Journal, 7*, 825–835.

Peckham, C. S., Senturia, Y. D., & Ades, A. E. (1987). Obstetrical and perinatal consequences of human immunodeficiency virus (HIV) infection: A review. *British Journal of Obstetrics and Gynecology, 94*, 403–407.

Penticuff, J. H. (1982). Psychologic implications in high-risk pregnancy. *Nursing Clinics of North America, 17*(1), 69–78.

Peterman, T. A., Cates, W., & Curran, J. W. (1988). The challenge of human immunodeficiency virus (HIV) and acquired immunodeficiency syndrome (AIDS) in women and children. *Fertility and Sterility, 49*(4), 571–581.

Pivnick, A., Jacobson, A., Eric, K., Mulvihill, M., Hsu, M. A., & Drucker, E. (1991). Reproductive decisions among HIV positive, drug using women: The importance of mother/child co-residence (Abstract W.C. 3227). In *VII International Conference on AIDS Abstract Book, 2* (p. 352). Florence, Italy.

Plourde, P. J., Plummer, F. A., Pepin, J., Agoki, E., Moss, G., Ombette, J., et al. (1992). Human immunodeficiency virus type 1 infection in women attending a sexually transmitted diseases clinic in Kenya. *Journal of Infectious Diseases, 166*, 86–92.

Poole, L. (1989). HIV infection in women. San Francisco: AIDS Knowledge Base from San Francisco General Hospital (online computer program)

Rogers, M. F. (1987). Controlling perinatally acquired HIV infection. *Western Journal of Medicine, 147*, 109–110.

Rudin, C., Lauper, U. & Biedermann, K., & Members of the Collaborative Study Group Swiss HIV and Pregnancy. (1991). HIV seroconversion during pregnancy (Abstract W.C. 3247). In *VII International Conference on AIDS Abstract Book, 2* (p. 357). Florence, Italy.

Schwarz, R. H. (1989). Human immunodeficiency virus and the obstetrician. *Postgraduate Obstetrics & Gynecology, 9*(1), 1–4.

Scofield, V., Rao, B., & Clisham, R. (June, 1991). Sperm as activating co-factors in AIDS transmission (Abstract W.C. 50). In *VII International Conference on AIDS Abstract Book, 2* (p. 35). Florence, Italy.

Scott, G. B., Fischl, M. A., Klimas, N., Fletcher, M. A., Dickinson, G. M., Levine, R. S., & Parks, W. P. (1985). Mothers of infants with the acquired immunodeficiency syndrome. *Journal of the American Medical Association, 253*(3), 363–366.

Selwyn, P. A., Carter, R. J., Schoenbaum, E. E., Robertson, V. J., Klein, R. S., & Rogers,

M. F. (1989a). Knowledge of HIV antibody status and decisions to continue or terminate pregnancy among intravenous drug users. *Journal of the American Medical Association, 261*(24), 3567–3571.

Selwyn, P. A., Schoenbaum, E. E., Davenny, K., Robertson, V. J., Feingold, A. R., Shulman, J. F., Mayers, M. M., Klein, R. S., Friedland, G. H., & Rogers, M. (1989b). Prospective study of human immunodeficiency virus infection and pregnancy outcomes in intravenous drug users. *Journal of the American Medical Association, 261*(9), 1289–1294.

Shaffer, N., Parekh, B. S., Pau, C. P., Abrams, E., Thomas, P., Krasinski, K., Bamji, M., Kaul, A., Schochetman, G., Rogers, M., George, J. R., & the NYC Perinatal HIV Transmission Collab. Study. (1991). Maternal antibodies to V3 loop peptides of gp 120 are *not* associated with lack of perinatal HIV-1 transmission (Abstract W.C. 48). In *VII International Conference on AIDS Abstract Book, 2* (p. 34). Florence, Italy.

Shannon, M., & Coats, B. (1990). Primary care of asymptomatic HIV positive pregnant women. Unpublished, UCSF/San Francisco General Hospital.

Stein, M. D., Piette, J., Mor, V., Wachtel, T. J., Fleishman, J., Mayer, K. H., & Carpenter, C. J. (1991). Differences in zidovudine (AZT) among symptomatic HIV-infected persons. *Journal of General Internal Medicine, 6*, 35–40.

Sunderland, A. (1990). Influence of human immunodeficiency virus infections on reproductive decisions. *Obstetrics and Gynecology Clinics of North America, 17*(3), 585–594.

Swift, E. L. (1988). Acquired immunodeficiency syndrome and perinatal procedures (Letter). *American Journal of Obstetrics & Gynecology, 154*(2), 785.

Swigar, M. E., Bowers, M. B., & Fleck, S. (1976). Grieving and unplanned pregnancy. *Psychiatry, 39*, 72–80.

Task Force on Pediatric AIDS. (1992). Perinatal human immunodeficiency virus (HIV) testing. *Pediatrics, 89*, 791–794.

Temmerman, M., Hawala, D., Ndinya-Achola, J. O., Plummer, F., & Piot, P. (1991). Maternal HIV infection and low CD4/CD8 ratio as risk factors for prematurity and stillbirth (Abstract M.C. 93). In *VII International Conference on AIDS Abstract Book, 1* (p. 46). Florence, Italy.

Tuomala, R. (1990). Human immunodeficiency virus education and screening of prenatal patients. *Obstetrics and Gynecology Clinics of North America, 17*(3), 571–583.

Ugen, K., Goedert, J. Boyer, J., Refaell, Y., Williams, W., Willoughby, A., et al. (1992, July). Vertical transmission of HIV-infection. VIII International Conference on AIDS, Amsterdam, the Netherlands, (PoA2085) 2:A17.

Ungvarski, P. (1990, November 12). Nursing management of opportunistic infections. Paper presented at the 3rd annual conference, Association of Nurses in AIDS Care, Seattle, Washington.

Uribe, P., Hernandez, M., De Zalduondo, Lamas, M., Hernandez, G. T. Chavez, Peon, F., & Sepulvada, J. (1991). HIV spreading and prevention strategies among female prostitutes (Abstract W.C. 3135). In *VII International Conference on AIDS Abstract Book, 2* (p. 329). Florence, Italy.

Valente, P., & Main, E. K. (1990). Role of the placenta in perinatal transmission of HIV. *Obstetrics and Gynecology Clinics of North America, 17*(3), 545–555.

VanDevanter, N. L., Grisoffi, A. B., Steilan, M., Scarola, M. E., Shipton, R. M., Teindler, C., & Pindyck, J. (1987). Counseling HIV antibody positive blood donors, *American Journal of Nursing, 87*, 1027–1030.

Viscarello, R. R. (1990a). AIDS, natural history and prognosis. *Obstetrics and Gynecology Clinics of North America, 17*(3), 607–616.

Viscarello, R. R. (1990b). Human immunodeficiency virus infection and pregnancy. *Resident & Staff Physician, 36*(7), 35–45.

Vogt, M. W., Witt, D. J., Craven, D. E., Byington, R., Crawford, D. F., Schooley, R. T., & Hirsch, M. S. (1986). Isolation of HTLV-III/LAV from cervical secretions of women at risk for AIDS. *Lancet 1*, 525–527.

Wetli, C. V., Roldan, E. D., & Fojaco, R. M. (1983). Listeriosis as a cause of maternal death: An obstetric complication of acquired immunodeficiency (AIDS). *American Journal of Obstetrics & Gynecology, 147*, 7–9.

Wiley, K., & Grohar, J. (1988). Human immunodeficiency virus and precautions for obstetric, gynecologic, and neonatal nurses. *Journal of Obstetric Gynecologic, and Neonatal Nursing, 17*(3), 165–168.

Williams, A. (1990). Reproductive concerns of women at risk for HIV infection. *Journal of Nurse-Midwifery, 35*(5), 292–298.

Wofsy, C. B., Cohen, J. B., Hauer, L. B., Padian, N. S., Michaelis, L. B., Evans, L. A., & Levy. J. A. (1986). Isolation of AIDS-associated retrovirus from genital secretions of women with antibodies to the virus. *Lancet, 1*, 527–529.

Working Group on HIV Testing of Pregnant Women and Newborns. (1990). HIV infection, pregnant women, and newborns: A policy proposal for information and testing. *Journal of the American Medical Association, 264*(18), 2416–2420.

World Health Organization. (1990). AIDS prevention: Guidelines for MCH/FP programme managers (Vol. 2., AIDS and maternal and child health, pp. 1–82). Geneva: WHO.

Zylke, J. (1991). Another consequence of uncontrolled spread of HIV among adults: Vertical transmission. *Journal of the American Medical Association, 265*, 1798–1799.

Part III

HIV Infection and AIDS in Children and Adolescents

7

Epidemiology of HIV Infection and AIDS in Children

Felissa L. Cohen

At the end of 1981, 189 cases of a newly recognized disorder now known as acquired immunodeficiency syndrome (AIDS) had been reported to the Centers for Disease Control (CDC). None of those cases were among children. In December 1982, the CDC published four case reports of infants under 2 years in New York, New Jersey, and California who had unexplained cellular immuno-deficiency and opportunistic infections. These reports also described features of another 18 young children with unusual cellular immunodeficiencies with and without opportunistic infections. At that time, the editorial note stated, "It is possible that these infants had the acquired immune deficiency syndrome (AIDS)" (Centers for Disease Control, 1982a, p. 667). In retrospect, clinicians have realized that they had been treating children with AIDS in the United States since the late 1970s (Oleske et al., 1983; Rubinstein, 1983; Rubinstein et al., 1983; Scott et al., 1984).

By the end of June 1992, there had been 3,898 cases of AIDS reported in children under 13 years of age. Less than one-third of the cases of pediatric AIDS diagnosed before 1988 were alive in late 1992. AIDS has become the ninth leading cause of death among children in the United States between the ages of 1 and 4 years. In New York State, AIDS was the leading cause of death among Hispanic children and the second leading cause of death among black children aged 1 to 4 years (Centers for Disease Control, 1992).

DEFINITION

The CDC has defined AIDS in children under 13 years of age for surveillance purposes with a revision in 1987 to place more emphasis on HIV testing (see Table 10.1) and has developed a classification system, described in Chapter 10. Two conditions in this definition are applicable only to children—lymphoid interstitial pneumonitis and recurrent serious bacterial infections ("Revision of the CDC," 1987). The World Health Organization (WHO) has adopted a provisional clinical case definition of pediatric AIDS (see Table 7.1). Clinicians generally believe that this latter definition is inadequate, missing children who die of acute illness. Although a WHO working group addressed some of these issues in 1989, adding "persistent or severe lower respiratory tract infection" as a major sign, they recommended the continued use of the original definition (Quinn, Ruff, & Halsey, 1991).

STATISTICS AND PATTERNS IN THE UNITED STATES

By June 30, 1992, 3,898 cases of pediatric AIDS (defined as children under 13 years of age) had been reported to the Centers for Disease Control. Of these, 2,039 (52.3%) had died. Pediatric cases presently account for about 1.7% of all cases of AIDS reported to the CDC. In children under 13 years, about 53% occurred in males and 47% in females. The slight overrepresentation of males mainly results from the category of hemophilia. Distribution of AIDS cases in children according to sex and age is shown in Table 7.2 (Centers for Disease Control, 1992).

In pediatric AIDS, the racial-ethnic distribution differs from that reported for adults. When both male and female adults are considered, the largest percentage of cases occurs in non-Hispanic whites. For all pediatric cases, black children account for about 53%, Hispanic children for about 25%, and white non-Hispanic children for 21%. The racial-ethnic distribution in pediatric AIDS, especially for those under 5 years of age, more closely parallels the distribution seen in adult women with AIDS (largely because of perinatal transmission) than the overall adult distribution. In children under 5 years of age, about 57% are black and in those between 5 and 12 years, about 36% are black (Centers for

TABLE 7.1 Provisional WHO Pediatric Clinical Case Definition of AIDS

Major Signs*	Minor Signs
Weight loss or failure to thrive	Generalized lymphadenopathy
	Oral thrush
Chronic diarrhea >1 month	
Chronic fever >1 month	Repeated common infections (otitis media, pharyngitis, etc.)
	Persistent cough
	Generalized dermatitis
	Confirmed maternal infection

*Persistent or severe lower respiratory infection was a recommended addition of a WHO working group in 1989 (Quinn, Ruff, & Halsey, 1991).

TABLE 7.2 Pediatric AIDS Cases in the United States by Sex and Age Group through June 1992

Age Group	Sex				Total
	Male		Female		
	N	%	N	%	
Under 5 years	1610	51.2	1532	48.8	3142
5–12 years	470	62.2	286	37.8	756
TOTAL:	2080	53.4	1818	46.6	3898

Source: Centers for Disease Control. HIV/AIDS Surveillance, July 1992. pp. 1–18.

Disease Control, 1992). The racial-ethnic distribution of AIDS according to age in children is shown in Table 7.3.

Pediatric cases of AIDS have been reported from 48 states and Puerto Rico. States that in 1992 had not yet reported a case of pediatric AIDS are North Dakota and Wyoming. The largest cumulative total numbers of pediatric cases come from New York, Florida, New Jersey, California, Texas, and Puerto Rico. Metropolitan areas reporting more than 60 cumulative pediatric AIDS cases are New York City; Miami; Newark; San Juan, Puerto Rico; Washington, D.C.; West Palm Beach; Los Angeles; Baltimore; Boston; Chicago; Ft. Lauderdale; Houston; Jersey City; and Philadelphia. These figures suggest that the majority of pediatric AIDS cases are from the large urban areas of the eastern United States. New York City reports the largest number of cases—940 as of June 30, 1992 (Centers for Disease Control, 1992). This number is more than four times the number reported by any other metropolitan area and represents a substantial

TABLE 7.3 Pediatric AIDS Cases in the United States by Age and Race-Ethnic Group through June 1992*

Race-Ethnic Group	Age Group Under 5 years		Age Group 5–12 years		Total*	
	N	%	N	%	N	%
White, non-Hispanic	531	16.9	278	36.8	809	20.8
Black, non-Hispanic	1826	58.2	274	36.3	2100	53.9
Hispanic	760	24.2	191	25.3	951	24.4
Asian, Pacific Islander	7	0.22	12	1.6	19	.5
American Indian, Alaskan Native	11	0.35	0	—	11	.3
Total:	3135	100	755	100	3890	100.0

*Excludes 8 cases whose race/ethincity is unknown.

Source: Centers for Disease Control, HIV/AIDS surveillance, July 1992, pp. 1–18.

health-care challenge for that city. As with racial-ethnic distribution, this distribution more closely parallels the distribution of reported AIDS in adult women than the overall distribution of cases of AIDS, again reflecting perinatal transmission from HIV-infected women of reproductive age.

WORLDWIDE STATISTICS AND PATTERNS

Little definitive information is available about AIDS and HIV infection among children in developing countries. In developed countries, pediatric AIDS constitutes about 2% of all cases of AIDS. In developing countries, however, where heterosexual transmission is the most important mode of acquisition, a greater proportion of women of reproductive age have been infected with HIV. Thus, in many of these developing countries, pediatric AIDS may comprise 15–20% of all AIDS cases (Quinn, Ruff, & Halsey, 1992). Part of the problem in obtaining accurate information about the extent of pediatric AIDS is due to the high infant mortality rate from diarrheal and respiratory infections. Some of the children who die from these causes may also be HIV-infected. In one study, in Burundi, 45% of the children between 2 and 29 months who were hospitalized for severe malnutrition were HIV-1 seropositive. In another study, in Haiti, about one-third of children with diarrhea who had been in a rehydration unit and who later died were HIV-1 seropositive (Quinn et al., 1991).

In early 1992, WHO estimated that there were at least 500,000 cases of pediatric AIDS worldwide. They believe this is an underestimate of the true numbers (World Health Organization, 1992).

Another area of risk for acquiring HIV infection in developing countries is through the practice of reusing needles and syringes for multiple injections, partially a result of cost factors and limited supplies. Infants receiving immunizations from reused needles and syringes may be placed at risk for HIV infection. WHO has recommended the use of a new needle and syringe for each injection. However, injectionists or lay persons who administer vitamins and other medications in some cultures rarely use disposable equipment or apply sterilization techniques (Quinn et al., 1991).

HIV SEROPREVALENCE

Various studies of the seroprevalence in newborns have been completed. These data tend to reflect the HIV infectivity status of the mother rather than the newborn because of the transfer of maternal antibodies to the newborn via the placenta. In New York State, mandatory newborn screening revealed an overall seroprevalence of 0.66%. In New York City, the seroprevalence rate was 1.25%; in upstate New York, 0.16%. These rates were higher in the zip-code areas with higher rates of drug use than in the rest of New York City, and among blacks (1.8%) and Hispanics (1.3%) than whites (0.13%) (Novick et al., 1989). Other studies conducted in New York City revealed HIV seroprevalence rates of 2.5% and 2.4% (Krasinski, Borkowsky, Bebenroth, & Moore, 1988; Landesman, Minkoff, Holman, McCalla, & Sijin, 1987).

A study of neonates admitted to the neonatal intensive-care unit at a Bronx, New York, hospital indicated that the prevalence of HIV infection during the study period was 11.6%. These data indicate that an intensive-care requirement for newborns may be an indication of HIV infection. Many of these infants had problems associated with maternal drug use and sexually transmitted diseases and were premature and small for gestational age (Hand et al., 1992).

A national population-based survey begun in 1988 and including 38 states and the District of Columbia estimated that in one 12-month period 1,800 infants acquired HIV infection in the United States. Assuming that the vertical transmission rate of HIV infection is 30%, then in 1989, approximately 1 in every 2,200 infants born in the United States was HIV-infected. The areas with the highest rate of perinatally acquired AIDS are Washington, D.C., New York, New Jersey, and Florida (Gwinn et al., 1991).

TRANSMISSION

Transmission to children can occur by exposure to HIV-infected secretions and fluids during sexual contact with an infected person, through injection of contaminated blood or blood products (e.g., via contaminated needles or apparatus or through a blood transfusion), or vertically from an infected mother. The latter mechanism accounts for the vast majority of cases of pediatric AIDS and is discussed below. The blood-borne route can include the multiple use of needles and syringes (particularly in developing countries, as discussed above) or through accidental needlesticks (e.g., from a discarded needle). For pediatric AIDS, the exposure categories as defined currently by the CDC do not acknowledge the possibility of AIDS in a child under 13 years of age due to injecting drug use or through sexual activity, either voluntary or forced. Presumably these might account for at least some of the cases in the "undetermined" category. In some countries, street children are particularly vulnerable to both drug use and sexual abuse. WHO estimates that depending upon the definition used, the number of street children in the world ranges from 10 million to 100 million. In Bogota, Colombia, for example, 95% to 100% of the 12,000 street children were involved in drug use daily (World Health Organization, 1992).

Sexual abuse or incest also poses a risk of HIV infection to children. Children are most frequently abused by someone they know, and often sexual abuse does not surface until a sexually transmitted disease (STD) is manifested (Schwarcz & Whittington, 1990). In the United States, at least 200,000 to 400,000 children per year may be subjected to sexual abuse (Krugman, 1991). While these figures may not add up to significant numbers in the transmission of HIV in this country at this time, this mechanism cannot be ignored. Little data are available regarding this method of transmission. The first report of possible infection with HIV, occurring during the sexual abuse of a 10-year-old female, was reported in 1986 (Leiderman & Grimm, 1986). One report noted that out of 15 sexually abused preadolescents seen in New Jersey, 3 (20%) were HIV-infected (Select Committee on Children, Youth and Families, 1988). Gutman and coworkers found that 14 of the 96 children (14.6%) who were HIV positive in their clinic were found on follow-up to have been sexually abused. In 10, the abuse was either a proven or potential source of HIV infection. Three of the abusers knew they were HIV positive at the time they sexually assaulted the child (Gutman et al., 1991). In another report, 18 children infected with HIV described no risk factors other than sexual abuse (Gellert & Durfee, 1989).

In countries where child prostitution is not uncommon, pediatric HIV infection may be acquired through sexual contact. Many of these children are homeless and are unaware of how to protect themselves from infection, even if they were capable of doing so ("AIDS and children," 1989). Further, recent news reports indicate that males seeking sexual gratification through prostitution are increasingly requesting children in an effort to protect themselves from HIV.

EXPOSURE CATEGORIES

As is true in adult and adolescent cases of AIDS, exposure categories for pediatric (below 13 years of age) cases of AIDS are arranged in a hierarchical, mutually exclusive manner. Thus cases with multiple characteristics that could be classified in more than one category are assigned to the group listed first. For pediatric AIDS, the major exposure categories in hierarchical order are:

1. hemophilia/coagulation disorders
2. mother with/at risk for HIV infection
3. receipt of blood transfusion, blood components, or tissue
4. undetermined

The distribution of pediatric cases of AIDS according to these exposure categories is shown in Table 7.4. The overwhelming majority of cases fall into the category of mother with/at risk for HIV infection. This percentage has steadily increased over the years for two reasons: (1) an increase in the number of women of childbearing age who have HIV infection; (2) a decrease in cases of AIDS acquired from blood transfusions. The latter change affects the categories of hemophilia/coagulation disorders and receipt of blood transfusions. However, while the relative number of cases of AIDS will continue to decrease in the blood transfusion category, most of the children with hemophilia who have already been infected with HIV have not yet progressed to full-blown AIDS (Pizzo, 1990). Whether they will ultimately be counted in the pediatric, adolescent, or adult categories depends upon the time it takes for their progression from HIV infection to full-blown AIDS. Each exposure category will be discussed below.

Hemophilia/Coagulation Disorder

In July 1982, the CDC first published reports of three cases of *Pneumocystis carinii* pneumonia (PCP) in three persons with hemophilia who had no identifiable risk factors for HIV infection other than receiving pooled factor VIII concentrates (Centers for Disease Control, 1982b). While the mechanism of infection for children with hemophilia appears to be through transfusion of contaminated blood products, hemophiliacs are allotted a separate exposure category by the CDC. In both children and adults, this category hierarchically precedes the category of receipt of blood transfusion. As of June 30, 1992, less than 5% of pediatric AIDS cases and less than 1% of adult AIDS cases fell in this category (Centers for Disease Control, 1992). In both groups, males are primarily affected because for both hemophilia A and hemophilia B, the mechanism for inheritance of the defective gene is X-linked recessive. Since males have only one X chromosome, only one copy of the gene for these types of hemophilia is necessary to produce manifestations necessitating management by administration of clotting-factor concentrates. Other coagulation disorders inherited by other mechanisms show a more equal sex distribution (Cohen, 1984).

Various prevalence studies have been conducted in persons with hemophilia, although little is reported specifically for children. In some study reports, up to 92% of persons with hemophilia A are seropositive for HIV, with estimates at about 50% for hemophilia B (Centers for Disease Control, 1987). Recombinant factor VIII is now being used for persons with hemophilia A, thus virtually eliminating HIV risk from the treatment. Desmopressin has been found to increase factor VIII in mild cases of hemophilia A and in persons with von Willebrand's disease (Eyster, 1991).

TABLE 7.4 Pediatric Cases of AIDS by Exposure Category as Reported to CDC through June 1992

Exposure category	N	%
Hemophilia/Coagulation disorders	179	4.6
Mother with/at risk for HIV infection	3315	85.0
Receipt of blood transfusion, blood components or tissue	300	7.7
Undetermined	104	2.7
Total:	3898	100.0

Source: Centers for Disease Control, HIV/AIDS Surveillance, July 1992, pp. 1–18.

Mother with/at Risk for AIDS or HIV Infection

Vertical Transmission. Perinatally acquired AIDS that is vertically transmitted from mother to child accounts for the majority of pediatric AIDS cases—approximately 85%. Several subgroups encompassed within this main exposure category are shown in Table 7.5. Injecting drug use plays an important role. Nearly 60% of all of the pediatric AIDS cases and nearly 70% of the cases in the subcategory result from the mother being an injecting drug user (IDU) or engaging in sexual activities with a known HIV-infected IDU (Centers for Disease Control, 1992).

Not all the infants born to mothers who are HIV-infected are infected with HIV. It has been difficult to determine immediately which infants are infected at or shortly after delivery because of the presence of maternal antibodies of the IgG class that are transplacentally acquired by the infant. The time it takes for the loss of these maternal antibodies can range from 45 to 421 days, with a mean of about 7 months; thus, actual diagnosis of HIV infection in infants below 12–15 months is currently difficult. Techniques such as the polymerase chain reaction (PCR), HIV culture, or viral antigen detection of infant-specific antigens of class IgM or IgA have been improving detection accuracy at an earlier age but have not yet been accepted as definitive (Arpadi & Caspe, 1991; Task Force on Pediatric AIDS, 1992). PCR is a technique for amplifying specific nucleic acid sequences by use of repeated cycles of DNA synthesis, thus allowing detection of a minute quantity of HIV-DNA, and has been used for the detection of other organisms as well. It holds promise for the reliable and rapid detection of HIV in infants (Peter, 1991; Petru et al., 1992). Recently, two

TABLE 7.5 Subcategories of the Pediatric Exposure Category "Mother with/at Risk for AIDS/HIV Infection" through June 1992

Subcategory	N	% of Subcategory	% of Total
Injecting drug use	1,561	47.1	40.1
Sex with injecting drug user	673	20.3	17.3
Sex with bisexual male	72	2.2	1.9
Sex with person with hemophilia	17	0.5	0.4
Born in Pattern-II country	264	8.0	6.8
Sex with person born in Pattern-II country	17	0.5	0.4
Sex with transfusion recipient with HIV infection	17	0.5	0.4
Sex with HIV-infected person, risk not specified	172	5.2	4.4
Receipt of blood transfusion, blood components, or tissue	70	2.1	1.8
Has HIV infection, risk not specified	452	13.6	11.6
Total of subcategory cases:	3,315		
Total of all pediatric AIDS cases:	3,898		

Source: Centers for Disease Control, HIV/AIDS Surveillance, July 1992, pp. 1–18.

research groups have described the use of the HIV-IgA immunoblot assay in early diagnosis with promising results. The sensitivity of this test was improved after the third month of life (Landesman et al., 1991; Quinn et al., 1991).

Currently, maternal-fetal transmission rates are reported to range from 10% to 52%, with an average rate of about 20–30% (Centers for Disease Control, 1991). The European Collaborative Study group in a study of 721 children born to HIV-infected predominantly white mothers detected a 14.4% vertical transmission rate (European Collaborative Study, 1992). Why some infants are HIV-infected while others remain uninfected is an extremely important question. Influences on the efficiency of vertical transmission may include the viral burden, characteristics of HIV, maternal time of acquisition of infection, antibody status, placental factors, genetic factors, or others, but are currently not understood. Those women with CD4+ counts less than 700 mm^3 or p24-antigenemia appeared to have an increased transmission risk (European Collaborative Study, 1992). A recent report suggests that some viral variants are more readily transmissible than others, an implication that is important for prevention approaches (Wolinsky et al., 1992).

While vertical transmission of HIV from an infected mother to her fetus or child is a recognized mode of transmission, the exact timing of HIV transmission is currently unknown. HIV has been isolated from fetal tissue as early as the eighth week of gestation and has been detected in vaginal and cervical secretions, amniotic fluid, placental tissue, colostrum, and breast milk (Lewis, Reynolds-Kohler, Fox, & Nelson, 1990; Mundy, Schinazi, Gerber, Nahmias, & Randall, 1987; Pizzo & Butler, 1991). Theoretically, then, the transmission of HIV could occur prenatally, at or around the time of delivery, and/or postnatally. In humans, no examples of viral infection of the fertilized egg through infected sperm or ova have been identified, although animal models for such transmission do exist (Andiman & Modlin, 1991). The eventual determination of the time (or times) of HIV transmission from the mother to her fetus/infant and factors determining subsequent infection might allow for the development of therapeutic interventions in that process. NIH has planned a clinical trial to administer anti-HIV-1 antibodies to pregnant women in hopes of blocking vertical transmission (Hooper, 1991). Another trial that is underway will examine the effect of zidovudine in vertical transmission prevention when given during pregnancy. An additional approach is to use prophylaxis against *Pneumocystis carinii* pneumonia (PCP) during pregnancy, although this is controversial (Heagarty & Abrams, 1992). Results of a retrospective collection of reports about HIV-infected women who received zidovudine in pregnancy revealed that it appeared well tolerated; however, it was not clear whether anemia and growth retardation seen in some infants could have been a direct or indirect result of such therapy (Sperling, Stratton et al., 1992).

A collaborative study of twins born to HIV-infected mothers looked at transmission. The risk of transmission was highest in firstborn vaginally delivered twins (50%), followed by firstborn caesarean delivery (38%) and secondborn delivery by either route (19%). The overall transmission rate was 32%. The authors speculate that passage through the birth canal may lead to some vertical HIV transmissions and that in vaginal deliveries, the firstborn twin may have greater exposure to potentially infectious secretions and blood than the second-born twin. The researchers suggest controlled clinical trials of caesarean delivery before membrane rupture as one way of reducing transmission (Goedert, Duliege, Amos, Felton, & Biggar, 1991). However, the effect of anesthesia and surgery on the maternal immune system must also be considered in weighing alternative actions (Fuith, Czarnecki, Wachter & Fuchs, 1992).

Another situation about which little information is available is the pregnancy outcome for a HIV seronegative female and a male partner who is HIV-positive. A study was done involving 11 couples in which the males were HIV-positive hemophiliacs and their long-term female partners were HIV-negative. Ten of the 11 women remained HIV-negative throughout pregnancy and delivered healthy uninfected infants. One woman remained seronegative but had a spontaneous abortion (Kraus, Brettler, Forsberg, & Sullivan, 1991).

Is There an HIV Malformation Syndrome?   Maternal infections of several types during pregnancy are known to often result in effects on the fetus that can include malformations, growth retardation, mental retardation, and other features. Rubella and cytomegalovirus infections are only two examples of viral infections that cause fetal damage when acquired congenitally. According to some researchers, the transplacental acquisition of HIV infection by the fetus in utero results in characteristic features (Iosub, Bamji, Stone, Gromisch, & Wasserman, 1987; Marion, Wiznia, Hutcheon, & Rubinstein, 1986; Marion, Wiznia, Hutcheon, & Rubinstein, 1987; Perro, 1987). Still other researchers and clinicians debate the existence of such a syndrome (Embree et al., 1989; Qazi, Sheikh, Fikrig, & Minkoff, 1988).

In 1986, Marion and colleagues described 20 infants and children who were HIV-infected and described as having similar characteristics. At that time, they called this syndrome the human T-cell lymphotropic virus type III (HTLV-III) embryopathy and have since used the terminology *fetal AIDS syndrome* to describe their findings (Marion et al., 1986; Marion et al., 1987). Others have used the terminology *HIV embryopathy syndrome* (Embree et al., 1989).

The growth and craniofacial abnormalities said to constitute this syndrome are listed in Table 7.6 in descending order of frequency. The identification of the fetal AIDS syndrome was initially based on subjective findings. Since that time, a more objective scoring system based on nearly 40 children with HIV infection has been devised (Marion et al., 1987).

Complicating issues are involved in ascertaining whether a congenital malformation syndrome resulting from in utero exposure to HIV exists. Many of the children studied in this regard have mothers who have used many drugs

TABLE 7.6 Features of the Proposed Fetal AIDS Syndrome

Growth failure (height and weight less than 3rd percentile for chronologic age)
Microcephaly (below 3rd percentile for chronologic age)
Prominent boxlike forehead
Short nose with flattened columella
Flat nasal bridge
Prominent triangular philtrum
Long palpebral fissures with obliquity of eyes
Blue sclerae of the eyes
Patulous lips
Hypertelorism (inner and outer canthal distances >95% for head circumference and age)

Sources: Iosub, Bamji, Stone, Gromisch, & Wasserman, 1987; Marion, Wiznia, Hutcheon, & Rubinstein, 1986, 1987.

during pregnancy, including alcohol, in whom nutrition was not optimal. Many of the features of the putative fetal AIDS syndrome are similar to those seen in the well-described fetal alcohol syndrome. Thus, it is very difficult to sort out the effects of a single agent in this complex intrauterine environment.

In 1989, researchers examined this problem in Kenya among a population of HIV-infected women in which none of the mothers was known to be an intravenous drug user and alcohol use was infrequent. The only consistent features found in their offspring were growth failure and microcephaly. However, in this study, infants were not differentiated as to those who were HIV-positive and those who were not, and infants were followed for periods ranging from two weeks to two and one-half years (Embree et al., 1989). These ages are younger than those of infants followed in other studies who were confirmed as HIV-infected. It is known that in other congenitally acquired infections such as syphilis, rubella, and cytomegalovirus infections, manifestations may not appear until later in childhood (Cohen, 1984). Whether the growth failure and microcephaly are acquired in utero or postnatally due to HIV effects on nutrition is not clear.

In summary, while there may be an HIV embryopathy syndrome, the evidence at this time is generally considered inconclusive. A reasonably consistent finding has been lower birth weights for infants born to HIV-positive mothers in many countries (Quinn et al., 1991).

Intrapartum Transmission.   Another possible time for the transmission of HIV from an infected mother to her infant is around the time of delivery. The infant is greatly exposed to maternal blood and fluids, and when separation of the placenta occurs at the time of delivery, maternal-infant transfusion takes place. A model for this type of viral transmission has already been observed in the case of the hepatitis-B virus and other viruses (Andiman & Modlin, 1991). Infection acquired in the intrapartum period is virtually impossible to detect in the newborn. At present, there is no evidence that altering the mode of delivery influences vertical transmission. However, strategies are being examined to affect this mode of transmission if it occurs. These include the administration of antiviral agents such as zidovudine in the intrapartum and postpartum periods and the use of hyperimmune anti-HIV immune globulin in the perinatal period (Andiman & Modlin, 1991).

Postnatal Transmission. The most obvious but not the only possible route of postnatal transmission of HIV from an infected mother to her infant is through breastfeeding. While colostrum and early milk contain higher concentrations of mononuclear cells such as macrophages, mature milk has also been shown to be capable of transmitting HIV. Many of the reports of postnatal mother to infant transmission through breastfeeding have been anecdotal. However, some of the strongest data came from case reports of women who became infected with HIV through postpartum blood transfusions, who then breastfed, and whose infants were subsequently found to be HIV-infected (Lepage et al., 1987; Stiehm & Vink, 1991; Weinbreck et al., 1988; Ziegler, Cooper, & Johnson, 1985).

By what mechanism does HIV cause infection in the infant through breast-feeding? The virus in the breast milk may penetrate the mucosa of the newborn or become attached to intestinal cells. The newborn does not have the protective gastric acid, thicker mucosa, and immunoglobulin A system that will later develop. Viral penetration may also occur through minute trauma in the oral cavity, pharynx, or gastrointestinal mucosa, allowing direct access to the blood-stream (Stiehm & Vink, 1991).

A recent prospective study of women and infants in Kigali, Rwanda, has demonstrated that HIV transmission occurred from mothers to their infants presumably by means of breastfeeding, even when mothers seroconverted at any time during lactation. Infants in this study acquired HIV as late as 15 and 18 months (Van de Perre et al., 1991). Others have challenged the validity of these findings (Espanol, Caragol, & Bertran, 1992; Jelliffe & Jelliffe, 1992). The European Collaborative Study (1992) found a twofold increase in the risk of infection among breastfed children of HIV-positive mothers, although the numbers in the study were small. Strong confirmation of the risk for HIV transmission to infants during breastfeeding was presented at the VIII International Conference on AIDS held in Amsterdam, the Netherlands, particularly if mothers become infected after giving birth, if HIV is detectable in the breastmilk and if they have depressed CD4+ cells ("HIV mother can . . .", 1992).

Breast-feeding has been advocated by the World Health Organization because of concern about infant morbidity and mortality, but the CDC has recommended that HIV-infected women avoid breastfeeding (CDC, 1985; WHO, 1987). At present, WHO still supports breastfeeding in countries where bottle-feeding with formula is associated with unacceptably high morbidity and mortality, often due to diarrhea and pulmonary infections from unsafe water ("Breastfeeding benefits usually outweigh," 1992). However, there is general consensus that when safe alternatives to breastfeeding exist, both seronegative mothers at high risk for HIV infection and mothers who are HIV-infected should be counseled against breast-feeding their infants (Pizzo & Butler, 1991; Van de Perre et al., 1991). Both positive and negative aspects of breast-feeding must be weighed according to a variety of factors. Some risk-benefit models have been developed (Lederman, 1992). The human adult T-cell leukemia virus (HTLV-I) is also known to be transmitted via breast-milk (Andiman & Modlin, 1991).

It is possible that postnatal transmission could occur through another route. It has been suggested that the very thin skin and mucous membranes of the neonate may pose a risk for viral entry (Cocchi & Cocchi, 1988).

Receipt of Blood Transfusion, Blood Components, or Tissue

The first recognized case of AIDS associated with a blood transfusion occurred in an infant and was reported by the CDC in December 1982. This white male infant had received exchange transfusions and other blood products for treatment of erythroblastosis fetalis in the spring of 1981. He died of *Pneumocystis carinii* pneumonia at 20 months. One of the blood donors for his multiple transfusions was found to have died of AIDS in August 1982 ("Possible Transfusion-associated," 1982). The percentage of cumulative transfusion-associated cases of pediatric AIDS in the United States was about 8.5%, as opposed to about 2.2% of adult AIDS cases in 1991 (Centers for Disease Control, 1992). If the proportion of AIDS cases that were transfusion-related are examined in the first 100,000 cases of AIDS compared with the second 100,000 cases in this country, there has been a decline from 11% to 5.6% among children ("The second 100,000 cases," 1992). The majority (about 70%) of transfusion-associated cases of pediatric AIDS were transfused in the first year of life (Jones, Byers, Bush, Oxtoby, & Rogers, 1992).

In the United States, although only about 2% of all transfusions are given to children, about 7% of all cases of transfusion-related AIDS has occurred in children. Reasons may include the following: (1) children, especially infants, have less mature immune systems, and thus may be more susceptible to infection; (2) children, especially infants, may receive a greater dose of virus relative to their body size; (3) children may be diagnosed more accurately and correctly; (4) children or infants may have a shorter incubation period; (5) infants or children may be more likely to receive transfusions from multiple donors (Centers for Disease Control, 1992; Cohen, 1991; Nicholas et al., 1989). One donor may provide blood for multiple pediatric units. One anecdote reveals that a unit of blood from a donor who subsequently was found to have AIDS was split into 16 pediatric units and given to 16 premature infants, all of whom ultimately died from AIDS (Nicholas et al., 1989).

Children acquiring HIV infection from a transfusion may have received that transfusion for an acute episode (such as trauma or surgery) or for treatment associated with a preexisting chronic disorder such as hemophilia or another coagulation disorder. However, for epidemiological reporting, CDC considers children who received transfusions for hemophilia or another coagulation disorder in a separate category.

Some of the chronic illnesses that often require transfusions include sickle cell disease, thalassemia, various congenital anemias, and leukemia. Less information is available about the prevalence of HIV infection among these other groups of children than is available for those who have hemophilia. In one study, of 1,800 chronically transfused patients with Cooley's anemia (thalassemia), 11% were HIV seropositive (Nicholas et al., 1989). Similar prevalences have been found in Europe. Among persons with congenital anemia, 15 of 197 multi-transfused individuals were HIV seropositive. In a retrospective study conducted in New York, 18 of 211 persons with leukemia who were treated from 1978 through 1984 were HIV seropositive (Eyster, 1991). In persons with sickle cell disease, HIV seroprevalence has been increasingly found (Girot & Lefrere, 1990).

For children acquiring HIV through transfusion, the time of acquisition is usually defined. For pediatric AIDS cases that are transfusion-associated, the median age at transfusion is less than 2 months. The median age at AIDS diagnosis is about 4 years, as opposed to a 1-year median diagnosis age for children with perinatally acquired AIDS (Jones et al., 1992). Most children receiving HIV-infected blood become seropositive (Cohen et al., 1991).

In developing countries in both Latin America and in Africa, the screening of donated blood is incomplete. In Africa, it is not uncommon for children to receive multiple transfusions, especially for acute malaria (Quinn et al., 1991, 1992). Thus, practitioners in the United States must be alert to children who may have received blood transfusions elsewhere (Feldman, Church, Mascola, & Sato, 1991).

It is estimated that as many as 300,000 neonates in the United States may receive transfusions annually, most frequently from multiple donors. The most frequent reason is birth weights under 1,500 grams. The potential risk for the transmission of HIV, other diseases (e.g., cytomegalovirus, hepatitis), and of noninfectious conditions (e.g., graft-vs.-host disease, iron overload) via transfusion is small for each exposure but increases for multiple transfusions. A recent review of neonatal transfusion practices concludes that there is little scientific basis underlying the present indications for transfusion of blood in neonates and offers guidelines for transfusion (Strauss, 1991).

With screening of blood for HIV antibody in place, the number of transfusion-associated cases of AIDS in children will decrease each year. Most of these will be newly diagnosed cases in which actual transmission will have occurred prior to March 1985 when widespread screening of the blood supply began; new cases due to transfusion of blood products will be extremely rare (Jones et al., 1992).

Undetermined

As in adults, this category includes those (1) who are lost to follow-up, (2) for whom no determination was made, (3) who are still under investigation, or (4) who have died before a determination was made about placement into the appropriate exposure category. For pediatric cases of AIDS the undetermined category represented a little over 2%, compared with nearly 4% in adult cases (Centers for Disease Control, 1992). As mentioned earlier, children, particularly older children, might have been exposed to HIV infection through sexual contact or through injecting drug use and therefore were not classified into the existing pediatric AIDS exposure categories. One must consider whether the existing exposure categories for children are limiting in planning appropriate educational and preventative activities, as they may restrict thinking in regard to the acquisition of HIV in children from sexual contact or from intravenous drug use. It is not pleasant to consider these exposure categories in children but may represent reality.

SUMMARY

The number of cases of pediatric AIDS and HIV infection continues to increase in the United States and the world. The major route of acquisition of HIV infection is vertical transmission from an infected mother to her child. In the United States, children of mothers with or at risk of AIDS comprise about 85% of pediatric AIDS cases. In the majority, injecting drug use has played some role in the mother's acquisition of HIV infection. A disproportionate percentage of black and Hispanic children comprise the pediatric AIDS population, and the greatest geographic concentration is in the northeastern United States and Florida. Children are affected by AIDS not only by direct HIV infection but also by the effects on their parents, siblings, and other relatives. The health and social implications of AIDS in children are an enormous and important challenge.

REFERENCES

AIDS and children: A family disease (pp. 1–20). (1989). London: The Panos Institute.

Andiman, W. A., & Modlin, J. F. (1991). Vertical transmission. In P. A. Pizzo & C. M. Wilfert (Eds.), *Pediatric AIDS* (pp. 140–155). Baltimore: Williams & Wilkins.

Arpadi, S., & Caspe, W. B. (1991). HIV testing. *Journal of Pediatrics, 119*, S8–S13.

Breast-feeding benefits usually outweigh HIV risk. (1992). *Global AIDS News, 2*, 4, 18.

Centers for Disease Control. (1982a). Unexplained immunodeficiency and opportunistic infections in infants—New York, New Jersey, California. *Morbidity and Mortality Weekly Report, 31*, 665–667.

Centers for Disease Control. (1982b.). *Pneumocystis carinii* pneumonia among persons with hemophilia. *Morbidity and Mortality Weekly Report, 31*, 365–367.

Centers for Disease Control. (1985). Recommendations for assisting in the prevention of perinatal transmission of human T-lymphocyte type III/lymphadenopathy-associated virus and acquired immunodeficiency syndrome. *Morbidity and Mortality Weekly Report, 34*, 721–732.

Centers for Disease Control. (1987). HIV infection and pregnancies in sexual partners of HIV-seropositive hemophilic men—United States. *Morbidity and Mortality Weekly Report, 36*, 593–595.

Centers for Disease Control. (1992). *HIV/AIDS Surveillance Report.* (1992, July), 1–18.

Chin, J. (1990). Current and future dimensions of the HIV/AIDS pandemic in women and children. *Lancet, 336*, 221–224.

Cocchi, P., & Cocchi, C. (1988). Postnatal transmission of HIV infection. *Lancet, 1*, 482.

Cohen, S. E., Mundy, T., Karassik, B., Lieb, L., Ludwig, D. D., & Ward, J. (1991). Neuropsychological functioning in human immunodeficiency virus type 1 seropositive children infected through neonatal blood transfusion. *Pediatrics, 88*, 58–68.

Cohen, F. L. (1984). *Clinical genetics in nursing practice.* Philadelphia: J. B. Lippincott.

Cohen, F. L. (1991). Etiology and epidemiology of HIV infection. In J. D. Durham & F. L. Cohen, *The Person with AIDS: Nursing perspectives* (pp. 1–59). New York: Springer.

Embree, J. E., Braddick, M., Datta, P., Muriithi, J., Hoff, C., Kreiss, J. K., Roberts, P. L., Law, B. J., Pamba, H. O., Ndinja-Achola, J. O., & Plummer, F. A. (1989). Lack of correlation of maternal human immunodeficiency virus infection with neonatal malformations. *Pediatric Infectious Disease Journal, 8*, 700–704.

Espanol, T., Caragol, I., & Bertran, J. M. (1992). Postnatal transmission of HIV infection. *New England Journal of Medicine, 326*, 642.

European Collaborative Study. (1992). Risk factors for mother-to-child transmission of HIV-1 infection. *Lancet, 339*, 1007–1012.

Eyster, M. E. (1991). Transfusion and coagulation factor-acquired human immunodeficiency virus infection. *Pediatric Infectious Diseases Journal, 10*, 50–56.

Ferdman, R. M., Church, J. A., Mascola, L., & Sato, J. K. (1991). Human immunodeficiency virus infections in children who received transfusions in Mexico. *Western Journal of Medicine, 155*, 547.

Fuith, L. C., Czarnecki, M., Wachter, H., & Fuchs, D. (1992). Mode of delivery in HIV-1 infected women. *Lancet, 339*, 1603.

Gellert, G. A., & Durfee, M. J. (1989). HIV infection and child abuse. *New England Journal of Medicine, 321*, 685.

Girot, R., & Lefrere, J. J. (1990). HIV infection and AIDS in thalassemia and sickle cell disease. *Haematologica, 75*(5), 128–131.

Goedert, J. J., Duliege, A-M, Amos, C. I., Felton, S., Biggar, R. J., & the International Registry of HIV-exposed Twins. (1991). High risk of HIV-1 infection for first-born twins. *Lancet, 338*, 1471–1475.

Gutman, L. T., St. Claire, K. K., Weedy, C., Herman-Giddens, M. E., Lane, B. A., Niemeyer, J. G., & McKinney, R. E., Jr. (1991). Human immunodeficiency virus transmission by child sexual abuse. *American Journal of Diseases of Children, 145*, 137–141.

Gwinn, M., Pappaioanou, M., George, J. R., Hannon, W. H., Wasser, S. C., Redus, M. A., Hoff, R., Grady, G. F., Willoughby, A., Novello, A. C., Petersen, L. R., Dondero, T. J. Jr., & Curran, J. W. (1991). Prevalence of HIV infection in childbearing women in the United States. *Journal of the American Medical Association, 265*, 1704–1708.

Hand, I. L., Wiznia, A., Checola, R. T., Kim, M. H., Noble, L. M., Daley, T. J., & Yoon, J. J. (1992). Human immunodeficiency virus seropositivity in critically ill neonates in the South Bronx. *Pediatric Infectious Disease Journal, 11*, 39–42.

Heagarty, M. C., & Abrams, E. J. (1992). Caring for HIV-infected women and children. *New England Journal of Medicine, 326*, 887–888.

HIV infected mother can infect baby through breast milk (1992, July 27). *Chicago Sun Times*, p. 11.

Hooper, C. (1991). NIH planning perinatal trial of HIV-1 antibodies. *The Journal of NIH Research, 3*, 35–36.

Iosub, S., Bamji, M., Stone, R. K., Gromisch, D. S., & Wasserman, E. (1987). More on human immunodeficiency virus embryopathy. *Pediatrics, 80*, 512–516.

Jelliffe, D. B., & Jelliffe, E. F. P. (1992). Postnatal transmission of HIV infection. *New England Journal of Medicine, 326*, 642–643.

Jones, D. S., Byers, R. H., Bush, T. J., Oxtoby, M. J., & Rogers, M. F. (1992). Epidemiology of transfusion-associated acquired immunodeficiency syndrome in children in the United States, 1981 through 1989. *Pediatrics, 89*, 123–127.

Katz, S. L., & Wilfert, C. M. (1989). Human immunodeficiency virus infection of newborns. *New England Journal of Medicine, 320*, 1687–1689.

Krasinski, K., Borkowsky, W., Bebenroth, D., & Moore, T. (1988). Failure of voluntary testing for human immunodeficiency virus to identify infected parturient women in a high-risk population. *New England Journal of Medicine, 318*, 185.

Kraus, E. M., Brettler, D. B., Forsberg, A. D., & Sullivan, J. L. (1991). Pregnancy in a cohort of long-term partners of human immunodeficiency virus-seropositive hemophiliacs. *Obstetrics and Gynecology, 78*, 735–738.

Krugman, R. D. (1991). Sexually transmitted diseases in childhood sexual abuse. *Pediatrics, 88*, 880.

Landesman, S., Minkoff, H., Holman, S., McCalla S., & Sijin, O. (1987). Serosurvey of human immunodeficiency virus infection in parturients: Implications for human immunodeficiency virus testing programs in pregnant women. *Journal of the American Medical Association, 258*, 2701–2703.

Landesman, S., Weiblen, B., Mendez, H., Willoughby, A., Goedert, J. J., Rubinstein, A., Minkoff, H., Moroso, G., & Hoff, R. (1991). Clinical utility of HIV-IgA immunoblot assay in the early diagnosis of perinatal HIV infection. *Journal of the American Medical Association, 266*, 3443–3446.

Lederman, S. A. (1992). Estimating infant mortality from human immunodeficiency virus and other causes in breast-feeding and bottle-feeding populations. *Pediatrics, 89*, 290–296.

Leiderman, M., & Grimm, K. T. (1986). A child with HIV infection. *Journal of the American Medical Association, 256*, 3094.

Lepage, P., Van de Perre, P., Carael, M., Nsengumuremyi, F., Nkurunziza, J., Butzler, J-P, & Sprecher, S. (1987). Postnatal transmission of HIV from mother to child. *Lancet, 2*, 400.

Lewis, S. H., Reynolds-Kohler, C., Fox, H. E., & Nelson, J. A. (1990). HIV-1 in trophoblastic and villous Hofbauer cells, and haematological precursors in eight-week fetuses. *Lancet, 335*, 565–568.

Marion, R. W., Wiznia, A. A., Hutcheon, R. G., & Rubinstein, A. (1986). Human T-cell lymphotropic virus type III (HTLV-III) embryopathy. *American Journal of Diseases of Children, 140*, 638–640.

Marion, R. W., Wiznia, A. A., Hutcheon, R. G., & Rubinstein, A. (1987). Fetal AIDS syndrome score. *American Journal of Diseases of Children, 141*, 429–431.

Mundy, D. C., Schinazi, D. C., Gerber, A. R., Nahmias, A. J., & Randall, H. W., Jr. (1987). Human immunodeficiency virus isolated from amniotic fluid. *Lancet, 2,* 459–460.

Nicholas, S. W., Sondheimer, D. L., Willoughby, A. D., Yaffe, S. J., & Katz, S. L. (1989). Human immunodeficiency virus infection in childhood, adolescence, and pregnancy: A status report and national research agenda. *Pediatrics, 83,* 293–308.

Novick, L. F., Berns, D., Strickof, R., Stevens, R., Pass, K., & Wethers, J. (1989). HIV seroprevalence in newborns in New York State. *Journal of the American Medical Association, 261,* 1745–1750.

Oleske, J., Minnefor, A., Cooper, R., Jr., Thomas, K., dela Cruz, A., Ahdieh, H. Guerrero, I., Joshi, V. V., & Desposito, F. (1983). Immune deficiency syndrome in children. *Journal of the American Medical Association, 249,* 2345–2349.

Perro, M. (1987). Dimorphism leading to a diagnosis of acquired immunodeficiency syndrome. American *Journal of Diseases of Children, 141,* 474.

Peter, J. B. (1991). The polymerase chain reaction: Amplifying our options. *Journal of Infectious Diseases, 13,* 166–171.

Petru, A., Dunphy, M. G., Azimi, P., Janner, D., Gallo, D., Hanson, C., Sohmer, P., & Stanley, M. (1992). Reliability of polymerase chain reaction in the detection of human immunodeficiency virus infection in children. *Pediatric Infectious Disease Journal, 11,* 30–33.

Pizzo, P. A. (1990). Pediatric AIDS: Problems within problems. *Journal of Infectious Diseases, 161,* 316–325.

Pizzo, P. A., & Butler, K. M. (1991). In the vertical transmission of HIV, timing may be everything. *New England Journal of Medicine, 325,* 593–598.

Possible transfusion-associated acquired immune deficiency syndrome (AIDS)—California. (1982). *Morbidity and Mortality Weekly Report, 31,* 652–655.

Qazi, Q. H., Sheikh, T. M., Fikrig, S., & Minkoff, H. (1988). Lack of evidence for craniofacial dysmorphism in perinatal human immunodeficiency virus infection. *Journal of Pediatrics, 112,* 7–12.

Quinn, T. C., Kline, R. L., Halsey, N., Hutton, N., Ruff, A., Butz, A., Boulos, R., & Modlin, J. F. (1991). Early diagnosis of perinatal HIV infection by detection of viral-specific IgA antibodies. *Journal of the American Medical Association, 266,* 3439–3442.

Quinn, T. C., Ruff, A., & Halsey, N. (1991). Special considerations for developing nations. In P. A. Pizzo & C. M. Wilfert (Eds.), *Pediatric AIDS* (pp. 714–744). Baltimore: Williams & Wilkins.

Quinn, T. C., Ruff, A., & Halsey, N. (1992). Pediatric acquired immunodeficiency syndrome: special considerations for developing nations. *Pediatric Infectious Disease Journal, 11,* 558–568.

Revision of the CDC surveillance case definition for acquired immunodeficiency syndrome. (1987). *Morbidity and Mortality Weekly Report, 36*(1S), 1S–15S.

Rubinstein, A. (1983). Acquired immunodeficiency syndrome in infants. *American Journal of Diseases of Children, 137,* 825–827.

Rubinstein A., Sicklick, M., Gupta, A., Bernstein, L., Klein, N., Rubinstein, E., Spigland, I., Fruchter, L., Litman, N., Lee, H., & Hollander, M. (1983). Acquired immuno-deficiency with reversed T_4/T_8 ratios in infants born to promiscuous and drug-addicted mothers. *Journal of the American Medical Association, 249,* 2350–2356.

Schwarcz, S. K., & Whittington, W. L. (1990). Sexual assault and sexually transmitted diseases: Detection and management in adults and children. *Reviews of Infectious Diseases, 12* (Suppl. 6), S682–S690.

Scott, G. B., Buck, B. E., Leterman, J. G., Bloom, F. L., & Parks, W. P. (1984). Acquired immunodeficiency syndrome in infants. *New England Journal of Medicine, 310,* 76–81.

Task Force on Pediatric AIDS. (1992). Perinatal human immunodeficiency virus (HIV) testing. *Pediatrics, 89*, 791–794.

The second 100,000 cases of acquired immunodeficiency syndrome—United States. (1992). *Morbidity and Mortality Weekly Report, 41*, 28–29.

Select Committee on Children, Youth and Families. (1988). *Continuing Jeopardy: Children and AIDS* (pp. 1–12). Washington, D.C.: GPO.

Sperling, R. S., Stratton, P., & members of the Obstetric-Gynecologic Working Group of the AIDS Clinical Trials Group of the National Institute of Allergy and Infectious Diseases. (1992). Treatment options for human immunodeficiency virus-infected pregnant women. *Obstetrics and Gynecology, 79*, 443–448.

Stiehm, E. R., & Vink, P. (1991). Transmission of human immunodeficiency virus infection by breast-feeding. *Journal of Pediatrics, 118*, 410–412.

Strauss, R. G. (1991). Transfusion therapy in neonates. *American Journal of Diseases in Children, 145*, 904–911.

Stricof, R. L., Kennedy, J. T., Nattell, T. C., Weisfuse, I. S., & Novick, L. F. (1991). HIV seroprevalence in a facility for runaway and homeless adolescents. *American Journal of Public Health, 81*, 50–53.

Van de Perre, P., Simonon, A., Msellati, P., Hitimana, D-G, Vaira, D., Bazubagira, A., Van Goethem, C., Stevens, A-M, Karita, E., Sondag-Thull, D., Dabis, F., & Lepage, P. (1991). Postnatal transmission of human immunodeficiency virus type 1 from mother to infant. *New England Journal of Medicine, 325*, 593–598.

Weinbreck, P., Loustaud, V., Denis, F., Vidal, B., Mounier, M., & de Lumley, L. (1988). Postnatal transmission of HIV infection. *Lancet, 1*, 482.

Wolinsky, S. M., Wike, C. M., Korber, B. T. M., Hutto, C., Parks, W. P., Rosenblum, L. L., Kunstman, K. J., Furtado, M. R., & Munoz, J. L. (1992). Selective transmission of human immunodeficiency virus type-1 variants from mothers to infants. *Science, 255*, 1134–1137.

World Health Organization. (1986). Acquired immunodeficiency syndrome (AIDS). *Weekly Epidemiological Record, 61*, 69–73.

World Health Organization. (1987). Breast-feeding/breastmilk and human immunodeficiency virus (HIV). *Weekly Epidemiologic Record, 62*, 245.

World Health Organization. (1992). Street children and drug abuse. *WHO Press*, February 12, 1992, pp. 1–2.

Ziegler, J. B., Cooper, D. A., Johnson, R. O. (1985). Postnatal transmission of AIDS-associated retrovirus from mother to infant. *Lancet, 1*, 896–898.

8

Epidemiology of HIV Infection and AIDS in Adolescents

Felissa L. Cohen

Adolescents are defined epidemiologically by the Centers for Disease Control (CDC) as persons 13 to 19 years of age. Adolescent cases of AIDS are reported by the CDC as part of the adult statistics rather than the pediatric statistics. Because of the variable and potentially lengthy incubation period, the occurrence of reported AIDS cases in the adolescent age range reflects both those who have acquired HIV infection before 13 years of age and those who have acquired it during the adolescent period. When examining the larger numbers of persons with AIDS in the age range of 20 to 29 years, it becomes apparent on the basis of what is known about the incubation period of HIV that many of them became infected with HIV during adolescence. To date, the rate of reported AIDS cases in adolescents is doubling every 14 months (Futterman & Hein, 1991). AIDS cases in adolescent females are increasing more rapidly than they are in adolescent males (Hirsch & Hincks, 1990).

Of particular concern to those who care for adolescents is the propensity of adolescents to take risks. Such risk behaviors may include those that make them vulnerable to acquiring HIV infection, such as experimentation with sex and injecting drugs. The use of substances such as marijuana and alcohol, while not directly HIV risk-related, can impair judgement and ability and therefore indirectly increase behavior more directly associated with HIV acquisition. Those adolescents who are runaways or are homeless are particularly vulnerable to HIV infection through risky behaviors.

STATISTICS AND PATTERNS IN THE UNITED STATES

By June 30, 1992, 872 AIDS cases in adolescents had been reported to the CDC. Of these, about 57% had died. Adolescent cases presently account for about 0.4% of the AIDS cases reported to CDC (Centers for Disease Control, 1991b, 1992).

In adolescents, about 72% of AIDS cases occurred in males and 28% in females. Distribution of AIDS cases in adolescents according to sex for one-year age intervals is shown in Table 8.1. Overall, less than 25% of adolescent AIDS cases are reported in persons 16 years of age or younger. The majority are reported in those between 17 and 19 years of age. With each increasing year of age, the percentage of the total adolescent AIDS cases increases.

Overall, about 45% of the adolescent AIDS cases are reported in whites, about 36% in blacks, and about 17.5% in Hispanics. For females, however, more than 75% of the adolescent AIDS cases occur in nonwhites, more than half being reported in black adolescent females and about 16% in Hispanic females. AIDS cases reported in minority teenagers exceeds their proportion in the adolescent population since the United States' population of adolescents between 13 and 19 years is composed of 14% black and 8% Hispanic persons (Millstein, 1990; Tucker & Cho, 1991). There is also a racial-ethnic variation in exposure categories. For black adolescents, the largest exposure categories are "men who have sex with men" and "heterosexual contact." For Hispanic adolescents, the largest exposure categories are "injecting drug use" and "men who have sex with men." For white adolescents, the largest exposure categories are "hemophilia-coagulation disorder" and "men who have sex with men" (Gayle & D'Angelo, 1991).

As of December 1991, adolescent cases of AIDS had been reported from 43 states, Washington D.C., and Puerto Rico. The largest cumulative total numbers of adolescent AIDS cases come from New York, Florida, California, Texas, New Jersey, Puerto Rico, Illinois, and Pennsylvania. Metropolitan areas reporting the highest cumulative totals are New York City; Los Angeles; San Juan, Puerto Rico; Chicago; Newark; Philadelphia; and Houston. As is the case for pediatric AIDS, New York City reports the largest number of cases, representing about 10% of the total (Centers for Disease Control, 1991, 1992).

TABLE 8.1 Percentage of AIDS Cases by Sex in Adolescents, as Reported to CDC

Age (Years)	Males	Females	Total
13	3.4	0.6	4.0
14	4.5	0.8	5.3
15	4.9	1.4	6.3
16	6.8	1.1	7.9
17	11.0	4.3	15.3
18	13.5	6.0	19.5
19	31.0	10.7	41.7

Source: Centers for Disease Control, Unpublished Data, October 30, 1991.

HIV SEROPREVALENCE

Various studies of HIV seroprevalence that include adolescents have been done; however, no general-population survey data similar to those collected in some locations such as New York State with general newborn screening are available.

In a study of blood samples drawn from adolescents presenting at a Washington, D.C., emergency room, it was reported that in 1987 the HIV seroprevalence rate was 4 per 1,000 samples; in 1991, it was reported as 13 per 1,000 samples—an alarming increase (Peck, 1991).

Mandatory HIV testing of adolescents is found in Job Corps and military applicants, and offers the major large-population surveys of adolescents. In the Job Corps, a federal training program for disadvantaged out-of-school youth, researchers found that the HIV seroprevalence rate was 3.6 per 1,000 overall. Seroprevalence increased with each year of age for those 16 to 21 years of age. Overall, seroprevalence was slightly higher in males than females, but the rate among those 16 and 17 years of age was higher for females. HIV seroprevalence rates increased with the size of the metropolitan statistical area and was highest in the Northeast, followed by the South. The seroprevalence rate per 1,000 was 5.3 for black, 2.6 for Hispanic, and 1.2 for white applicants (St. Louis et al., 1991).

A blinded HIV seroprevalence study was conducted at Children's National Medical Center in Washington, D.C., among adolescents 13 to 19 years of age who were having blood drawn for other routine indications. Overall, the seroprevalence in this group was 0.37%. Females had a prevalence of 0.47%, and adolescents 18 and 19 years had a prevalence of 0.56% (D'Angelo, Getson, Luban, & Gayle, 1991).

Among military adolescent applicants, the HIV seroprevalence was less than that found for Job Corps applicants; the overall HIV seropositivity was 0.34 per 1,000. Marked geographic differences were found, with the highest state prevalences found in Delaware and Maryland and in urban counties of Maryland, Texas, New York, and Washington, D.C., with the lowest prevalences in the north-central states. By race and ethnicity, prevalences were 1.06, 0.31, and 0.18 per 1,000 applicants for black, Hispanic, and white teenagers, respectively (Burke et al., 1990).

HIV seroprevalence studies have been conducted in runaway adolescents. In studies in New York City and San Francisco, 5.3% and 8.2%, respectively, were HIV seropositive (Shalwitz, Goulart, Dunnigan, & Flannery, 1990; Stricof, Kennedy, Nattell, Weisfuse, & Novick, 1991). In the New York study, HIV seroprevalence rates were higher for males than females and increased with age. Hispanics had the highest seroprevalence (6.8%), followed by whites (6.0%) and blacks (4.6%) (Stricof et al., 1991).

TRANSMISSION

Adolescents acquire HIV in the same ways as adults—through the exchange of HIV-contaminated body fluids and/or blood or blood products, primarily through risky sexual activities, injecting drug use, and transfusions. However, if the age at AIDS diagnosis is examined, younger adolescents tend to reflect pediatric patterns of HIV acquisition, whereas patterns in older adolescents more closely follow those in adults. Therefore, aspects of transmission discussed in Chapters 1, 3, and 7 are relevant to adolescents and will not be repeated here.

Risk-taking Behaviors

It is well known that adolescence is a time of risk taking. Also during this time there is a change in thinking from concrete to abstract and from perceptions of invulnerability to reality. Some of this risk taking is reflected in the top three causes of death among adolescents in the United States—suicide, homicide, and accidents (Futterman & Hein, 1991). This risk taking frequently extends to experimentation with sex and drugs (including alcohol), often increasing the teenager's risk for HIV infection. The vast majority of adolescents are apparently aware of the type of high-risk behaviors that lead to HIV transmission, but this knowledge does not necessarily translate into behavioral changes (Tucker & Cho, 1991; see Chapter 9).

Sexual Transmission

In the United States today, more adolescents have initiated sexual intercourse at younger ages than ever before. The CDC reports that despite AIDS prevention campaigns, in 1988 a larger percentage of teenagers were initiating sexual intercourse at younger ages than in 1982 ("Progress toward Achieving," 1990). In a 1989 study of sexual behavior of high school students at 42 sites in the United States, it was revealed that depending on the site, between 27% and 76% (median 56%) of participants had begun sexual intercourse by 18 years of age ("HIV-related Knowledge," 1990). By age 20, 80% of males and 70% of females will have initiated sexual intercourse. The majority do not use condoms during their first sexual intercourse, and many have multiple partners (Futterman & Hein, 1991; Millstein, 1990). In the previously mentioned study, between 7% and 40% of students (median 21%) reported having four or more sexual partners ("HIV-related Knowledge," 1990). White students were more likely than black or female Hispanic students to have used condoms during last sexual intercourse (41.7%, 36.7%, and 28.1%, respectively). In the same study, condom use was higher for male students in all the ethnic groups (Centers for Disease Control, 1992). Among 10th-grade boys in a survey done in Washington, D.C.,

66% reported that they had had four or more sexual partners to date (Peck, 1991). Males initiate this activity earlier than females, and black adolescents begin sexual activity earlier than white adolescents (DiClemente et al., 1992; "HIV-related Knowledge," 1990; Millstein, 1990). Both gay male adolescents and female adolescents may engage in sexual relations with an older partner, thus increasing their risk of exposure to HIV because of higher HIV prevalence rates in older age groups. As discussed in Chapter 7, adolescents may also be subjected to sexual abuse or incest, placing them at risk for acquiring HIV infection.

The type of sexual activity engaged in by adolescents may also pose HIV-related risks. About 2.5 million cases of sexually transmitted diseases (STDs) are reported among adolescents each year, representing about 25% of all reported STDs. Nationally, 15- to 19-year-olds have the highest rates of gonorrhea, syphilis, chlamydia, and hospitalization for pelvic inflammatory disease (Kipke, Futterman, & Hein, 1990). Most adolescents do not use condoms. At least 1 million pregnancies occur among adolescents each year in the United States (Tucker & Cho, 1991). Worldwide, it is believed that 1 in 20 teenagers contracts a STD each year (Hirsch & Hincks, 1990). The type of sexual practices among teenagers may also place them at risk. In one study of urban Hispanic and black teenagers, about 25% acknowledged anal intercourse. For vaginal intercourse, 23% said they used condoms always or often, and about 11% did so for anal intercourse. The age at first intercourse was 11 to 18 (mean 14.8 years), and 22.5% reported that they were sexually active by 13 years of age (Jaffe, Seehaus, Wagner, & Leadbeater, 1988). In another study of middle-class teenagers attending a clinic, 2% of females and 8% of males stated that they used condoms consistently when engaging in sexual intercourse (Kegeles, Adler, & Irwin, 1988).

Most adolescents engage in sexual intercourse, and most have more than one partner in their lifetime. Yet if asked, they may consider themselves monogamous, even if that state only lasts for a few weeks (Hein, 1991). This practice of serial monogamy is not the same as having only one sexual partner but may be so considered by the adolescent. Many teenagers will protect themselves against pregnancy, but fewer protect themselves against STDs, including HIV. Further, teenagers who have acquired HIV are unlikely to be aware of their infection, as they are often asymptomatic. Therefore, they are unaware that they are putting a sexual partner at risk. Even if they are aware of an HIV-positive status, it may be nearly impossible for them to find a way to tell their partner that they are HIV-infected. Condom use is one of the most important means for adolescents to reduce HIV transmission by sexual contact (Hein, 1991).

Factors influencing transmission rates among adolescents are largely unexplored. It has been suggested that the state of physical development of the female reproductive tract during adolescence may play a role in facilitating HIV transmission. Such physical factors might include early anovulatory cycles, early lack of progesterone, more permeable cervical mucous, and histological characteristics of tissue in early puberty (Futterman & Hein, 1991).

Runaways, the Homeless, and Sexual Transmission

In the United States, about 1 million teenagers are runaways and about 250,000 adolescents are homeless. Many of these engage in what has been called "survival sex," or the exchange of sex for money, food, drugs, companionship, or shelter. Of the approximately 900,000 adolescents engaged in prostitution, about two-thirds are female and one-third are male. Nearly four-fifths of adolescent female prostitutes are believed to be runaways. Their sexual relationships tend to be with high-risk partners and are usually unprotected by condom use (Futterman & Hein, 1991; Hirsch & Hinck, 1990). Among male homeless or street youths, many may be gay or bisexual and may have left home because of their sexual orientation (Kruks, 1991).

Among runaway adolescents in two shelters in New York City, the majority had been sexually active with a median of two sexual partners in the last three months, usually without condom use. Those 15 years of age and younger were less likely to be sexually active than older adolescents (Rotheram-Borus, Koopman, Haignere, & Davies, 1991). Among street youth in Brazil, the Dominican Republic, and Mexico, HIV seropositivity may range from 2% to 10%. In Thailand, one study reports that 6% of known HIV-seropositive persons are female prostitutes between 15 and 20 years (Hirsch & Hincks, 1990).

Transmission in the Athletic Setting

An area that has attracted relatively less attention regarding HIV transmission is sports competition. There are two concerns: (1) possible exposure to HIV contaminated blood and body fluids during contact sports; (2) the practice of needle and/or syringe sharing when illicitly injecting drugs, including anabolic steroids to increase body mass (Nemechek, 1991). The Committee on Sports Medicine and Fitness of the American Academy of Pediatrics (1991) has issued recommendations regarding HIV in the athletic setting. They emphasize that there only is one report of possible HIV transmission during an athletic event—an undocumented one from Italy involving a soccer collision. However, it remains theoretically possible that HIV transmission could occur during sports in which bleeding and skin abrasions (such as in wrestling and football) often occur. The recommendations of the American Academy of Pediatrics for the athletic setting are given in Table 8.2.

TABLE 8.2 Human Immunodeficiency Virus (Acquired Immunodeficiency Syndrome [AIDS] Virus) in the Athletic Setting

The American Academy of Pediatrics recommends that

1. Athletes infected with HIV should be allowed to participate in all competitive sports. This advice must be reconsidered if transmission of HIV is found to occur in the sports setting.
2. A physician counseling a known HIV-infected athlete in a sport involving blood exposure, such as wrestling or football, should inform him of the theoretical risk of contagion to others and strongly encourage him to consider another sport.
3. The physician should respect a HIV-infected athlete's right to confidentiality. This includes not disclosing the patient's status of infection to the participants or the staff of athletic programs.
4. All athletes should be made aware that the athletic program is operating under the policies in recommendations 1 and 3.
5. Routine testing of athletes for HIV infection is not indicated.
6. The following precautions should be adopted:
   a. Skin exposed to blood or other body fluids visibly contaminated with blood should be cleaned as promptly as is practical, preferably with soap and warm water. Skin antiseptics (e.g., alcohol) or moist towelettes may be used if soap and water are not available.
   b. Even though good hand washing is an adequate precaution, water-impervious gloves (latex, vinyl, etc.) should be available for staff to use if desired when handling blood or other body fluids visibly contaminated with blood. Gloves should be worn by individuals with nonintact skin. Hands should be washed after glove removal.
   c. If blood or other body fluids visibly contaminated with blood are present on a surface, the object should be cleaned with fresh household bleach solution made for immediate use as follows: 1 part bleach in 100 parts of water, or 1 tablespoon bleach to 1 quart water (hereafter called "fresh bleach solution"). For example, athletic equipment (e.g., wrestling mats) visibly contaminated with blood should be wiped clean with fresh bleach solution and allowed to dry before reusing.
   d. Emergency care should not be delayed because gloves or other protective equipment are not available.
   e. If the caregiver wishes to wear gloves and none are readily available, a bulky towel may be used to cover the wound until an off-the-field location is reached where gloves can be used during more definitive treatment.
   f. Each coach and athletic trainer should receive training in first aid and emergency care and be provided with the necessary supplies to treat open wounds.
   g. For those sports with direct body contact and other sports where bleeding may be expected to occur:
      i. If a skin lesion is observed, it should be cleansed immediately with a suitable antiseptic and covered securely.
      ii. If a bleeding wound occurs, the individual's participation should be interrupted until the bleeding has been stopped and the wound is both cleansed with antiseptic and covered securely or occluded.
   h. Saliva does not transmit HIV. However, because of potential fear on the part of those providing cardiopulmonary resuscitation, breathing (Ambu) bags and oral airways for use during cardiopulmonary resuscitation should be available in athletic settings for those who prefer not to give mouth-to-mouth resuscitation.

(continued)

Table 8.2 (*continued*)

i. Coaches and athletic trainers should receive training in prevention of HIV transmission in the athletic setting; they should then help implement the recommendations suggested above.

Used with permission of the American Academy of Pediatrics: Committee on Sports Medicine and Fitness, (1991), Human immunodeficiency virus (acquired immunodeficiency syndrome [AIDS] virus) in the athletic setting, *Pediatrics, 88*, 640–641.

EXPOSURE CATEGORIES

For adolescent cases of AIDS, exposure categories are arranged in a hierarchical mutually exclusive manner and are the same as for adults, as discussed in Chapter 1. The distribution of adolescent cases of AIDS according to these exposure categories is shown in Table 8.3. The distribution varies from that seen in adults, as shown in Figure 8.1. There are also differences between younger and older adolescents. A comparison of younger (13–15 years) and older (16–19 years) adolescents by exposure category is shown in Table 8.4. Each exposure category is discussed below.

Men Who Have Sex with Men

While this category encompasses the majority of all reported adult cases of AIDS in the United States, this is not true among adolescents. About 25% (all males) are classified into this category, and if those from the combined category of "men who have sex with men" and "injecting drug user" are considered, about 29% of all adolescent cases have a component of male-to-male sexual trans-

TABLE 8.3 U.S. Adolescent AIDS Cases by Exposure Category and Sex, as Reported to the CDC (in percent)

Exposure categories	Male Cases % of Total	Female Cases % of Total	Total
Men who have sex with men	26.2	—	26.2
Injecting drug use	5.6	4.6	10.2
Men who have sex with men and inject drugs	4.3	—	4.3
Hemophilia/coagulation disorder	30.0	0.5	30.5
Heterosexual contact	2.0	12.0	14.0
Recipient of transfusion of blood, blood components, or tissue	3.7	3.8	7.5
Other/undetermined	3.2	3.3	6.5

Source: Centers for Disease Control, Unpublished Data, October 30, 1991.

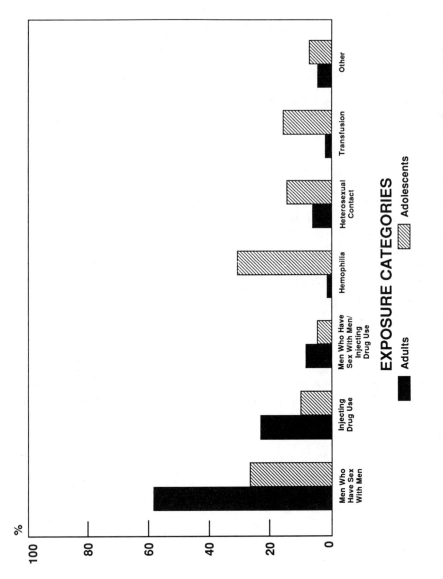

FIGURE 8.1 Comparison of adults and adolescents on exposure categories for AIDS.

TABLE 8.4 Comparison of Distribution of Younger and Older Adolescents by Exposure Category (in percent)

Exposure Category	Adolescent Age Group	
	13–15 years	16–19 years
Men who have sex with men	6.1	29.9
Injecting drug use	3.1	12.6
Men who have sex with men and use injecting drugs	0	5.1
Hemophilia/coagulation disorder	65.3	24.1
Heterosexual contact	5.1	15.4
Transfusion recipient	17.3	5.7
Other/undetermined	3.1	7.2
Totals:	100.0	100.0

Source: Centers for Disease Control, Unpublished data, October 30, 1991.

mission (Centers for Disease Control, 1992). One study indicates that between 17% and 35% of adolescent males have had same-sex experiences resulting in orgasm and that their partners are usually older (Futterman & Hein, 1991). The fact that male adolescents often have older partners may put them at even greater risk for HIV acquisition because the older their partner, the more likely he is HIV-positive. Because the youth may not wish to be thought of as unsophisticated, he may engage in even greater risky behaviors and may not practice behaviors such as safe sex or condom use.

Because of peer pressure and other factors, gay male adolescents may engage in both homosexual and heterosexual behavior, the latter to hide a gay identity (Futterman & Hein, 1991). This puts the heterosexual partner at unknown risk. Coping with these stresses may lead to dysfunction and even attempted suicide, and may also keep those who need help from the appropriate education and services (Kruks, 1991; Remafedi, 1987). More older than younger adolescents have been classified into this category (see Table 8.4).

Injecting Drug Users

The category of injecting drug use (IDU) encompasses drugs used for self-injection that were not prescribed by a physician or licensed medical practitioner. These may include drugs injected intravenously or subcutaneously or "skin-popped." The drug used may vary from heroin to cocaine to amphetamines to anabolic steroids. In the 42-site study previously described, 1–5% of high school students reported injecting cocaine, heroin, or other illegal drugs ("HIV-related Knowledge," 1990). In a 1987 study, the proportion of students reporting having injected illegal drugs ranged from 2.8% to 6.3% ("HIV-related beliefs," 1987). IDU alone accounts for nearly 13% of AIDS cases in adolescents, and

when combined with the category "men who have sex with men and use injecting drugs," another 4.2% is added to the IDU effects (see Table 8.3). Among
cases of AIDS in female adolescents, about 22% of female adolescents are classified into this exposure category. As discussed in Chapter 3, IDU for women
also has implications for indirect HIV risk through sexual transmission. This
category is more important for older than younger adolescents.

Men Who Have Sex with Men and Inject Drugs

This category combines the two preceding ones. About 4% of all cases of AIDS
in adolescents are classified to this exposure category (Centers for Disease
Control, 1992).

Hemophilia/Coagulation Disorder

The majority of overall adolescent AIDS cases are classified into this exposure
category, accounting for about 30% of all cases. Primarily males are affected,
as explained in the previous chapter. Among adolescent females, very few cases
have been assigned to this exposure category, making it a minor one for adolescent females, as shown in Table 8.3 (Centers for Disease Control, 1992). Teenagers with hemophilia who are HIV-infected may still engage in the risky sexual
behaviors that are commonly seen in adolescents. In one study, only 1 of 9 male
teenagers with hemophilia who were engaged in sexual intercourse consistently
used condoms (Overby, Lo, & Litt, 1989). This category is more important in
younger adolescents (see Table 8.4).

Heterosexual Contact

As shown in Table 8.3, overall, this exposure category encompasses about 14%
of adolescent AIDS cases. However, for female adolescents, this category is the
most important one. Nearly 50% of AIDS cases in female adolescents can be
classified into this exposure category. Only 2.5% of the male adolescent cases
are so classified (Centers for Disease Control, 1992). Male IDUs have been
identified as the sexual partners in about 60% of all female heterosexually
acquired cases (Gayle & D'Angelo, 1991). More older than younger adolescents
are classified into this category (see Table 8.4). Aspects of sexual transmission
among teenagers have been extensively discussed above.

Receipt of Blood Transfusion, Blood Components, or Tissue

The percentage of cumulative transfusion-associated cases of adolescent AIDS
in the United States was about 6.3%, compared to about 8% of the pediatric
and about 2% of adult AIDS cases in 1992 (Centers for Disease Control, 1992).

The percentages of the adolescent cases classified as transfusion-associated are nearly equally distributed between male and female adolescents, as shown in Table 8.3.

Other/Undetermined

For adolescents, similar numbers of males and females are classified into this category, accounting for about 7% of all cases of adolescent AIDS (see Table 8.3; Centers for Disease Control, 1992). Components of this category are discussed in Chapter 1.

CONCLUSION

AIDS cases reported in adolescents 13 to 19 years currently account for less than 0.5% of all AIDS cases reported in the United States. However, many of the cases reported among those 20 to 29 years (accounting for about 20% of all cases) were probably acquired during adolescence. Epidemiologically, the most important exposure category for all adolescents is "hemophilia-coagulation disorder." For female adolescents, the most important category is heterosexual contact. Characteristics of adolescents include getting into high-risk situations and/or engaging in risk-taking behaviors. These behaviors may be reflected in experimentation with sex and drugs (including alcohol) in ways that place the adolescent at risk for the acquisition of HIV infection. For some adolescents schools can be an effective source of prevention efforts, but for those not in school other efforts are needed.

REFERENCES

Burke, D. S., Brundage, J. F., Goldenbaum, M., Gardner, L. I., Peterson, M., Visintine, R., Redfield, R. R., & the Walter Reed Retrovirus Research Group. (1990). Human immunodeficiency virus infections in teenagers. *Journal of the American Medical Association, 263*, 2074–2077.

Centers for Disease Control. (1991, October 31). Unpublished data.

Centers for Disease Control. (1992). *HIV/AIDS Surveillance*, July 1992, 1–18.

Centers for Disease Control. (1992). Sexual behavior among high school students—United States, 1990. *Morbidity and Mortality Weekly Report, 40*, 885–888.

Committee on Sports Medicine and Fitness. (1991). Human immunodeficiency virus [acquired immunodeficiency syndrome (AIDS) virus] in the athletic setting. *Pediatrics, 88*, 640–641.

D'Angelo, L. J., Getson, P. R., Luban, N. L. C., & Gayle, H. D. (1991). Human immunodeficiency virus infection in urban adolescents: Can we predict who is at risk? *Pediatrics, 88*, 982–986.

DiClemente, R. J., Durbin, M., Siegel, D., Krasnovsky, F., Lazarus, N., & Comacho, T. (1992). Determinants of condom use among junior high school students in a minority, inner-city school district. *Pediatrics, 89,* 197–202.

Futterman, D., & Hein, K. (1991). Medical Management of Adolescents. In P. A. Pizzo & C. M. Wilfert (Eds.), *Pediatric AIDS* (pp. 546–550). Baltimore: Williams & Wilkins.

Gayle H. D., & D'Angelo, L. J. (1991). The epidemiology of AIDS and HIV infection in adolescents. In P. A. Pizzo & C. M. Wilfert (Eds.), *Pediatric AIDS* (pp. 38–50). Baltimore: Williams & Wilkins.

Hein, K. (1991). Risky business: Adolescents and human immunodeficiency virus. *Pediatrics, 88,* 1052–1054.

Hirsch, J., & Hincks, J. (1990, December). Young women and AIDS: A worldwide perspective. Washington, DC: Center for Population Options (unpaginated).

HIV-related beliefs, knowledge, and behaviors among high school students. (1987). *Morbidity and Mortality Weekly Report, 37,* 717–721.

HIV-related knowledge and behaviors among high school students—selected U. S. sites. (1990). *Morbidity and Mortality Weekly Report, 39,* 385–397.

Jaffe, L. R., Seehaus, M., Wagner, C., & Leadbeater, B. J. (1988). Anal intercourse and knowledge of acquired immunodeficiency syndrome among minority-group female adolescents. *Journal of Pediatrics, 112,* 1005–1007.

Kegeles, S. M., Adler, N. E., & Irwin, C. E. (1988). Sexually active adolescents and condoms: Changes over one year in knowledge, attitudes and use. *American Journal of Public Health, 78,* 460–461.

Kipke, M. D., Futterman, D., & Hein, K. (1990). HIV infection and AIDS during adolescence. *Medical Clinics of North America, 74*(5), 1149–1167.

Kruks, G. (1991). Gay and lesbian homeless/street youth: Special issues and concerns. *Journal of Adolescent Health, 12,* 515–518.

Millstein, S. G. (1990). Risk factors for AIDS among adolescents. *New Directions for Child Development. 50,* Winter, 3–15.

Nemechek, P. M. (1991). Anabolic steroid users—another potential risk group for HIV infection. *New England Journal of Medicine, 325,* 357.

Overby, K, J., Lo, B., & Litt, I. F. (1989). Knowledge and concerns about acquired immune-deficiency syndrome and their relationship to behavior among adolescents with hemophilia. *Pediatrics, 83,* 204–210.

Peck, P. (1991, October 2). AIDS rate soars for urban teens. *Chicago Sun-Times,* pp. 1, 24.

Progress toward achieving the 1990 objectives for the nation for sexually transmitted diseases. (1990). *Morbidity and Mortality Weekly Report, 39,* 53–57.

Remafedi, G. (1987). Adolescent homosexuality. Psychosocial and medical implications. *Pediatrics, 79,* 331–337.

Rotheram-Borus, M. J., Koopman C., Haignere, C., & Davies, M. (1991). Reducing HIV sexual risk behaviors among runaway adolescents. *Journal of the American Medical Association, 266,* 1237–1241.

St. Louis, M. E., Conway, G. A., Hayman, C. R., Miller, C., Petersen, L. R., & Dondero, T. J. (1991). Human immunodeficiency virus infection in disadvantaged adolescents. *Journal of the American Medical Association, 266,* 2387–2391.

Shalwitz, J., Goulart, M., Dunnigan, K., & Flannery, D. (1990, June). Prevalence of sexually transmitted diseases (STD) and HIV in a homeless youth medical clinic in San Francisco (Abstract S. C.571). In *Final Program and Abstracts of the Sixth International Conference on AIDS* (vol 3, p. 231), San Francisco.

Stricof, R. L., Kennedy, J. T., Nattell, T. C., Weisfuse, I. S., & Novick, L. F. (1991). HIV seroprevalence in a facility for runaway and homeless adolescents. *American Journal of Public Health, 81*(Suppl.), 50–53.

Tucker, V. L., & Cho, C. T. (1991). AIDS and adolescents. *Postgraduate Medicine, 89*(3), 49–53.

9

Prevention of HIV Infection in Adolescents

Margaret Beaman

The epidemiology of HIV infection and AIDS in adolescents has been discussed in Chapter 8. This chapter outlines adolescent AIDS risk behavior and its correlates, reviews various theoretical approaches, discusses successful interventions, and suggests methods of evaluation.

ADOLESCENT RISK BEHAVIORS AND CORRELATES

Although many teens report a change in their behaviors since they heard of the AIDS epidemic, adolescents as a group still practice high-risk sexual behavior (Bruce, Shrum, Trefethen, & Slovik, 1990; Centers for Disease Control, 1990; DiClemente, Forrest, Mickler, & Principal Site Investigators, 1990; Fisher & Misovich, 1990; McNally & Mosher, 1991). Since 1987, select schools across the country have conducted annual sexual behavior surveys of students aged 13 to 18 years (Centers for Disease Control, 1990). In 1989, the rates of sexual intercourse among these students ranged from 56% in Iowa to 76% in Washington, D.C. More males had sexual intercourse (55–90%) than females (43–64%), and a greater percentage of males had four or more sexual partners (21–67%) compared to females (10–20%). Of the adolescents surveyed, few reported very high-risk behavior; 5–10% reported anal intercourse, and 2–5% reported injecting drugs. More females reported injecting drugs than males (Beaman & Strader, 1989; Catania et al., 1989; Centers for Disease Control, 1990).

More studies of adolescent sexual behavior have been conducted in relation to pregnancy and childbearing. Many factors are associated with both the initiation of intercourse and the use of condoms by adolescents (Hayes, 1987). Sexual activity by adolescents increases with age and regardless of gender, intercourse is generally initiated with someone older. Physical maturity affects age at first intercourse for boys more than girls. Since girls reach puberty between 10 and 14 years (mean = 12.5), and boys reach puberty between 12 and 16 years (mean = 14), girls are more vulnerable to first intercourse almost two years before boys (Murray & Zenter, 1989). Age might merely be an overt measure of the adolescent's level of cognitive development, which is rarely measured (Sachs, 1985). Cognitive development, however, was the most significant predictor of sexual behavior in Sachs's sample of black adolescent girls.

Racial differences in adolescent sexual behavior have been found. Regardless of age, sexual activity is highest among blacks (Hayes, 1987). Pregnancy rates of black teens outrank those of Hispanics and whites (Kalmuss, 1986). More white teens than black or Hispanic teens practiced birth control; however, condom use among blacks outranks use among white or Hispanics in some studies (Rickert, Jay, Gottlieb, & Bridges, 1989; Sonenstein, Pleck, & Ku, 1989).

Older teens tend to use contraception at first intercourse; 50% use a condom (Hayes, 1987). Younger teens are not prepared for contraception at first intercourse and continue to practice contraception inconsistently. In AIDS-related studies, less than 50% of all teen respondents reported using condoms (Baldwin & Baldwin, 1988; Bruce et al., 1990; Catania et al., 1989; Katzman, Mulholland, & Sutherland, 1988; Rickert et al., 1989; Thurman & Franklin, 1990). Moreover, condom use is poor among teens at highest risk for AIDS: those with a number of serial partners (DiClemente, Durbin, Siegel, Krasnovsky, Lazarus, & Comacho, 1992; Kegeles, Adler, & Irwin, 1988; Sonenstein et al., 1989), those who have sex with a prostitute, and those with personal or partners' use of injecting drugs (Sonenstein et al., 1989). In one study of female adolescents, those who engaged in other risky behaviors such as substance use were less likely to use condoms (Orr et al., 1992). The sex partner has a strong influence on the sexual behavior of adolescents. The more ardent the relationship, the more likely and frequently an adolescent will have intercourse. The sex partner also influences condom use and intentions to use condoms (Fishbein & Middlestadt, 1989; Kegeles et al., 1988; Jemmott & Jemmott, 1990, 1991; Strader & Beaman, 1989). Those who communicate with their partner are more apt to use condoms (Beaman & Strader, 1989; Bruce et al., 1990; Strader & Beaman, 1989; Weisman et al., 1989); however, this communication must deal with specific activity of the couple, not merely general risk.

Adolescent sexual risk is also highly associated with the use of alcohol, marijuana, and cocaine (Fisher & Misovich, 1990; Fullilove & Fullilove, 1989; Hingson, Strunin, Berlin, & Heerin, 1990; Nemoto, Brown, Foster, & Chu, 1990). Social behaviors associated with alcohol, drugs and sexual activity are weapon use, fighting, truancy, and tobacco use (Kulbok, Earls, & Montgomery, 1988).

Other sociopsychological variables affect age at first intercourse and contraception (Hayes, 1987). Personal and family religiosity influence young teens to postpone first intercourse; peer acceptance of intercourse encourages inception of intercourse. High school dropouts and the economically deprived are more sexually active. Adolescents with higher grades and career goals and those in two-parent families wait longer to have sexual intercourse and are more likely to practice contraception. However, neither economic status nor religiosity affect contraception (Hayes, 1987).

Studies of adolescents in the child welfare or juvenile system indicate they are at increased risk of AIDS because of their lack of knowledge about sexuality, early initiation of intercourse, poor use of contraception, and history of sexual abuse (DiClemente, Lanier, Horan, & Lodico, 1991; Melchert & Burnett, 1990; Polit, Morton & White, 1989; Vermund, Alexander-Rodriquez, Macleod, & Kelley, 1990).

Although most adolescents are knowledgeable about AIDS, they overestimate the risk through casual contact and underestimate their personal sexual risk of AIDS (Baldwin & Baldwin, 1988; Bruce et al., 1988; DiClemente, Boyer, & Morales, 1988; DiClemente et al., 1990; DiClemente, Zorn, & Temoshok, 1986; Helgerson, Petersen, & AIDS Education Study Group, 1988; Katzman et al., 1988; Kegeles et al., 1988; McNally & Mosher, 1991; Nagy, Hunt, & Adcock, 1990; Thurman & Franklin, 1990; Walter, Vaughan, & Cohall, 1991). Increased knowledge about AIDS and risk behavior is not accompanied by increased HIV prevention behavior (Baldwin & Baldwin, 1988; Beaman & Strader, 1989; Ehrhardt, 1988; Fisher & Mosovich, 1990; Katzman, Mulholland, & Sutherland, 1988; Sonenstein et al., 1989; Thurman & Franklin, 1990). This apparent contradiction might be due to a behavioral threshold effect (Becker & Joseph, 1988). Significant behavior changes are seen only with improvements in low-level knowledge and attitudes. Since adolescents have high levels of AIDS knowledge, one would not expect related improvement in behavior. Thus education alone is an insufficient intervention.

Studies of alcohol and substance use indicate a difference in the correlates of trial use and abuse. While knowledge, attitudes, and behavioral intentions have more effect on trial use, the relationships with family, school, and peers have more effect on abuse (Elliott, Huizinga, & Ageton, 1985; Johnson, Pentz et al., 1990). Therefore, AIDS prevention interventions should be planned for all three arenas. Many programs occur in schools, but the family is often not included. Parents should receive educational materials to increase their knowledge about substances and resources to help their children resist peer pressure. Older teens can be given ideas to discuss with their family and then the class. The National Institute for Alcohol and Drug Abuse, National Institutes of Health, has compiled a list of suitable materials for various age groups.

LEVELS OF RISK AND PREVENTION SETTINGS

Hein (1989a) characterizes levels of risk as three concentric circles (see Figure 9-1). The largest circle represents the majority of adolescents who have no risk behaviors or few risk behaviors, and thus they are at low risk for AIDS. Almost

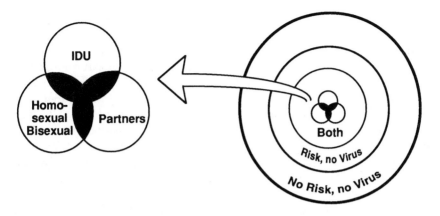

FIGURE 9.1 Circles of risk.

From "AIDS in adolescence: Exploring the challenge" by K. Hein, 1989, *Journal of Adolescent Health Care, 10*, p. 14S. Adapted by permission.

all young adolescents who are not sexually active fall into this circle. As teens become sexually active, they move to the middle circle. Both these circles may be reached through school classes and formal and informal youth organizations. The teens in the inner circle are sexually active and practice high-risk behaviors of male-male intercourse, use drugs, or share high-risk behavior with infected partners who are older. They form a "bridge" of exposure to the general adolescent population. Many of these teens live in urban areas and are black and Hispanic. Some are HIV positive. A small percentage of these adolescents can be reached through the school or established community agencies. However, the majority are school dropouts, runaways, homeless, unemployed or working as prostitutes, and/or selling drugs. The following settings work with adolescents in the inner circle: foster care, the welfare and juvenile system, drug treatment centers, general mental health care, adolescent behavior programs, and community shelters (Hein, 1989a; Rotherman-Borus, Koopman, Haignere, & Davies, 1991). Education in these settings must deal with reality and instill hope for a better future for these youngsters. Even then, behavior change will be slow (Bowen & Michal-Johnson, 1990).

Each of these settings would emphasize a different level of prevention to complement the level of risk of the teen participants (Flora and Thoresen, 1988, 1989). Primary prevention of AIDS involves interventions to maintain healthy behavior, prevent or reduce high-risk behavior, and learn decision-making skills. Secondary prevention incorporates early recognition of an HIV infection, diagnosis and treatment of associated diseases. After a positive diagnosis, individuals need assistance to maintain a healthy lifestyle for themselves and eliminate viral exposure to others. Tertiary prevention includes maintenance of present health status and function to deter further complications of the disease. Adolescent primary and secondary prevention tactics would differ from those used for adults, while tertiary prevention efforts would be similar.

All three levels or circles of risk described by Hein (1989a) need primary prevention, which entails general information about AIDS to recognize types of activities that are risky and casual contact that is safe, as well as training to make safe decisions. Sexually active teens at the midlevel of risk particularly need to be taught communication skills to know their sex partners and methods to make better decisions about their sexual activity (Ford & Norris, 1991). They must be given resources for future use, such as hotlines where anonymous questions can be answered, clinics sensitive to adolescents, and agencies for more specific counseling and testing for HIV.

In addition to primary prevention, HIV seronegative teens in the smaller circle need to understand the importance of being tested for HIV as a secondary AIDS prevention measure. Such a test can recognize early seroconversion. Early diagnosis means early treatment and prolonged life, and a possible break in the transmission of the virus by the HIV-infected person. Details should include test-site alternatives, the process of testing and counseling, the meaning of a negative or positive result, sources of assistance if the test is positive. Such information will clarify any misperceptions teens may have about the tests, alleviate any fear about the process, and prepare them to make a personal decision about being tested. A significant adult, preferably a parent or family member, should help the teen make the decision (Levine & Bayer, 1989). If the test is positive, this individual can provide support and assist with follow-up.

THEORETICAL MODELS FOR AIDS PREVENTION

Several models of adult health behavior or its components have been used with varying degrees of success to *explain* adolescent sexual risk behavior: the Health Belief Model (Becker & Joseph, 1988), the Theory of Reasoned Action (Fishbein & Middlestadt, 1989), and Self-Efficacy (Bandura, 1990). However, few interventions to *change* behavior have been grounded in a theory. Extensive cardiovascular health promotion research with young people indicates a theoretical foundation increases program effectiveness (Stone, Perry, & Luepker, 1989). Theory can guide an intervention to target significant behavioral determinants. In addition, providers are more likely to find reliable instruments to measure change in the determinants as well as the behavioral outcomes.

Since the determinants of adult and adolescent risk behavior are not the same, separate adolescent models need to be devised (Yarcheski & Mahon, 1989). An adolescent model should consider physical, emotional, and cognitive developmental factors and the influence of the peer group (Brown, DiClemente, & Reynolds, 1991; Montgomery et al., 1989). Physical maturity affects adolescents' self-perception and social interactions; cognitive development affects their ability to make decisions about risk taking (Irwin & Millstein, 1986).

Stiffman and colleagues (1991) have developed an adolescent AIDS risk-behavior model based on multivariate analysis of longitudinal interview data from a stratified random sample of 602 adolescents. Peers influenced risk behavior, but analysis indicated that only personal alcohol and drug abuse had significantly strong negative influences on risk taking, followed by the number of life stressors and suicidal ideas. Social relationships and achievement orientation did not influence behavior. Unfortunately, as knowledge of AIDS risk increased, so did the risk behaviors. The results of initial testing of this model indicate a need for interventions to address life stressors, substance abuse, and depression.

Two other models include key adolescent variables. The School-Based Health Promotion Model addresses four adolescent behavioral influences: physical, psychological, personal and social health (Perry, 1984). The Health for All nursing model addresses not only the biological, sociological, and environmental factors associated with risk behavior but the medical, technologic, and organizational factors that affect prevention and treatment efforts (Talashek, Tichy, and Salmon, 1989). Both these models are suitable for AIDS prevention efforts with adolescents but need to be tested.

Flora and Thoresen (1988) combine threads of several theories into three educational approaches to improve adolescent AIDS risk behavior: (1) programs based on cognitive-affective theories include knowledge about the disease and risks, self-talk with positive statements about the new behavior, and self-efficacy to increase ability to perform low-risk behavior; (2) behavioral theories stress behavior-outcome expectancies, social skills to resist peers and talk to sex partner, and personal behaviors to substitute for high risk; (3) environmental theories encourage social support of others, behavioral incentives, and social modeling by older peers or video examples.

PROGRAM GUIDELINES

General AIDS Education in Schools

Up to age 18, most adolescents can be reached with primary prevention through the schools. The Centers for Disease Control (CDC) has published guidelines for AIDS education in the schools (CDC, 1988; 1992) and many states have mandated such education. Ideally, education policies and programs should be planned by all parties involved. The program should be incorporated into existing health education. The regular classroom teachers should teach elementary-school children; health educators should teach older children; all should be trained and receive periodic updating. Depending on the school nurses' role, they might be involved in actual delivery of the education or be responsible for training the health educators or teachers. Content should be age-specific. The benefits of sexual abstinence and sex within marriage need to be taught along with skills to avoid risky behavior. Time and educational resources should be available for program development as well as presentation, and periodic evaluation of the process and outcome should take place. Several schools that have implemented successful programs suggest the AIDS education policy should be broad, with a simple purpose statement (Lohrman, 1988). An advisory committee of teachers, parents, administrators, clergy, students, and health-care personnel, especially the school nurse, should be appointed early to assist in planning (Brainerd, 1989). The school programs that coordinate their efforts with other community efforts report the best outcomes (Allensworth & Symons, 1989).

AIDS prevention education during early adolescence should be integrated into the rest of the curriculum (Pies, 1988). Young adolescents need concrete facts about their bodies, the transmission of the HIV virus, and behavior that will put them at risk. These facts can be presented, along with problem-solving exercises involving everyday situations such as communicating personal feelings to parents and peers and negotiating with parents and peers about difficult situations, including risk taking. These exercises will strengthen self-confidence and prepare teens to make independent decisions.

AIDS prevention education for high school students must focus even more on decision making and more specific sex and drug education and skill training (Schinke, Botvin, Orlandi, Schilling, & Gordon, 1990). These concepts can be integrated into family life or health classes (Quackenbush, 1988). However, if teachers feel unprepared to give specific facts about HIV infection and transmission, medical, nursing, health-education, and other health professional students can assist in the education (Johnson et al., 1988).

The topic of AIDS can be incorporated in several classroom activities. A variety of methods will help hold the interest of the group and meet the different learning needs of individuals. Every method reinforces information learned in another medium, and repetition is important for retention (Flora & Thoresen, 1989). An English class, for example, might read and react to a story about teens who take risks and suffer the consequences. Another alternative is writing an essay on the upsetting aspects of AIDS (Brown, Nassau, & Levy, 1990). A social-studies class could collect articles about the AIDS epidemic in their area; biology students could focus on the difference between cold viruses and HIV. Along with classroom activity, self-instruction reinforces classroom learning and increases peer discussion (Schinke, Gordon, & Weston, 1990). Students can take home assignments for peer and family discussions. Books used as resources should be written with the adolescent in mind (Blake, 1990). Resources should be available to families who want more information.

Education should emphasize the value of health and the health risk of certain sexual behaviors (Lohrman, 1988). Program educators need to teach teens how to make decisions through identification of the problem and the alternatives, analysis of the potential result of each alternative, and evaluation of their final choice (Kerr, 1990). The emphasis must be on the individual's responsibility for his or her welfare and respect for each individual's personal choice within the peer group or a more intimate relationship. Assertiveness and refusal skills are also important components of AIDS education. Allensworth and Symons (1989) add the need to learn social action, such as lobbying for after-school activities to fill free time or action to assist persons with AIDS.

Debate is another tool that might be used for a challenging intellectual interchange (Hein, 1989). The preparatory research by each team will be as educational as the debate itself. Members of the group who act only as observers should not feel left out. The leaders could assist them in preparing questions for each team. They could observe and report on the nonverbal activity that takes place among the debaters.

Students who report inability to tolerate homosexuals or persons with AIDS should be challenged to examine their beliefs and accept a different viewpoint (Bruce et al., 1990). More complex real-life examples can be used for discussion. To help personalize the risk for AIDS, young persons with AIDS should present their stories, if not in person, then on videotapes available through the American Red Cross and the National AIDS Information Clearinghouse (see address later in this chapter).

In addition to videotapes, other media must be used as interventions. High school and college students obtain their AIDS information from many sources: TV and radio, followed by magazines, newspapers, or pamphlets, with little information from parents or teachers (Fisher & Misovich, 1990; Helgerson, Petersen, & AIDS Education Study Group, 1988). When the school AIDS programming is strong, more students report the school as an educational source (Miller & Downer, 1988). Schools also can keep the community informed of the school activities through the TV, radio, and newspaper media (Black & Jones, 1988). This maintains parental confidence and prevents misconceptions about the role of the school. The Division of Adolescent and School Health at the CDC provides technical assistance for prevention programs (Centers for Disease Control, 1991; Jorgensen & Herring, 1990).

All educational materials in every media must be carefully worded. Adolescents can misperceive their risk for AIDS unless all words are clearly defined (Hamilton, 1988). Even survey questions should be clarified upon completion to avoid misinterpretation of responses the teen believes are correct (Skurnick, Johnson, Quinones, Foster, & Louria, 1991).

There is rarely controversy over drug use or sexual abstinence content. However, religious and parental authority conflicts often arise over the teaching of safe sexual behaviors, such as condom usage or sexual alternatives to intercourse (Reis & Seidl, 1989). Sexual abstinence is recognized as the only way to prevent AIDS, but previous research with homosexual males strongly indicates this advice is rarely followed. Monogamy is the next safest sexual behavior, but teens often interpret this to mean one partner at a time rather than one lifetime partner. Although parents express fear that expanded sex education will encourage sexual promiscuity, research demonstrates sex education does not significantly affect initiation of sexual activity (Marsiglio & Mott, 1986; Taylor-Nicholson, Wang, & Adame 1989).

Some high schools have instituted condom distribution through school-based clinics or vending machines. Although these programs to control the spread of HIV are surrounded by much debate and controversy, they must be evaluated to determine their impact. At least two outcome measures must be considered: age at first intercourse and condom use. If the program is effective, age at first intercourse must remain stable, and condom use should increase. Such programs must be accompanied by strong education to provide (1) knowledge about sexual health as well as AIDS, (2) decision-making skills to determine readiness to be sexually active, and (3) communication skills to convey their decision to others and negotiate safe sexual practices.

Not all adolescents are having intercourse, but all need to be taught to make decisions about potentially risky behavior. To make sound decisions, students need complete information, their questions answered honestly, and encouragement to discuss material with their parents. The facts about the effectiveness of various methods of contraception in preventing AIDS can serve to underscore the importance of communication before having sex, and the need for shared decisions, which may be a new gender role for some teens (Melchert & Burnett, 1990). Regardless of the age when the education starts, providers must be role models for students, accepting the students' views and allowing them room to explore alternatives and gradually make changes (Hein, 1989).

Special Groups

Interventions to counter sexual and injecting drug use behaviors of black and Hispanic minorities must be culturally sensitive (De La Cancela, 1989; DiClemente & Houston-Hamilton, 1989; Marin, 1989; Mays & Cochran, 1988; Schilling et al., 1989; Singer, 1991). These adolescents need empowerment skills to make healthy choices (De La Cancela, 1989). Those residing in urban neighborhoods need peer role models and a social network of other teens who will support healthy behavior choices (DiClemente & Houston-Hamilton, 1989). Teen leaders should be identified to assist in the communitywide prevention efforts. The parents and extended families of black and Hispanic teens ideally should be involved in planning and participation in adolescent programs, especially those outside school. Various formal and informal community organizations can assist with outreach projects for youth who are no longer in school (DiClemente

& Houston-Hamilton, 1989; Freudenberg, Lee, & Silver, 1989; Johnson, Williams, & Kotarba, 1990; Marin, 1989). Without instilling fear, these groups of teens need to be informed that their risk for AIDS equals or exceeds that of whites (DiClemente & Houston-Hamilton, 1989).

To disseminate AIDS information, skits, plays and appropriate music have been used (Bowser, Fullilove, & Fullilove, 1990; DiClemente & Houston-Hamilton, 1989; Kotarba, Williams, & Johnson, 1991; Marin, 1989; Rushing & Stohr, 1991). Written material should be in the appropriate language. Students should evaluate educational material for accuracy, acceptance, and cultural sensitivity (D'Augelli & Kennedy, 1989). Posters in the neighborhood may not be read, since reading them is a public activity, but newspapers and radio can be attended to in private (Marin, 1989). The church will reach some black youths and may not be appropriate to reach others (DiClemente & Houston-Hamilton, 1989). A large sex education program in several black, white, and multiracial Illinois churches has proven to be quite effective (Isberner & Wright, 1988).

Such programs emphasize the role of the family and the community. The sense of family responsibility should be stressed when working with Hispanic youth (Marin, 1989). Ethnic pride is strengthened through the use of cultural specific materials that empower minority students to choose a healthy lifestyle (Schinke et al., 1990). Schinke and colleagues recommend hourly programs every week for 12–15 weeks with semiannual reinforcement.

Other groups of teens both in and out of school need special consideration. Personnel from agencies serving teens in foster care or the juvenile system, runaways, homeless, prostitutes, and known substance abusers must not wait until young people at high risk come to talk about AIDS. Neither adolescents themselves nor social service personnel can always identify high-risk behaviors (Stiffman, Earls, Robins, & Jung, 1988). Because AIDS-related behaviors are private, they are difficult to identify. Such agencies must determine their interest level and ability to offer prevention programs. Planners should investigate the possibilities for programming with the local and state health departments or neighborhood clinics. Agency personnel could be trained to offer the program. In some areas, the service could be offered on-site by experts from another agency, or clients can be referred for classes or individual counseling elsewhere.

To determine which adolescents need special assistance or referral, baseline assessments should be conducted. The adolescents must understand how the information will be used and who has access to it. Survey respondents must be assured of privacy and confidentiality (U.S. Preventive Services Task Force, 1990). The greater the level of trust between the program leaders and participants, the more honest the responses will be and the more likely the program will be a success. One screening tool available in English and Spanish is the Problem Oriented Screening Instrument for Teenagers, developed by the National Institute of Drug Abuse (NIDA) (Rahdert, 1991). One clinical study indicates adolescents are reluctant to report high-risk behavior (Paperny et al., 1991). The young respondents were more willing to answer in the strong affirmative to questions about risk behavior when queried by computer versus face-to-face interview. They were also more ready to receive information about their risks via the computer.

Adolescents at moderate risk for AIDS might work in small groups. The mathematic explanations of the logarithmic exposure of multiple partners cannot be understood by young teens who are unable to think abstractly. Games and role-plays have been devised to teach these concepts (Illinois Department of Children and Family Services & Midwest AIDS Training and Education Center, 1991). For up-to-date material, the CDC-sponsored National AIDS Information Clearinghouse (301-762-5111 or 1-800-458-5231) has access to a data base on organizations and educational material. Program planners should be able to identify written material, films, videotapes, and games that have been produced for a variety of age groups with particular risks, needs, and interests. School material information can be obtained by calling the CDC at (404) 488-5372 or writing to the Centers for Disease Control, Division of Adolescent and School Health, 1600 Clifton Rd., Mail Stop K-31, Atlanta, GA 30333.

For group activities, the leader must be sensitive to the levels of comprehension of the group as well as the confidence levels of the participants. Self-assessment for comprehension and discussion should follow the exercise to explore attitudes and feelings of the group members. Role-playing is another one-on-one activity that can be achieved in groups. Role-play is like a dress rehearsal for life experience. Therefore the "play" should be as real as possible, with a sense of the actual pressures teens have to take risks (Flora & Thoresen, 1988). The counselor-leader and the individual client or one of the participants can role-play various situations where the adolescent will be making a decision related to drugs or sex. In the group setting, the participants can react, critique, and suggest. Early in the group meetings, written comments might be easier for the participants. In individual counseling sessions, the client can report his or her feelings to the counselor. In group or individual sessions, positive attitudes and behavior should be reinforced. The adolescent needs help to determine how to deal with the negative feelings the situation aroused.

Role-play in front of a group is difficult, even for professionals who are among their peers. Over time, however, adolescents can feel comfortable in group role-playing activities. Such activities, however, should not be undertaken until the group members know one another. Persons at greatest risk should be referred for one-to-one counseling by someone who is trained to work with adolescents. They are more vulnerable than adults because of their developmental level and lack of skill and power to make decisions about their actions. Such counseling sessions begin with a more in-depth assessment (U.S. Preventive Service Task Force, 1990). A Comprehensive Assessment Battery has been developed by

NIDA for this purpose (Rahdert, 1991). Personal risks identified are reviewed with each individual. For each risk, safer behaviors should be suggested and alternatives discussed.

EVALUATION

In every setting, evaluation is an important component of any prevention program, and should be part of initial planning and budgeting (Flora & Thoresen, 1989; Rugg, O'Reilly, & Galavotti, 1990; Valdiserri, 1989). The U.S. Conference on Mayors (1990) has published some clear guidelines for evaluation of AIDS prevention programs. Most program evaluations focus on the process of the intervention such as the number of participants and their characteristics, compared to the characteristics of the target population. The information is used to determine how to increase participation. Class content or client visits can be evaluated by an unbiased observer and/or surveys of clients. The climate of the agency, especially staff-client relationships, has a positive effect on the client outcomes (Nathanson & Becker, 1985).

Process evaluation remains important, but future funding will demand evaluation of outcomes. The unit of outcome analysis is dependent upon the level of the intervention (Flora & Thoresen, 1989). If the individual is the target for preventive counseling to change behavior, individual participants should be surveyed. Individual learning from educational programs is frequently evaluated with a pretest and a posttest. For the most accurate results, these two tests should be alternate forms. A delayed posttest aids in determining the level of retention and the timing of needed reinforcement of the learning. Curriculum effectiveness often decreases after six weeks (Yarber, 1988). A comparison group with similar characteristics would also strengthen the evaluation. Sometimes it is necessary to evaluate subgroup differences to determine where the program needs improvement (Brown, Fritz, & Barone, 1989).

If the prevention effort is aimed at the media to provide more human-interest stories on the effects of AIDS on teens, the readership should be surveyed to ascertain the effect of the stories. Perhaps a teen sexually transmitted disease (STD) program was initiated to address a surge in STD rates among teenagers. If a teen STD program is started, post program data should include the adolescent STD rate for the target population. Any questionnaire that is used to evaluate knowledge, attitudes, or behavior must be valid (represent accurate content) and reliable (internally and externally consistent). The results will be only as good as the data collected. The CDC continually updates facts about AIDS, so any knowledge questionnarie should reflect current information.

For evaluating decision making and communication, Ross, Caudle, and Taylor (1989) have developed a scale to measure AIDS-related interpersonal activities. The internal consistency reliability of the questionnaire is strong but has yet to be tested for predictive validity following communication education. This questionnaire might be useful as a post-test to measure changes in tension or anxiety with interpersonal activity.

SUMMARY

Although adolescents are knowledgeable about AIDS, they continue to practice high-risk behavior. The risks are greatest among the urban poor, especially black and Hispanic youth. Primary prevention programs are targeted toward all teens and offered in school settings to prevent the initiation of AIDS risk behaviors. Secondary prevention programs are added for teens who already practice high-risk behavior with persons who are HIV-positive. Family planning and STD clinics and community outreach programs for troubled youth are likely settings. Adolescents with known risk should be referred for counseling and HIV testing to maintain their health status and prevent further transmission of the virus. Adolescent, parent, and community leader involvement in program planning increases the cultural sensitivity of the programs.

Prevention programs with a theoretical basis are more effective. Education alone, however, is inadequate to prevent HIV transmission. Students need to learn how to communicate with their parents, peers, and sex partners; how to be assertive; and how to make healthy decisions. A variety of methods and media will hold teens' interest and match their cognitive levels and individual learning styles (Sy, Richter, & Copello, 1989). The method of evaluation must match the level of the program and include process and outcome variables. Research is needed to document the behavioral effectiveness of AIDS interventions. If results were made public, alternative methods could be compared.

REFERENCES

Allensworth, D., & Symons, C. (1989). A theoretical approach to school-based HIV prevention. *Journal of School Health, 59*, 59–65.

Baldwin, J., & Baldwin, J. (1988). AIDS information and sexual behavior on a university campus. *Journal of Sex Education and Therapy, 14*(2), 24–28.

Bandura, A. (1990). Perceived self-efficacy in the exercise of control over AIDS infection. *Evaluation and Program Planning, 13*(1), 9–17.

Beaman, M., & Strader, M. K. (1989). STD patient's knowledge about AIDS and attitudes toward condom use. *Journal of Community Health Nursing, 6*(3), 5–16.

Becker, M., & Joseph, J. (1988). AIDS and behavioral change to reduce risk: A review. *American Journal of Public Health, 78*, 394–410.

Black, J., & Jones, L. (1988). HIV infection: Educational programs and policies for school personnel. *Journal of School Health, 58*, 317–322.

Blake, J. (1990). *Risky times: How to be AIDS smart and stay healthy: A guide for teenagers.* New York: Workman.

Bowen, S. P., & Michal-Johnson, P. (1990). A rhetorical perspective for HIV education with black urban adolescents. *Communication Research, 17,* 848–866.

Bowser, B., Fullilove, M., & Fullilove, R. (1990). African-American youth and AIDS high-risk behavior. *Youth & Society, 22*(1), 54–66.

Brainerd, E. (1989). HIV in the school setting: The school nurse's role. *Journal of School Health, 59,* 316–317.

Brooks-Gunn, J., Boyer, C., & Hein, K. (1988). Preventing HIV infection and AIDS in children and adolescents. *American Psychologist, 43,* 958–964.

Brown, L., Fritz, G., & Barone, V. (1989). The impact of AIDS education on junior and senior high school students: A pilot study. *Journal of Adolescent Health Care, 10,* 386–397.

Brown, L., DiClemente, R., & Reynolds, L. (1991). HIV prevention for adolescents: Utility of the health belief model. *AIDS Education and Prevention, 3*(1), 50–59.

Brown, L., Nassau, J., & Levy, V. (1990). "What Upsets Me Most About AIDS is . . .": A Survey of Children and Adolescents. *AIDS Education and Prevention, 2,* 296–304.

Bruce, K., Shrum, J., Trefethen, C., & Slovik, L. (1990). Students' attitudes about AIDS, homosexuality, and condoms. *AIDS Education and Prevention, 2,* 220–234.

Catania, J., Dolcini, M., Coates, T., Kegeles, S., Greenblatt, R., Puckette, S., Corman, M., & Miller, J. (1989). Predictors of condom use and multiple partnered sex among sexually active adolescent women: Implications for AIDS related health intervention. *The Journal of Sex Research, 20,* 514–524.

Centers for Disease Control. (1988). Guidelines for effective school health education to prevent the spread of AIDS. *Journal of School Health, 58,* 142–148.

Centers for Disease Control. (1990). HIV-related knowledge and behaviors among high school students—selected U.S. sites, 1989. *Morbidity and Mortality Weekly Report, 39*(3), 385–397.

Centers for Disease Control. (1991a, July). *HIV/AIDS prevention.*

Centers for Disease Control. (1991b). The HIV/AIDS epidemic: The first 10 years. *Morbidity and Mortality Weekly Report, 40*(22), 362.

Cobliner, W. G. (1981). Prevention of adolescent pregnancy: A developmental perspective. *Birth Defects, 17*(3), 35–47.

Curran, J. W., Jaffe, H. W., Hardy, A. M., Morgan, W. M., Selik, R. M., & Dondero, T. J. (1988). Epidemiology of HIV infection and AIDS in the United States, *Science, 239,* 610–616.

D'Augelli, A. R., & Kennedy, S. (1989). Evaluation of AIDS prevention measures for university women. *AIDS Education and Prevention, 1*(2), 134–140.

De La Cancela, V. (1989). Minority AIDS prevention: Moving beyond cultural perspectives towards sociopolitical empowerment. *AIDS Education and Prevention, 1*(2), 141–153.

DiClemente, R., Boyer, C., & Morales, E. (1988). Minorities and AIDS: Knowledge, attitudes and misconceptions among black and Latino adolescents. *American Journal of Public Health, 78,* 55–57.

DiClemente, R., Forrest, K., Mickler, S., & principal site investigators. (1990). College students' knowledge and attitudes about AIDS and changes in HIV-preventive behaviors. *AIDS Education and Prevention, 2*(3), 201–212.

DiClemente, R., & Houston-Hamilton, A. (1989). Health promotion strategies for prevention of human immunodeficiency virus infection among minority adolescents. *Health Education, 20,* 39–43.

DiClemente, R. J., Zorn, J., & Temoshok, L. (1986). Adolescents and AIDS: A survey of knowledge, attitudes and beliefs about AIDS in San Francisco. *American Journal of Public Health, 76,* 1443–1445.

DiClemente, R., Durbin, M., Siegel, D., Krasnovsky, F., Lazarus, N., & Comacho, T. (1992). Determinants of condom use among junior high school students in a minority, inner-city school district. *Pediatrics, 89,* 197–202.

DiClemente, R., Lanier, M., Horan, P., & Lodico, M. (1991). Comparisons of AIDS knowledge, attitudes, and behaviors among incarcerated adolescents and a public school sample in San Francisco. *American Journal of Public Health, 81,* 628–630.

Ehrhardt, A. (1988). Preventing and treating AIDS: The expertise of the behavioral sciences. *Bulletin of the New York Academy of Medicine, 64,* 513–519.

Elliott, D. S., Huizinga, D., & Ageton, S. S. (1985). *Explaining delinquency and drug abuse.* Newbury Park, CA: Sage.

Fishbein, M., & Middlestadt, S. E. (1989). Using the theory of reasoned action as a framework for understanding and changing AIDS-related behaviors. In V. M. Mays, G. W. Albee, & S. F. Schneider (Eds.), *Primary prevention of AIDS: Psychological approaches.* Newbury Park, CA: Sage.

Fisher, J. D., & Misovich, S. J. (1990). Evaluating college students AIDS related behavioral responses attitudes, knowledge and fear. *AIDS Education and Prevention, 2*(4), 322–337.

Flora, J., & Thoresen, C. (1988). Reducing the risk of AIDS in adolescents. *American Psychologist, 43,* 965–970.

Flora, J., & Thoresen, C. (1989). Components of a comprehensive strategy for reducing the risk of AIDS in adolescence. In V. Mays, G. Albee, & S. Schneider (Eds.), *Primary Prevention of AIDS: Psychosocial Approaches.* Newbury Park, CA: Sage.

Ford, K., & Norris, A. (1991). Urban African-American and Hispanic adolescents and young adults: Who do they talk to about AIDS and condoms? *AIDS Education and Prevention, 3*(3), 197–206.

Freudenberg, N. (1989). *Preventing AIDS: A guide to effective education for the prevention of HIV infection.* Washington, DC: American Public Health Association.

Freudenberg, N., Lee, J., & Silver, N. (1989). Black and latino community organizations respond to the AIDS epidemic: A case study in one new neighborhood. *AIDS Education and Prevention, 1*(1), 12–21.

Fullilove, M. T., & Fullilove, R. E. (1989). Intersecting epidemics: Black teen crack use and sexually transmitted diseases. *Journal of the American Medical Women's Association, 44,* 146–147.

Hamilton, M. (1988). Masculine generic terms and misperception of AIDS risk. *Journal of Applied Social Psychology, 18,* 1222–1240.

Hayes, C. (Ed.). (1987). *Risking the future: Adolescent sexuality, pregnancy and childbearing* (Vol. 1). Washington, DC: National Academy Press.

Hein, K. (1989a). AIDS in adolescence: Exploring the challenge. *Journal of Adolescent Health Care, 10* (Suppl.), 10–35.

Hein, K. (1989b). Problem behaviors and AIDS. *Bulletin of the New York Academy of Medicine, 65*(3), 356–366.

Helgerson, S., Petersen, L., & AIDS Education Study Group. (1988). Acquired immuno-deficiency syndrome and secondary school students: Their knowledge is limited and they want to learn more. *Pediatrics, 81,* 350–355.

Hingson, R., Strunin, L., Berlin, B., & Heeren, T. (1990). Beliefs about AIDS, use of alcohol and drugs, and unprotected sex among Massachusetts adolescents. *American Journal of Public Health, 80,* 295–299.

Holman, R., Gomperts, E., Jason, J., Abildgaard, C., Zelasky, M., & Evatt, B. (1990). Age and human immunodeficiency virus infection in persons with hemophilia in California. *American Journal of Public Health, 80,* 967–969.

Illinois Department of Children and Family Services and Midwest AIDS Training and Education Center (1991). *HIV and adolescents: Training manual for youth services.* Chicago: Author.

Irwin, C. E., & Millstein, S. G. (1986). Biopsychosocial correlates of risk-taking behaviors during adolescence. *Journal of Adolescent Health Care, 7* (Suppl.), 82–96.

Isberner, F., & Wright, W. R. (1988). Sex education in Illinois churches: The octopus program. *Journal of Sex Education and Theory, 14,* 29–33.

Jemmott, L. S., & Jemmott, J. B. (1990). Sexual knowledges, attitudes and risky sexual behavior among inner-city black male adolescents. *Journal of Adolescent Research, 5,* 346–369.

Jemmott, L. S., & Jemmott, J. B. (1991). Applying the theory of reasoned action to AIDS risk behavior: Condom use among black women. *Nursing Research, 40,* 228–234.

Johnson, C. A., Pentz, M. A., Weber, M. D., Dwyer, J. H., Baer, N., McKinnon, D. P., Hansen, W. B., & Flay, B. R. (1990). Relativeness of comprehensive community programming for drug abuse prevention with high-risk and low-risk adolescents. *Journal of Consulting and Clinical Psychology, 58,* 447–456.

Johnson, J., Sellow, F., Campbell, A., Haskell, E., Gay, A., & Bell, B. (1988). A program using medical students to teach high school students about AIDS. *Journal of Medical Education, 63,* 522–530.

Johnson, J., Williams, M., & Kotarba, J. (1990). Proactive and reactive strategies for delivering community-based HIV prevention services: An ethnographic analysis. *AIDS Education and Prevention, 2*(3), 191–200.

Jorgensen, C. M., & Herring, L. W. (1990). Communication skills for HIV prevention at state and local levels. *Public Health Reports, 105,* 262.

Kalmuss, D. (1986). Contraceptive use: A comparison between ever- and never-pregnant adolescents. *Journal of Adolescent Health Care, 7,* 332–337.

Katzman, E., Mulholland, M., & Sutherland, E. (1988). College students and AIDS: A preliminary survey of knowledge, attitudes and behavior. *Journal of American College Health, 37*(3), 127–130.

Kegeles, S., Adler, N., & Irwin, C. (1988). Sexually active adolescents and condoms: Changes over one year in knowledge, attitudes and use. *American Journal of Public Health, 78,* 460–461.

Kerr, D. (1990). Students need skills to prevent HIV infection. *Journal of School Health, 60,* 39.

Kipke, M., Futterman, D., & Hein, K. (1990). HIV infection and AIDS during adolescence. *Medical Clinics of North America, 74*(5), 1149–1167.

Klitzner, M. (1989). AIDS prevention and education: Recommendations of the work group. *Journal of Adolescent Health Care, 10,* 45S–47S.

Kotarba, J. A., Williams, M. L., & Johnson, J. (1991). Rock music as a medium for AIDS intervention. *AIDS Education and Prevention, 3*(1), 47–49.

Kulbok, P., Earls, F., & Montgomery, A. (1988). Life style and patterns of health and social behavior in high-risk adolescents. *Advances in Nursing Science, 11*(1), 22–35.

Levine, C., & Bayer, R. (1989). The ethics of screening for early intervention in HIV disease. *American Journal of Public Health, 79,* 1661–1667.

Lohrmann, D. (1988). AIDS education at the local level: The pragmatic issues. *Journal of School Health, 58,* 330–334.

Marin, G. (1989). AIDS prevention among Hispanics: Needs, risk behaviors, and cultural values. *Public Health Reports, 104,* 411–415.

Marsiglio, W., & Mott, F. (1986). Impact of sex education on sexual activity, contraceptive use and premarital pregnancy among American teenagers. *Family Planning Perspectives, 18*(4), 151–161.

Mays, V. M., & Cochran, S. D. (1988). Issues in the perception of AIDS risk and risk reduction activities by black and Hispanic/Latina women. *American Psychologist, 43,* 949–957.

McNally, J., & Mosher, W. (May/1991). AIDS-related knowledge and behavior among women 15–44 years of age: United States, 1988. *Advance Data,* No. 200.

Melchert, T., & Burnett, K. (1990). Attitudes, knowledge, and sexual behavior of high-risk adolescents: Implications for counseling and sexuality education. *Journal of Counseling & Development, 68*(3), 293–298.

Miller, L., & Downer, A. (1988). AIDS: What you and your friends need to know—a lesson plan for adolescents. *Journal of School Health, 58,* 137–141.

Montgomery, S. B., Joseph, J. B., Becker, M. H., Ostrow, D. G., Kessler, R. C., & Kirscht, J. P. (1989). The Health Belief Model in understanding compliance with preventive recommendations for AIDS: How useful? *AIDS Education and Prevention, 1,* 303–323.

Moss, G., & Kreiss, J. (1990). The interrelationship between human immunodeficiency virus infection and other sexually transmitted diseases. *Medical Clinics of North America, 74*(6), 1647–1660.

Murray, R., & Zentner, J. (1989). *Nursing assessment & health promotion strategies through the life span* (4th ed.). East Norwalk, CT: Appleton & Lange.

Nagy, S., Hunt, B., & Adcock, A. (1990). A comparison of AIDS and STD knowledge between sexually active alcohol consumers and abstainers. *Journal of School Health, 60,* 276–279.

Nathanson, C., & Becker, M. (1985). The influence of client-provider relationships on teenage women's subsequent use of contraception. *American Journal of Public Health, 75,* 33–38.

Nemoto, S., Brown, L., Foster, K., & Chu, A. (1990). Behavioral risk factors of human immunodeficiency virus infection among intravenous drug users and implications for preventive interventions. *AIDS Education and Prevention, 2,* 116–126.

Novick, L. (1991). HIV seroprevalence surveys: Impetus for preventive activities. *American Journal of Public Health, 81* (Suppl.), 61–63.

Orr, D. P., Langefeld, C. D., Katz, B. P., Caine, V. A., Dias, P., Blythe, M., et al. (1992). Factors associated with condom use among sexually active female adolescents. *Journal of Pediatrics, 120,* 311–317.

Paperny, D., Aono, J., Lehman, R., Hammar, S., & Risser, R. (1990). Computer-assisted detection and intervention in adolescent high-risk health behaviors. *Journal of Pediatrics, 116,* 456–462.

Perry, C. L. (1984). A conceptual approach to school-based health practice. *School Health Research, 4,* 33–38.

Petosa, R., & Wessinger, J. (1990). The AIDS education needs of adolescents: A theory-based approach. *AIDS Education and Prevention, 2,* 127–136.

Pies, C. (1988). AIDS education in school settings: Grades 7–9. In M. Quackenbush, M. Nelson, & K. Clark (Eds.), *The AIDS challenge: Prevention, education for young people.* Santa Cruz, CA: Network.

Polit, D., Morton, T., & White, C. (1989). Sex, contraception and pregnancy among adolescents in foster care. *Family Planning Perspective, 21,* 203–208.

Quackenbush, M. (1988). AIDS education in school settings: Grades 10–12. In Quackenbush, M., Nelson, M., & Clark, K. (Eds.), *The AIDS Challenge: Prevention Education for Young People.* Santa Cruz, CA: Network.

Rahdert, E. (Ed.). (1991). The adolescent assessment/referral system manual. DHHS pub. no. 91-1735.

Reis, J., & Seidl, A. (1989). School administrators, parents, and sex education: A resolvable paradox? *Adolescence, 24,* 639–645.

Remafedi, G. (1988). Preventing the sexual transmission of AIDS during adolescence. *Journal of Adolescent Health Care, 9*, 139–143.

Rickert, V., Jay, M., Gottlieb, A., & Bridges, C. (1989). Adolescents and AIDS: Female's attitudes and behaviors toward condom purchase and use. *Journal of Adolescent Health Care, 10*, 313–316.

Ross, M., Caudle, C., & Taylor, J. (1989). A preliminary study of social issues in AIDS prevention among adolescents. *Journal of School Health, 58*(7), 308–311.

Rotherman-Borus, M., Koopman, C., Haignere, C., & Davies, M. (1991). Reducing HIV sexual risk behaviors in runaway adolescents. *Journal of the American Medical Association, 266*, 1237–1241.

Rugg, D., O'Reilly, K., & Galavotti, C. (1990). AIDS prevention evaluation: Conceptual and methodological issues. *Evaluation and Program Planning, 13*, 79–89.

Rushing, J., & Stohr, E. (Eds.). (1991). AIDS theater project for youth debuts. *American Red Cross Outlook, 1*(2), 5.

Sachs, B. (1985). Contraceptive decision-making in urban, black female adolescents: Its relationship to cognitive development. *International Journal of Nursing Studies, 22*(2), 117–126.

Schilling, R., Schinke, S., Nichols, S., Zavas, L., Miller, S., Orlandi, M., & Botvin, G. (1989). Developing strategies for AIDS prevention research with black and Hispanic drug users. *Public Health Reports, 104*, 2–11.

Schinke, S., Botvin, G., Orlandi, R., Schilling, R., & Gordon, A. (1990). African-American and Hispanic-American adolescents, HIV infection, and preventive intervention. *AIDS Education and Prevention, 2*(4), 305–313.

Schinke, S., Gordon, A., & Weston, R. E. (1990). Self-instruction to prevent HIV infection among African-American and Hispanic-American adolescents. *Journal of Consulting and Clinical Psychology, 58*, 432–436.

Singer, M. (1991). Confronting the AIDS epidemic among IV drug abusers: Does ethnic culture matter? *AIDS Education and Prevention, 3*(3), 258–283.

Skurnick, J., Johnson, R., Quinones, M., Foster, J., & Louria, D. (1991). New Jersey high school students' knowledge, attitudes, and behavior regarding AIDS. *AIDS Education and Prevention, 3*, 21–30.

Sonenstein, F., Pleck, J., & Ku, L. (1989). Sexual activity, condom use and AIDS awareness among adolescent males. *Family Planning Perspectives, 21*, 152–158.

Stiffman, A., Cunningham, R., Earls, F., & Dore, P. (1991). Change in AIDS risk behaviors from adolescence to adulthood. In *Science Challenging AIDS: Conference Proceedings, 7th International Conference on AIDS* (pp. 214–225). Basel Switzerland, Karger.

Stiffman, A., Earls, F., Robins, L., & Jung, K. (1988). Problems and help seeking in high-risk adolescent patients of health clinics. *Journal of Adolescent Health Care, 9*, 305–309.

Stone, E., Perry, C., & Leupker, R. (1989). Synthesis of cardiovascular behavioral research for youth health promotion. *Health Education Quarterly, 16*, 155–169.

Strader, M. K., & Beaman, M. L. (1989). College student knowledge about AIDS and attitudes toward condom use. *Public Health Nursing, 6*, 62–66.

Sy, F., Richter, D., & Copello, A. G. (1989). Innovative educational strategies and recommendations for AIDS prevention and control. *AIDS Education and Prevention, 1*, 53–56.

Talashek, M., Tichy, A., & Salmon, M. (1989). The AIDS pandemic: A nursing model. *Public Health Nursing, 6*, 182–188.

Taylor-Nicholson, M., Wang, J., & Adame, D. (1989). Impact of AIDS education on adolescent knowledge, attitudes and perceived susceptibility. *Health Values, 13*(5), 3–7.

Thurman, Q., & Franklin, K. (1990). AIDS and college health: Knowledge, threat and prevention at a Northeastern University. *American Journal of College Health, 38*, 179–184.

United States Conference of Mayors. (1990, December). Evaluation for HIV/AIDS prevention programs, technical assistance reports. Washington, DC: Author.

U.S. Preventive Services Task Force. (1990, April). Counseling to prevent HIV infection and other sexually transmitted diseases. *American Family Planning, 41*, 1179–1187.

Valdisseri, D. (1989). *Preventing AIDS: The design of effective programs.* New Brunswick, NJ: Rutgers University Press.

Vermund, S., Alexander-Rodriquez, T., Macleod, S., & Kelley, K. (1990). History of sexual abuse in incarcerated adolescents with gonorrhea or syphilis. *Journal of Adolescent Health Care, 11*, 449–452.

Vermund, S., Hein, K., Gaffe, H., Cary, J., Thomas, P., & Drucker, E. (1989). Acquired immunodeficiency syndrome among adolescents. *American Journal of Diseases of Children, 143*, 1220–1225.

Walter, H., Vaughan, R., & Cohall, A. (1991). Psychosocial influences on acquired immunodeficiency syndrome—risk behaviors among high school students. *Pediatrics, 88*, 846–852.

Weisman, C., Nathanson, C., Ensminger, M., Teitelbaum, M., Robinson, J. C., & Plichta, S. (1989). AIDS knowledge, perceived risk and prevention among adolescent clients of a family planning clinic. *Canadian Journal of Public Health, 21*, 213–218.

Yarber, W. (1988). Evaluation of the health behavior approach to school STD education. *Journal of Sex Education and Theory, 14*(1), 33–38.

Yarcheski, A., & Mahon, N. (1989). A causal model of positive health practices: The relationship between approach and replication. *Nursing Research, 38*, 88–93.

10

The Clinical Spectrum and Treatment of HIV Infection in Children and Adolescents

Carolyn Burr

The clinical spectrum of HIV disease presents a challenge to providers caring for infants, children, and adolescents infected with HIV. For infants and young children, the damage caused by the virus can be rapid and devastating. The infant's immature immune system has not had the opportunity to encounter, recognize, and protect the body from invading organisms before that ability is undermined by HIV. Other unique aspects of HIV disease in infants and children stem from epidemiology, diagnosis, clinical progression, and treatment as these impact upon clinical management.

Clinical manifestations of HIV disease in adolescents more closely follow the patterns of disease in adults than those in children, but psychosocial issues and growth and development concerns particularly influence the care and management of infected adolescents. This chapter provides an overview of the clinical spectrum of HIV disease in infants, children, and adolescents and discusses treatment and management issues.

CLASSIFICATION OF CHILDREN WITH HIV INFECTION

A surveillance definition for pediatric AIDS that specified particular diagnoses as AIDS indicators was developed by the CDC and has undergone several revisions (Centers for Disease Control, 1987a). The most recent proposed revision of the AIDS definition includes any HIV-infected person with a CD4 count of less than 200 mm³, as discussed in Chapter 1. The AIDS-indicator conditions for pediatric AIDS are shown in Table 10.1. They are similar to those in adults, except that lymphoid interstitial pneumonitis (LIP) and recurrent multiple bacterial infections are applicable only to children under 13 years of age.

Table 10.1 AIDS-Indicator Diagnoses in the 1987 CDC Revised Surveillance Definition for Pediatric AIDS

Multiple or recurrent bacterial infections[a]
Candidiasis of the trachea, bronchi, or lungs[b]
Candidiasis of the esophagus[b,c]
Coccidioidomycosis, disseminated or extrapulmonary[a]
Cryptococcosis, extrapulmonary[b]
Cryptosporidiosis, chronic intestinal[b]
Cytomegalovirus disease (other than liver, spleen, nodes) onset at >1 month of age[b]
Cytomegalovirus retinitis (with loss of vision)[b,c]
HIV encephalopathy[a]
Chronic herpes simplex ulcer (>1 month duration) or pneumonitis or esophagitis, onset at >1 month of age[b]
Histoplasmosis, disseminated or extrapulmonary[a]
Isosporiasis, chronic intestinal (>1 month duration)[a]
Kaposi's sarcoma[b,c]
Lymphoid interstitial pneumonitis[b,c]
Lymphoma, primary brain[b]
Lymphoma (Burkitt's, or immunoblastic sarcoma)[a]
Mycobacterium avium complex or *Mycobacterium kansasii*, disseminated or extrapulmonary[b]
Mycobacterium tuberculosis or acid-fast infection (species not identified), disseminated or extrapulmonary[a]
Pneumocystis carinii pneumonia[b,c]
Progressive multifocal leukoencephalopathy[b]
Toxoplasmosis of brain, onset at >1 month of age[b,c]
Wasting syndrome due to HIV[a]

[a]Requires laboratory evidence of HIV infection (1987 addition).
[b]If indicator disease is diagnosed definitively (e.g., by biopsy or culture) and there is no other cause of immunodeficiency, laboratory documentation of HIV infection is not required.
[c]Presumptive diagnosis of indicator disease is accepted if there is a laboratory evidence of HIV infection (1987 addition).

While the definition of AIDS in children is important for tracking the epidemic, it does not delineate the range of HIV disease. In 1987, the CDC developed a classification system for children that better describes the clinical spectrum of HIV disease in infants and children, as shown in Table 10.2 (Centers for Disease Control, 1987b). Class P-0 (indeterminate infection) is used to classify infants under 15 months who are born to HIV-infected mothers but whose definitive diagnosis of HIV is not yet confirmed. Class P-1 includes infants and children with asymptomatic HIV infection with or without abnormal immune function. Symptomatic children are classified as P-2, with a range of subclasses that detail the symptomatology. The P-2 class is much broader than the definition of AIDS. It includes failure to thrive in subclass A and AIDS-defining conditions in subclasses B, C, D-l, D-2, and E-l. This classification system offers clinicians a systematic approach to tracking HIV manifestations in children.

IMMUNOLOGICAL CHANGES
IN THE CHILD WITH HIV INFECTION

As discussed in Chapter 1, T4 lymphocytes are the principal target of HIV, and their depletion is the hallmark of HIV infection. T4 cells not only play a critical role in the body's cell mediated immunity by providing a direct defense against specific invading organisms but also play a crucial role in the immunoregulation of the body's humoral or B-cell immunity, which produces antibodies against infectious agents. As HIV infection progresses, the individual loses the ability to mount an effective immune response through either cell-mediated or humoral defenses. For many HIV-infected infants and children, the effect of HIV on the immune system is seen rapidly. The infant's immature immune system has not fully developed and has not had the opportunity to encounter and develop antibodies against invading bacteria. Thus, infants and children with HIV have a very high incidence of bacterial infections such as meningitis, sepsis, and recurrent otitis media. Bacterial infections are seen less commonly in HIV-infected adults whose immune systems were mature and intact prior to HIV infection.

Hypergammaglobulinemia (very high levels of immunoglobulin G [IgG], immunoglobulin M [IgM], and immunoglobulin A [IgA]) is seen in over 90% of HIV-infected children and was one of the early markers of the disease (Oleske et al., 1983; Rubinstein et al., 1983). These high levels do not reflect appropriate antibody production; thus, many HIV-infected children are unable to mount an antibody response to infection or immunization. The reason for the hypergammaglobulinemia is not clear but seems to reflect dysfunction of the humoral immune system from lack of T-cell regulation. The immune dysfunction caused by HIV leaves the child vulnerable to common infectious agents, opportunistic infections, and the development of tumors.

THE CLINICAL SPECTRUM

HIV disease in children often presents with constitutional symptoms that may not initially be recognized as HIV-associated. Failure to thrive, with poor growth in both height and weight, often below the fifth percentile, is common. Unexplained fever and diarrhea are frequent symptoms. Lymphadenopathy (cervical, inguinal, and axillary), parotitis, hepatomegaly, and splenomegaly are common constitutional symptoms reflecting immune dysfunction. Chronic nasal discharge and chronic, recurrent otitis media unresponsive to conventional therapy may also be present. Oral candidiasis (thrush) and *Candida* diaper dermatitis that do not respond to routine treatment are also common early manifestations. As HIV disease progresses, the virus attacks other organs causing damage and dysfunction in the central nervous system, heart, lungs, kidneys, and gastrointestinal system.

Table 10.2 CDC Classification System for HIV in Children

Class P-O: Indeterminate infection

Infants <15 months born to infected mothers but without definitive evidence of HIV infection or AIDS

Class P-1: Asymptomatic infection

Subclass A   Normal immune function
Subclass B   Abnormal immune function: hypergammaglobulinemia, T4 lymphopenia, decreased T4:T8 ratio, or absolute lymphopenia
Subclass C   Immune function not tested

Class P-2: Symptomatic infection

Subclass A   Nonspecific findings ($\geq$2 for $\geq$2 months): fever, failure to thrive, generalized lymphadenopathy, hepatomegaly, splenomegaly, enlarged parotid glands, persistent or recurrent diarrhea
Subclass B   Progressive neurologic disease: loss of developmental milestones or intellectual ability, impaired brain growth, or progressive symmetrical motor deficits
Subclass C   Lymphoid interstitial pneumonitis
Subclass D   Secondary infectious diseases
    Category D-1   Opportunistic infections in the CDC case definition
      Bacterial: mycobacterial infection (noncutaneous, extrapulmonary, or disseminated); nocardiosis
      Fungal: candidiasis (esophageal, bronchial, or pulmonary), coccidioidomycosis, disseminated histoplasmosis, extrapulmonary cryptococcosis
      Parasitic: *Pneumocystis carinii* pneumonia, disseminated toxoplasmosis with onset $\geq$1 month of age, chronic cryptosporidiosis or isosporiasis, extraintestinal strongyloidiasis
      Viral: cytomegalovirus disease (onset $\geq$1 month of age), chronic mucocutaneous/disseminated herpes (onset $\geq$1 month age), progressive multifocal leukoencephalopathy
    Category D-2   Unexplained, recurrent, serious bacterial infections (2 or more in a 2-year period): sepsis, meningitis, pneumonia, abscess of an internal organ, bone/joint infections
    Category D-3   Other infectious diseases: including persistent oral candidiasis, recurrent herpes stomatitis ($\geq$2 episodes in 1 year), multidermatomal or disseminated herpes zoster
Subclass E   Secondary cancers
    Category E-1   Cancers in the AIDS case definition: Kaposi's sarcoma, B- cell non-Hodgkin's lymphoma, or primary lymphoma of brain
    Category E-2   Other malignancies possibly associated with HIV
Subclass F   Other conditions possibly due to HIV infection: including hepatitis, cardiopathy, nephropathy, hematologic disorders, dermatologic diseases

Perinatally Acquired HIV Infection

The epidemiological aspects of vertically transmitted HIV disease are discussed fully in Chapter 7. Infants born to HIV-infected mothers will have transplacentally acquired IgG antibody to HIV, whether or not they are truly HIV infected. Screening of these young infants for HIV antibodies by enzyme-linked immunosorbent antibody testing (ELISA) or Western blot will yield a positive test result, but these positive results actually reflect the mother's HIV-positive antibody status. During the first months of life, generally by 15 months but occasionally as late as 24 months, the infant loses maternal antibody. The uninfected infant will then test negative for HIV antibody. An infant born to an HIV-positive mother who has two negative antibody tests by Western blot after 15 months (including at least one after 24 months) is considered uninfected with HIV and should be followed in the same manner as any other infant for primary health-care needs.

However, the infant born to an HIV-positive mother will continue to need attentive follow-up from the health-care provider. Infants born to HIV-positive mothers who remain asymptomatic should be followed closely, particularly for physical findings such as abnormal growth, motor, or cognitive development; frequent mild or moderate infections such as otitis media, thrush, or eczema; and lymphadenopathy, LIP or organomegaly (Healy, 1992). Because the infant's mother is HIV-infected, and the father, siblings, or other family members may also be infected, providers must carefully monitor and appropriately intervene to promote this infant's health and development. In offering family-centered care, providers should refer the mother for her HIV-related care and help the family access other needed services from day care and respite to entitlements and psychosocial support. The long-term impact on uninfected infants born into HIV-affected families is not known, but early interventions aimed at promoting family stability and the healthy development of all family members would seem to be a critical first step.

The HIV-infected infant will begin to make his or her own antibody to HIV and will remain HIV-positive on antibody screening. The perinatally HIV-infected infant often begins to show symptoms of HIV infection very early in life, although two types of clinical courses are commonly observed. In the first, onset is early, before 1 year, and immunodeficiency and its sequelae develops rapidly. Typically, PCP is the presenting illness in these children, although wasting syndrome and encephalopathies are seen. Mortality is high. In the second course, children may remain asymptomatic for years, gradually showing signs and symptoms. LIP and other lymphoproliferative disorders are part of this clinical picture (Wilfert, 1991). The median age for AIDS diagnosis is 12 months, although children continue to be diagnosed well into childhood. Experts believe the median age at diagnosis is more likely to be 3 years when all factors are considered (Oxtoby, 1991). Thus, children with risk factors for HIV who begin to show HIV-related symptoms should be carefully evaluated, regardless of age.

With time, HIV-infected children become increasingly symptomatic, and most will ultimately meet the CDC-defined criteria for AIDS. The AIDS diagnosis may be helpful in establishing a child's eligibility for certain types of services, such as Medicaid model waiver programs, which are tied to the diagnosis of AIDS rather than HIV infection. The diagnosis of AIDS may be less helpful clinically since it represents the end point of a classification system rather than a staging system. For example, a child with lymphoid interstitial pneumonitis (LIP) meets the CDC definition of AIDS but has a far better prognosis than a child classified as AIDS because of *Pneumocystis carinii* pneumonia (PCP); thus it is imperative that providers discuss with families a child's clinical status and disease progression (Scott et al., 1989). Families are often stunned to learn that their child "has AIDS" when they thought the child "only had 'the virus.'" The clinical implications of reaching an AIDS diagnosis for a child must be clearly and repeatedly discussed with the family.

Diagnosis of HIV Infection in Infants and Children

Using the CDC classification system for pediatric HIV disease, infants under 15 months are classified as "indeterminate" until their infection status can be definitively determined or they meet other criteria for HIV classification. The dilemma of the indeterminate infant has increased the difficulty of effectively monitoring and treating these at-risk infants. Technologies that offer definitive diagnosis of HIV infection in infants are becoming increasingly available. Testing is discussed in Chapter 1.

Polymerase chain reaction (PCR), increasingly used in neonates, detects viral DNA by amplifying the HIV-DNA to detect presence of the virus. It requires only 1–3 ml. of blood and can be completed in a day. It is 50–60% sensitive in the neonatal period and 90+% sensitive in the postneonatal samples (Rogers et al., 1989.) However, standardization of the PCR technique is still underway, and it is available from only selected commercial or research laboratories. PCR may also fail to detect the truly infected infant.

Continued research holds the promise of early definitive diagnosis of HIV in infants. Until that is routinely available, indeterminate infants require careful monitoring of their immune function, growth, development, and health status to be alert to changes that can indicate HIV infection. At present, the diagnosis of HIV infection should be made using a combination of laboratory evaluation and assessment of the child. A confirmed positive HIV antibody screening by ELISA and Western blot provides laboratory evidence of HIV infection in children over 24 months, as it does in adults. Laboratory evaluation should also include immunoglobulins, lymphocyte subsets (T-4, T-8, T-4/T-8 ratio), and a complete blood count. The medical history should carefully evaluate growth, developmental milestones, recurrent or serious infections, and nutritional status, while physical examination should identify specific and constitutional symptoms associated with HIV infection. This battery of information will provide a basis for counseling the family on the child's HIV status and current health state.

Hemophilia/Coagulation Disorders and Transfusion/Blood Product-Acquired HIV Infection

The majority of persons who acquired HIV through contaminated blood or blood products are believed to have already come to the attention of the health-care system. As discussed in Chapter 7, most children in this category have had other health conditions, such as prematurity, hemophilia, or cardiac disease, that necessitated their receiving blood or blood products. Many of their families were already facing the possibility of chronic or life-threatening illness for their children when they were confronted with the diagnosis of HIV infection. Both the families and their infected child may display anger at the health-care system for this additional burden.

Management of HIV infection can be complicated by any prior underlying health problem. Determining whether neurologic symptoms, for example, are secondary to prematurity or HIV infection may be difficult. A child with cardiac disease may be failing to thrive from cardiac and/or HIV-related causes.

Children with transfusion-acquired HIV present with symptomatology similar to that of those with perinatally acquired HIV. However, opportunistic infections such as toxoplasmosis and cryptococcal meningitis, which represent reactivation of primary infection, are seen more frequently since these children were older when they acquired HIV. Septic arthritis, loss of antibodies to factor VIII, and increased bleeding potential caused by immune thrombocytopenia are three HIV complications peculiar to children with hemophilia (Ragni, 1989). Damage caused by previous joint bleeds increases the likelihood of bacterial infection in these joints. Hemophiliacs who have developed antibodies to infused factor VIII necessitating higher and higher doses may lose that antibody, allowing lower doses of factor VIII to be used with more effect. Immune thrombocytopenia occurs in other patients with HIV but is more likely to cause bleeding in the presence of the preexisting coagulation disorder. In persons with hemophilia, AIDS is now the leading cause of death and has accounted for 50% of the deaths since 1984 (Ragni, 1989).

Adolescents

Knowledge of the clinical spectrum of HIV in adolescents is still evolving. The natural history of HIV infection in adolescents may more closely resemble HIV in adults than children (Futterman & Hein, 1991). While the majority of adolescents with AIDS are classified into the exposure category of hemophilia/coagulation disorders (acquiring HIV through transfusions), a growing percentage have been exposed through sexual or drug-using behaviors, particularly in older adolescents (see Chapters 8 and 9). Because the incubation period of HIV in adolescents is believed to be long, many young people infected with HIV as adolescents will not become symptomatic until they are young adults.

Adolescents with blood product-acquired HIV may have been offered counseling and HIV testing through their health-care services since their risk was known, especially if they received blood transfusions as part of the therapy for a chronic health condition. However, families may choose not to have the adolescent tested, and he or she may first come to attention when already showing HIV-related symptoms and/or conditions. For a variety of reasons, including socioeconomic ones, adolescents with HIV acquired through sexual or drug-using behaviors are less likely to enter the health-care system for testing and counseling and may also be quite ill before HIV is diagnosed.

Once the adolescent begins receiving care, developmental and lifestyle issues may affect care. Adolescents may be reluctant to comply with drug-treatment regimens because they do not believe they are ill or do not want to be reminded of their HIV infection (Futterman & Hein, 1991). In the chaotic life of adolescents living on the street, often needing food as well as shelter, compliance with medications and medical follow-up is likely to be a low priority.

CLINICAL MANIFESTATIONS AND INTERVENTIONS
Recurrent Bacterial Infections

Bacterial infections are a common and frequent complication of HIV disease in children. Unlike HIV-infected adults, a child's immune system has not encountered and made antibodies to invading organisms prior to HIV infection. When it does occur, the quality of antibody response is often defective (Pelton & Klein, 1991). Bacteremia, meningitis, and pneumonia are common with *Streptococcus pneumoniae, Haemophilus influenzae* type b, group B *Streptococcus*, and *Salmonella* as the most frequent causative organisms (Pelton & Klein, 1991). Chronic and recurrent otitis media and sinusitis are common and difficult to treat. Infections of the urinary tract, gastrointestinal tract, and soft tissues also occur regularly. Antibiotic therapy should be based on the sensitivity of isolates and generally must be of longer duration than usual in non-HIV-infected children.

Infection with *Mycobacterium avium* complex (MAC) represents late-stage disease in persons with AIDS. MAC can disseminate widely, progressing to the blood and multiple organs. Symptoms include weight loss, anorexia, diarrhea, chills, night sweats, and elevated liver-function tests. A study of 11 children with MAC in blood or stool found that the prognosis after diagnosis was poor with a median survival of nine months (Hoyt, 1991). Treatment of MAC has not been very successful with regimens of multiple TB drugs, showing little improvement in controlling symptoms. Azithromycin, a new antibiotic related to erythromycin, has shown promise as an effective agent. Drug-treatment studies in children with HIV are now under way.

Intravenous Immunoglobulin (IVIG)

Early in the AIDS epidemic, children with HIV were treated with intravenous immunoglobulin (IVIG) because of their frequent and often overwhelming bacterial infections and their similarity in presentation to children with congenital immunodeficiencies (Oleske, 1991, personal communication.) The National Institute of Child Health and Human Development (NICHD) conducted a multicenter placebo-controlled study of IVIG in 372 HIV-infected children. Researchers concluded that IVIG significantly increased the period during which children were free of infection and decreased the number of serious and minor bacterial infections for children with CD4 counts over 200 mm^3 (Mofenson et al., 1992; NICHD IVIG Study Group, 1991). Overall guidelines for determining which children would benefit most from IVIG have not yet been established, but many clinicians base their treatment protocol on a child's history of recurrent or serious bacterial infections and evidence that the child does not make effective antibody.

IVIG is given at a dose of 300 to 400 mg/kg of body weight every three to four weeks (Buckley & Schiff, 1991). Common reactions to IVIG include abdominal or back pain, nausea, headache, chills, fever, myalgia, or fatigue. These can be prevented by slowing the rate of infusion of IVIG or by pretreating with aspirin. True anaphylaxis to IVIG is rare (Buckley & Schiff, 1991).

Immunizations

Another critical tool in preventing infection is childhood immunizations (see Table 10.3). Children with HIV should receive routine childhood immunizations, with two exceptions. Oral polio vaccine should not be given to children who are HIV seropositive or HIV-infected since it poses a risk to the child and other immunocompromised family member who might come in contact with the vaccine virus that is shed in the infant's stool. Inactivated polio vaccine (IPV) should be given instead.

Although the measles, mumps, and rubella (MMR) vaccine is a live attenuated virus, it should be given according to the most current recommended schedule since it poses much less risk than the risk of severe or fatal illness from exposure to the wild-type measles virus. Recent outbreaks of measles have emphasized the need for vigilance in keeping immunizations current. Because of the dysfunction of the humoral immune system caused by HIV, some children may not make antibody to immunizations. Antibody levels for measles, for example, should be measured four to six weeks after immunization and the immunization repeated if protective antibody is not detected. If a child consistently fails to make protective antibody to immunizations, passive protection through intravenous immunoglobulin should be considered. Pneumococcal vaccine and hepatitis B vaccine should also be given to children with HIV.

Table 10.3 Modified Immunization Schedule for Infants with HIV Infection

Age	Immunizations*
2 months	IPV, DPT, and PRP-OMP (Merck) or HbOC (Praxis) and HBV**
4 months	IPV, DPT, and PRP-OMP (Merck) or HbOC (Praxis) and HBV
6 months	DPT, HbOC (Praxis), HBV
12 months	PRP-OMP (Merck)
15 months	IPV, MMR, HbOC (Praxis), DPT***
24 months	Pneumococcal vaccine

*HBV = hepatitis B vaccine
DPT = diphtheria and tetanus toxoids and pertussis vaccine;
IPV = inactivated poliovirus vaccine; MMR = live virus measles, mumps, and rubella;
PRP-OMP = *Haemophilus influenzae* type b conjugate vaccine; (Merck)
HbOC = *Haemophilus influenzae* type b conjugate vaccine (Praxis)
**HBV may be given at birth, a second dose at 1–2 months, and a third at 6 to 18 months.
***4th DPT may be given at 18 months.

Source: Centers for Disease Control (1991). Hepatitis B virus: a comprehensive strategy for eliminating transmission through universal childhood vaccination. Recommendations of the Immunizations Practices Advisory Committee. *Morbidity and Mortality Weekly Report*, *40*, 784–786; Committee on Infectious Diseases, American Academy of Pediatrics (1991). Report of the Committee on Infectious Diseases. (21st Edition) (1991). (Elk Grove Village, IL: American Academy of Pediatrics).

Opportunistic Infections (OIs)

Pneumocystis carinii pneumonia (PCP). PCP is the most common opportunistic infection in infants and children with HIV. It often represents the presenting disease of HIV infection and is associated with high morbidity and mortality in children. *P. carinii* is a ubiquitous organism, classified as either a fungus or a protozoan. Exposure to *P. carinii* is thought to occur early in life in healthy children, causing an asymptomatic infection (Husson & Pizzo, 1990.) Organisms persist in a latent state in the healthy host, but with serious compromise of cell-mediated immunity, *P. carinii* pneumonia (PCP) occurs.

PCP was diagnosed in 39% of the children with AIDS reported to the CDC through 1990 (Centers for Disease Control, 1991) and is most commonly diagnosed between three and six months of age (Hughes, 1991). PCP is a particularly devastating illness for infants since it takes advantage of the infant's immature immune system and usually represents primary infection rather than disease reactivation. Thirty-five percent of children with PCP die within two months of diagnosis (Centers for Disease Control, 1991).

PCP presents with cough, tachypnea, fever, and dyspnea, and a chest X ray showing bilateral diffuse alveolar disease. Diagnosis is made by identification of the organism in induced sputum or specimens obtained by bronchoalveolar lavage or, rarely, from open lung biopsy. Rapid treatment with antibiotics is essential. Trimethoprim-sulfamethoxazole (TMP-SMX, Septra, Bactrim) given intravenously is the recommended initial treatment. Once the pneumonia is resolving, oral medication can be given for a full course of three weeks of antibiotic therapy. Adverse effects to TMP-SMX may be seen, including a transient erythematous rash, which usually resolves when the drug is stopped. TMP-SMX then can be readministered without recurrence of the rash. More serious side effects such as urticaria, Stevens-Johnson syndrome, neutropenia, and anemia are possible but are seen less often in children than in adults (McSherry, Wright, Oleske, & Connor, 1988).

Pentamidine can be given intravenously for two to three weeks to patients who are intolerant to TMP-SMX or fail to respond. Adverse effects in children include hepatic and renal toxicity, hypo- or hyperglycemia, hypotension, rash, thrombocytopenia, and anemia, and are seen frequently (Hughes, 1991).

Experience gained from treating children with cancer and adults with AIDS has shown that PCP is preventable. Guidelines for PCP prophylaxis in children have been developed by a working group convened by the National Pediatric HIV Resource Center (CDC, 1991). The strongest predictors for PCP in children were found to be (1) age under 1 year and (2) reduction in the CD4+ count well below that normal for age (Connor et al., 1991; Kovacs et al., 1991). Accordingly, the guidelines recommend prophylaxis for HIV-positive infants under 12 months with a CD4+ count less than 1,500 mm³, for children 12 to 23 months with a CD4+ count less than 750 mm³, for children 24 months to 5 years with a CD4+ count less than 500 mm³, and for children over 6 years with a CD4+ count less than 200 mm³. TMP-SMX is recommended as the first choice for prophylaxis with aerosolized pentamidine and dapsone as alternatives. Careful monitoring of the child's CD4+ cell count and response to treatment are detailed in the guidelines.

Early identification of infants at risk for HIV offers the greatest hope for prevention of PCP and should be part of "a comprehensive program of medical and social services, which includes HIV education, counseling and voluntary antibody testing (with consent) in the obstetric prenatal setting, and access to care for both the HIV-infected woman and her newborn" (Centers for Disease Control, 1991).

Fungal Infections.   The most common yeast-type fungus to infect children with HIV is *Candida albicans*. This organism colonizes all infants in the early weeks of life. However, in HIV-infected children, oral candidiasis (thrush) can be recurrent and difficult to treat with standard therapy. Patchy white plaques occur on the mucous membrane of the mouth, palate, and gingiva, causing pain with eating or sucking. The infection can spread to the esophagus, causing retrosternal pain and dysphagia. *Candida* diaper dermatitis, while common, often requires vigilant treatment to control. Disseminated candidiasis leading to critical illness can be difficult to diagnose and may be recognized only on autopsy.

Treatment for *Candida* can include topical or oral therapies. Topical preparations such as nystatin may be the initial therapy. When this is ineffective or esophagitis is present, an oral drug such as ketoconazole is indicated (van't Wout, 1991). Ketoconazole is an oral antifungal agent active against a variety of yeasts and in doses up to 5 mg/kg/day generally tolerated well by children (Walsh & Butler, 1991). It has variable absorption dependent on gastric acidity. Orally administered fluconazole has shown good effectiveness against *Candida* and *Cryptococcus*, but studies in children investigating safety, tolerance, and clinical efficacy are not yet complete (Walsh & Butler, 1991). Intravenous amphotericin B continues to be the recommended drug for disseminated candidiasis.

Diseases caused by other fungi such as *Cryptococcus neoformans*, *Histoplasma capsulatum*, and *Coccidioides immitis*, while seen in adults with HIV, are unusual in children. As children live longer, and in adolescents, these agents may play a larger role.

Viral Infections.   The herpes viruses—herpes simplex types 1 and 2, varicella zoster virus, cytomegalovirus, and Epstein-Barr virus—are ubiquitous in humans and especially problematic in children with HIV infection. Varicella, for example, can cause more extensive or atypical chickenpox as well as recurrent or prolonged infection. HIV-infected children exposed to chickenpox should receive varicella immune globulin to prevent or ameliorate the varicella infection. HIV-infected children with varicella or with herpes zoster are frequently hospitalized for treatment with intravenous acyclovir, as are children who have primary gingivostomatitis caused by the herpes simplex virus.

Cytomegalovirus (CMV) may represent congenital or primary disease in children. Clinical manifestations include interstitial pneumonia, gastrointestinal symptoms, and encephalitis. Although rare in children, reactivation of CMV as retinitis has occurred. Treatment with ganciclovir has shown benefit (Henderly, Freeman, Causey, & Rao, 1987). However, ganciclovir can be used with zidovudine only with careful monitoring of hematologic toxicity because of the risk of bone-marrow suppression.

Lymphoid Interstitial Pneumonitis (LIP)

Lymphoid interstitial pneumonitis is an AIDS-defining condition in children with HIV whose etiology is not yet established but which may be related to Epstein-Barr infection. Infiltration of lymphocytes in the interstitium of the lung leads to interference with oxygen–carbon dioxide exchange and hypoxemia. Distinctive changes occur on chest X ray. Children experience cough and ultimately, clubbing, dyspnea, and hypoxemia. Treatment with oral corticosteroids and of superimposed bacterial infections improves symptoms. Children with LIP often have other evidence of significant lymphoproliferative disease such as hepatomegaly, splenomegaly, lymphadenopathy, and parotitis (Grubman, Conviser, & Oleske, 1992).

Neurologic Manifestations

Central nervous system (CNS) manifestations occur early and frequently in children with HIV disease. The exact mechanism of damage to the CNS is not known, but is believed to involve both direct effect by viral products and immune-mediated tissue damage as the body tries to clear the virus (Brouwers et al., 1991.) More than 90% of HIV-infected infants or children eventually show some degree of central nervous system dysfunction although problems such as prematurity, frequent hospitalization, psychosocial problems and family stress may compound effects caused by HIV alone (Prober & Gershon, 1991).

The wide range of neurologic manifestations includes a progressive encephalopathy in which children lose developmental milestones or fail to attain new ones; develop progressive motor dysfunction such as change in gait and loss of head control; and may develop rigidity, hypertonicity, and hyperreflexia. Older children may experience loss of cognitive function manifested as poor school performance or experience attention deficits and emotional lability (Brouwers et al., 1991). About 25% of children have a static encephalopathy characterized by cognitive delay and motor deficits without loss of previous developmental milestones.

A child's loss of developmental milestones is an emotionally difficult problem for families and health-care providers. Antiretroviral therapy such as with zidovudine or dideoxyinosine (ddI) has been shown to improve, sometimes dramatically, the neurologic functioning of children with HIV, although deterioration can recur with time (see chapter 2).

CNS lymphoma is also seen in children with HIV, as are cerebrovascular accidents. Opportunistic infections of the CNS, such as toxoplasmosis, occur primarily in older children and adolescents.

Failure to Thrive

Failure to thrive (FTT) is frequently a presenting symptom of HIV children with height and weight below the fifth percentile. Other children may grow along an appropriate curve for a time, then begin to fail to grow appropriately. A number of factors play a role in FTT, including gastrointestinal dysfunction, such as the presence of OI's in the mouth or in the lower GI tract and neurologic dysfunction, which can complicate feeding. Chronic diarrhea and wasting are often seen in the absence of proven infectious agents. Biopsies in such cases have shown villi atrophy and chronic inflammation of the GI tract (McLoughlin, 1988).

Early and vigorous nutritional interventions can be helpful in preventing or halting weight loss. Dietary evaluation and counseling by a nutritionist, and evaluation for dysphagia by a speech pathologist or feeding specialist, are crucial to planning an intervention (Bentler & Stanish, 1987; Pressman & Morrison, 1988). High-calorie, nutrient-dense snacks and dietary supplements, along with family teaching, are the initial interventions. In children with neurologic dysfunction or those who cannot take in the needed calories, feeding via nasogastric tube can be instituted. If oral feeding is inadequate or is contraindicated, parenteral feedings can be used. Families can usually be taught to manage nasogastric or parenteral feedings and with proper professional support, carry on these interventions at home.

Organ System Failure

As HIV disease progresses, HIV attacks additional body systems, leading to kidney dysfunction, heart disease, hematologic problems, and electrolyte imbalances in addition to the lung and GI problems already described (Wiznia & Nicholas, 1990.) This multisystem failure provides a challenge in management. A child may receive medication for cardiac disease, hypertension, and kidney disease while receiving one or more antiviral medications. The pharmacolgic implications and the child's multiproblem status may prove overwhelming for the family.

Pain Management

Children with HIV infection suffer from pain for many reasons. Failure to assess and treat pain can lead to missed diagnoses and missed opportunities. A retrospective chart review of 150 HIV-infected children at Children's Hospital AIDS Program in Newark found that HIV-related pathology causes several types of pain: acute, chronic and recurrent intermittent. (Czarniecki & Oleske, 1991). Pain can be associated with infections such as abscesses; otitis and meningitis; opportunistic infections such as MAC, *Cryptosporidium*, herpes, and *Candida*; and severe dental disease, tumors, organomegaly and spasticity. Children report all types of pain—headache, abdominal cramps, leg pain, chest pain, pain on swallowing. Pain may also be iatrogenic. Multiple venipunctures and other procedures are frequent causes of pain.

The appropriate use of nonsteroidal antiinflammatory agents, muscle relaxants, and opioids can effectively control pain. Nonpharmacologic interventions such as hypnosis and guided imagery can also be beneficial. In one of my experiences, one 5-year-old girl with disseminated MAC was withdrawn, silent, lethargic, and believed to be depressed. When given oral methadone, she became active, sociable, and cheerful. Barriers to good pain management in HIV patients have included concerns about parental drug abuse, extended family resistance to opioids because of a history of drug abuse in the child's immediate family, and difficulty assessing pain in encephalopathic children.

Antiretroviral Therapy

As knowledge of the HIV and its life cycle has increased, research has been aimed at developing agents that would interrupt the life cycle of HIV and prevent its destruction of CD4+ cells. Initial trials of antiretroviral agents were carried out initially in adults and only later in children. Thus, access to antiretroviral agents for children was limited before 1990.

Zidovudine (azidothymidine, AZT, Retrovir, ZDV) was the first antiretroviral licensed in the United States for children. Studies of AZT in children symptomatic with HIV, begun in 1986, found improvements in weight, appetite, hepatosplenomegaly, lymphadenopathy, CD4 count, and neurodevelopmental status (Pizzo et al., 1988.) Improvements in IQ and adaptive behaviors were maintained after 12 months of AZT therapy (Brouwers et al., 1990.) A study of 88 children with advanced HIV disease on intermittent oral doses of AZT found improvements in weight gain, improvement in cognitive function, stabilization of CD4 count, and reduction of immunoglobulin levels (NIH/NIAID AIDS Clinical Trials Group Protocol 043 Team, 1990). Based on these studies, AZT was licensed by the FDA in May 1990 for use in children with symptomatic HIV infection and those with significant immunosuppression. The recommended dose of AZT for children 3 months to 13 years is $180mg/m^2$ given orally every 6 hours (Connor & McSherry, 1991). Anemia and neutropenia, the common toxic effects, may necessitate a dose reduction and should be regularly monitored with complete blood counts and differential.

Dideoxyinosine (ddI) is active against HIV *in vitro* and has shown evidence of antiretroviral activity without significant hematologic toxicity. It is not stable in an acid environment, however, and must be given orally with antacids. Principal side effects are pancreatitis and peripheral neuropathy (Connor & McSherry, 1991). A study of 43 children at the National Cancer Institute have shown a reduction in p24 antigen and increased CD4 lymphocyte count (Butler et al., 1991). The positive neurodevelopmental effects of ddI may not be as consistent as those of AZT (Connor & McSherry, 1991). The FDA approved ddI for both adults and infants over 6 months with advanced HIV infection in 1991 (Nightingale, 1991).

Other antiretroviral therapies such as ddC (dideoxycytidine) are undergoing clinical trials, and the use of combinations or alternating regimens of antiretrovirals is under investigation ("Combinations of AZT and ddI," 1992; Pizzo et al., 1990). Therapeutic interventions that interfere with the virus's ability to attach to CD4+ molecules or inhibit viral replication in other ways are being explored (Connor & McSherry, 1991). Information about current investigational drug trials can be obtained by calling the NIAID AIDS Clinical Trials Information Service at 1-800-TRIALS-A.

The advent of treatment of HIV infection holds important promise for infants, children, and adolescents. With the decreased mortality and increased quality of life that treatment brings, HIV infection becomes increasingly like other childhood chronic illnesses such as cystic fibrosis and sickle cell disease.

SERVICES TO INFECTED CHILDREN AND THEIR FAMILIES

Pediatric HIV disease, like other childhood chronic illnesses, has an impact on the entire family. For children with perinatally transmitted HIV, multiple family members are often affected, and families may face multigeneration illness and loss. Services for children with HIV must be family-centered, comprehensive, and coordinated if they are to address the complex needs of these families adequately (see Chapter 11). Community-based services such as outpatient care, respite, transportation services, psychosocial support, and others, help ensure that families can stay intact and receive services primarily at home rather than in expensive, disruptive inpatient or institutional settings. By adopting this model of family-centered, community-based care, providers can help HIV-affected families and children, wherever they are in the clinical spectrum of HIV disease, maintain an appropriate level of wellness.

REFERENCES

Bentler, M., & Stanish, M. (1987). Nutrition support of the pediatric patient with AIDS. *Journal of the American Dietetic Association, 87*, 488–491.

Brouwers, P., Belman, A., & Epstein, L. G. (1991). Central nervous system involvement: Manifestations and evaluation. In P. A. Pizzo & C. M. Wilfert (Eds.), *Pediatric AIDS* (pp. 318–335). Baltimore: Williams & Wilkins.

Brouwers, P., Moss, H., Wolters, H., Eddy, J., Balis, F., Poplack, D. G., & Pizzo, P. (1990). Effect of continuous-infusion zidovudine therapy on neuropsychologic functioning in children with symptomatic human immunodeficiency virus infection. *Journal of Pediatrics, 117*, 980–985.

Buckley, R., & Schiff, R. (1991). The use of intravenous immune globulin in immuno-deficiency diseases. *New England Journal of Medicine, 325*, 110–117.

Butler, K. M., Husson, R. N., Balis, F. M., Brouwers, P., Eddy, J., El-Amin, D., Gress, J., Hawkins, M., Jarosinski, P., Moss, H., Poslack, D., Santacroce, S., Venzon, D., Wiener, L., Wolters, P., & Pizzo, P. A. (1991). Dideoxyinosine in children with symptomatic human immunodeficiency virus infection. *New England Journal of Medicine, 324*, 137–144.

Centers for Disease Control. (1981). Pneumocystis pneumonia—Los Angeles. *Morbidity and Mortality Weekly Report, 30*, 250–252.

Centers for Disease Control. (1987a). Revision of the CDC surveillance case definition for acquired immunodeficiency syndrome. *Morbidity and Mortality Weekly Report, 36* (Suppl. 1s), 1s–15s.

Centers for Disease Control. (1987b). Classification system for human immunodeficiency virus (HIV) Infection in children under 13 years of age. *Morbidity and Mortality Weekly Report, 35*, 225–235.

Centers for Disease Control. (1991). The HIV/AIDS epidemic: The first 10 years. *Morbidity and Mortality Weekly Report, 40*, 357–363.

Combination of AZT and ddI tested in children with HIV infection. (1992 Winter–Spring). *Clinical Research, 4–5*, 14.

Committee on Infectious Diseases, American Academy of Pediatrics (1991). Report of the committee on infectious diseases. Twenty-second edition. Elk Grove Village, IL: American Academy of Pediatrics.

Connor, E., Bagarazzi, M., McSherry, G., Holland, B., Boland, M., Denny, T., & Oleske, J. (1991). Clinical and laboratory correlates of *Pneumocystis carinii* pneumonia in children infected with HIV. *Journal of the American Medical Association, 265*, 1693–1697.

Connor, E., & McSherry, G. (1991). Antiviral treatment of human immunodeficiency virus infection in children. *Seminars in Pediatric Infectious Diseases, 2*, 285–300.

Czarniecki, L., & Oleske, J. (1991). Pain in children with HIV infection (Abstract). *Journal of Pain and Symptom Management, 6*, 177.

Evans, J. L., Chapman, E., Caldwell, B., & Luban, N. (1991). Clinical outcome of transfusion associated HIV in children. In *7th International Conference on AIDS Abstract Book*, June 1991 (Abstract M.C. 3355, vol. 1, p. 387). Florence, Italy.

Eyster, M. E. (1991). Transfusion and coagulation factor-acquired human immunodeficiency virus infection. *Pediatric Infectious Disease Journal, 10*, 50–56.

Fischl, M. A., Richman, D. D., Grieco, M. H., et al. The AZT Collaborative Working Group. (1987). The toxicity of azidothymidine (AZT) in the treatment of patients with AIDS and AIDS-related complex. *New England Journal of Medicine, 317*, 192–197.

Futterman, D., & Hein, D. (1991). Medical management of adolescents. In P. A. Pizzo & C. M. Wilfert (Eds.), *Pediatric AIDS* (pp. 531–545). Baltimore: Williams & Wilkins.

Goedert, J., Kessler, C. M., Aledort, L. M., et al. (1989). A prospective study of human immunodeficiency virus type 1 infection and the development of AIDS in subjects with hemophilia. *New England Journal of Medicine, 321*, 1141–1148.

Grubman, S., Conviser, R., & Oleske, J. (1992). HIV infection in infants, children, and adolescents. In G. Wormser (Ed.), *AIDS and Other Manifestations of HIV Infection* (pp. 201–216). New York: Raven Press.

Gwinn, M., Pappaioanou, M., George, J. R., et al. (1991). Prevalence of HIV infection in childbearing women in the United States. *Journal of the American Medical Association, 265*, 1704–1708.

Healy, B. (1992). Helping children infected with human immunodeficiency virus. *Journal of the American Medical Association, 267*, 1319.

Henderly, D. E., Freeman, W. R., Causey, D. M. & Rao, N. A. (1987). Cytomegalovirus retinitis and response to therapy with ganciclovir. *Ophthalmology, 94*, 425–434.

Hoyt, L. (1991, February). Atypical mycobacterial infection in pediatric AIDS. Paper presented at the 5th National Pediatric AIDS Conference, Washington, D.C.

Hughes, W. (1991). *Pneumocystis carinii* pneumonia. *Pediatric Infectious Disease Journal, 10*, 391–399.

Husson, R. N., & Pizzo, P. A. (1990). Lung disease in children with HIV. *Journal of Critical Illness, 5*, 440–458.

Kovacs, A., Frederick, T., Church, J., Eller, A., Oxtoby, M., & Mascola, L. (1991). CD4 T-lymphocyte counts and *Pneumocystis carinii* pneumonia in pediatric HIV infection. *Journal of the American Medical Association, 265*, 1698–1703.

McLoughlin, L. (1988). Nutrition and gastrointestinal disease in acquired immunodeficiency syndrome. *Topics in Clinical Nutrition, 3*, 72–76.

McSherry, G., Wright, M., Oleske, J., Connor, E. (1988). Frequency of serious adverse reactions to trimethoprim-sulfamethoxazole and pentamidine among children with human immunodeficiency virus (Abstract 1357). Paper presented at the Interscience Conference on Antimicrobial Agents and Chemotherapy.

Mofenson, L. M., Moye, J., Jr., Bethel, J., Hirschhorn, R., Jordan, C., Nugent, R., et al. (1992). Prophylactic intravenous immunoglobulin in HIV-infected children with CD4+ counts of 0.20×10^9/L or more. *Journal of the American Medical Association, 268*, 483–488.

National Institute of Child Health and Human Development Intravenous Immunoglobulin Study Group. (1991). Intravenous immune gobulin for the prevention of bacterial infections in children with symptomatic human immunodeficiency virus infection. *New England Journal of Medicine, 325*, 73–80.

NIH/NIAID AIDS Clinical Trials Group Protocol 043 Team. (1990). Safety and efficacy of zidovudine in children with AIDS of severe AIDS-related complex (Abstract 105). *Pediatric Research, 27,* 178a.

Nightingale, S. L. (1991). Didanosine (DDI) approved for advanced HIV infection. *Journal of the American Medical Association, 266,* 2528.

Oleske, J. (1991). Personal communication.

Oleske, J., Minnefor, A., Cooper, R., Jr., Thomas, K., dela Cruz, A., Ahdieh, H., Guerrero, I., Joshi, V. V., & Desposito, F. (1983). Immune deficiency syndrome in children. *Journal of the American Medical Association, 249,* 2345–2349.

Oxtoby, M. J. (1991). Perinatally acquired human immunodeficiency virus. *Pediatric Infectious Diseases Journal, 9,* 609–619.

Pelton, S. I. & Klein J. O. (1991). Bacterial diseases in infants and children with infections due to HIV. In P. A. Pizzo & C. M. Wilfert (Eds.), *Pediatric AIDS* (pp. 199–208). Baltimore: Williams & Wilkins.

Pizzo, P. A., Butler, K., Balis, F. Brouwers, E., Hawkins, M., Eddy, J., & Einloth, M. (1990). Dideoxycytidine alone and in an alternating schedule with zidovudine in children with symptomatic human immunodeficiency virus infection. *Journal of Pediatrics, 117,* 799–808.

Pizzo, P. A., Eddy, J., Falloon, J., Balis, F. M., Murphy, R. F., Moss, H. et al. (1988). Effect of continuous intravenous infusion of zidovudine (AZT) in children with symptomatic HIV infection. *New England Journal of Medicine, 319,* 889–896.

Pressman, H., & Morrison, S. (1988). Dysphagia in the pediatric AIDS population. *Dysphagia, 2,* 166–169.

Prober, C. G., & Gershon, A. A. (1992). Medical management of newborns and infants born to human immunodeficiency virus-seropositive mothers. *Pediatric Infectious Disease Journal, 10,* 684–695.

Ragni, M. V. (1989). Medical aspects of hemophilia and AIDS. *FOCUS: A Guide to AIDS Research, 4*(5).

Rogers, M. F., Ou, C-Y, Kilbourne, B., & Schochetman, G. (1991). Advances and problems in the diagnosis of HIV infection in infants. In P. A. Pizzo & C. M. Wilfert (Eds.), *Pediatric AIDS* (pp. 159–174). Baltimore: Williams & Wilkins.

Rogers, M., Ou, C-Y, Rayfield, M., Thomas, P. A., Schoenbaum, E. E., Abrams, E., et al. (1989). Use of the polymerase chain reaction for early detection of the proviral sequences of human immunodeficiency virus in infants born to seropositive mothers. *New England Journal of Medicine, 320,* 1649–1654.

Rosenberg, Z. F., & Fauci, A. S. (1991). Immunopathology and pathogenesis of HIV infection. In P. A. Pizzo & C. M. Wilfert (Eds.), *Pediatric AIDS* (pp. 82–94). Baltimore: Williams & Wilkins.

Rubinstein, A., Sislick, M., Gupta, A., Bernstein, L., Klein, N., Rubinstein, E. et al. (1983). Acquired immunodeficiency with reversed T_4/T_8 ratios in infants born to promiscuous and drug-addicted mothers. *Journal of the American Medical Association, 249,* 2340–2345.

Schmitt, F. A., Bigley, J. W., McKinnis, R., Logue, P. E., Evans, R. W., Drucker, J. L., & AZT Collaborative Working Group. (1988). Neuropsychological outcome of zidovudine (AZT) treatment of patients with AIDS and AIDS-related complex. *New England Journal of Medicine, 319,* 1573–1578.

Scott, G., Hutto, C., Makuch, R., Mastrucci, M., O'Connor, T., Mitchell, C., Trapido, E., & Parks, W. (1989). Survival in children with perinatally acquired human immunodeficiency virus type 1 infection. *New England Journal of Medicine, 321,* 1791–1796.

van't Wout, J. (1991). Candidiasis: pathogenesis & therapy. *Opportunistic Infections: Pathogenesis & Therapy.* Proceedings of the satellite symposium conducted at the 7th International Conference on AIDS, Florence, Italy.

Volberding, P. A., Lagakos, S. W., Koch, M. A., Pettinelli, C., Myers, M. W., Booth, D. K. et al. (1990). Zidovudine in asymptomatic human immunodeficiency virus infection: a controlled trial in persons with fewer than 500 CD4-positive cells per cubic millimeter. *New England Journal of Medicine, 332,* 941–949.

Walsh, T. J., & Butler, K. M. (1991). Fungal infections complicating pediatric AIDS. In P. A. Pizzo & C. M. Wilfert (Eds.), *Pediatric AIDS* (pp. 225–244). Baltimore: Williams & Wilkins.

Wilfert, C. M. (1991). HIV infection in maternal and pediatric patients. *Hospital Practice, 26*(5), 55–67.

Wiznia, A., & Nicholas, S. (1990). Organ system involvement in HIV-infected children. *Pediatric Annals, 19,* 475–481.

Working Group on PCP Prophylaxis in Children. (1991). Guidelines for prophylaxis against *Pneumocystis carinii* pneumonia for children infected with human immunodeficiency virus. *Morbidity and Mortality Weekly Report, 40* (RR-2), 1–13.

Part IV
Perspectives on Selected Issues Affecting Women and Children

11

Family and Living Issues for HIV-Infected Children

Wendy Nehring, Katherine Malm, and Donna Harris

Pediatric HIV infection affects every individual having contact with the infected child, including immediate family, extended family, friends, neighbors, health workers, and social service personnel. As the number of children affected by HIV grows, so will the impact of this pediatric condition on society. Not only are such demographic variables as race and socioeconomic status factors in treatment and outcome, but a subset of children with both HIV infection and hemophilia creates special challenges for society and the health-care community (see Chapter 10). Each family has unique features, underscoring rapid changes in American families over the past two decades. Unfortunately, the literature on pediatric HIV infection has tended to focus on the medical issues of HIV infection, descriptions of sample care plans, and descriptions of clinic programs rather than on research around such family issues as the impact of HIV infection and AIDS on the family, the child's environment, care of the child, placement of the child, and educational issues.

IMPACT ON THE FAMILY

Pediatric HIV infection often touches more than one member of the family (see Chapter 2) and is disproportionately a disease of the poor and minority groups, mainly black and Hispanic. Figure 11.1 illustrates the ecological system of the child with HIV infection. As noted, this disease affects how the child is educated, how his or her family is viewed, and how society responds.

At present, children with HIV infection are living longer because of better treatments and quality of care, especially in the home setting, leading to the view by some that pediatric HIV infection is a chronic illness (Abrams & Nicholas, 1990). It is also known that neurological complications of HIV infection in children usually result in developmental disabilities and the loss of acquired developmental milestones (Cohen, Mundy et al., 1991; Schmitt, Seeger,

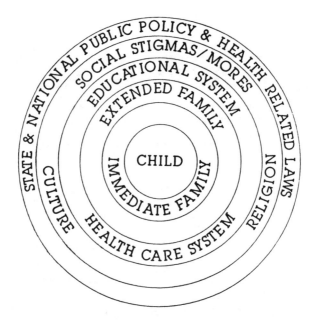

FIGURE 11.1 The ecological system of the child with HIV infection.

Kieciz, Enenhel, & Jacobi, 1991). Furthermore, once the child becomes symptomatic, death will be the eventual outcome. Thus the elements of a terminal disease are present (Dailey, 1991). All of these factors characterize the picture of the child with AIDS (see Figure 11.2).

Families having children with *developmental disabilities* speak of chronic sorrow, lessened expectations, slowed developmental milestones, marital problems, and the child's being "different" (Crnic, Friedrich, & Greenberg, 1983). Families of children with *chronic illness* speak of altered self-images, behavior problems, decreased social interactions, altered daily routines, isolation, financial problems, and the "sick role" (Meyers & Weitzman, 1990). Emotional, financial, and social issues are concerns in children with terminal cancer (Dailey, 1991). Pediatric HIV infection encompasses all of these concerns. In addition, pediatric AIDS is a progressive, multisystem disease having acute exacerbations, involves other family members, and largely affects an already disenfranchised segment of society.

Other members of the child's immediate family, including one or both parents, are often HIV-infected and may be ill or have died from complications of the disease. Siblings may also be infected with HIV. The diagnosis of HIV infection in family members and the possibility of death are frightening but nec-

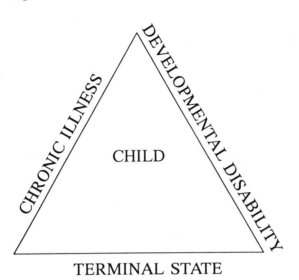

FIGURE 11.2 Pediatric AIDS/HIV health effect.

essary discussion topics. Often the unaffected siblings are forgotten in concerted efforts to acquire medical care and social supports for the affected family members. It is important to understand the feelings and thoughts these "unaffected" children may have regarding their family member's illness. Common fears involve death, infection of other members, and financial problems. Feelings of anger, abandonment, guilt, and loneliness also occur. Therefore, the noninfected siblings must be assured that their feelings are heard and attended to. Misinformation should be corrected, including self-blame. Older unaffected siblings of children with HIV infection are often observed to function as parental caregivers, and role-reversal may occur. Parents should be encouraged to spend "special" time with each child, attend to the developmental needs of each child, keep to a normal routine, not favor any one child, and pay particular attention to any school problems that may develop in uninfected children (Waterbury, 1991).

Siblings who have been asked about their reactions to having a brother or sister with HIV infection have reported that they told only those who would understand or that they did not tell anyone. They also believed and hoped for the recovery of their family members (Cohen, Nehring, Malm, & Harris, 1991). Further exploration of sibling response is needed to have a fuller understanding of family relationships when a member is infected with HIV.

In a recent study of families having adult members infected with HIV, subjects were asked to identify their major concerns. The major concerns reported were the uncertainty regarding the future, a desire to maintain physical and/or psychological health, social unacceptability, fatigue, and weight loss (Longo, Spross, & Locke, 1990). The concerns were similar among participants in a pilot study of seven families with a child who was perinatally infected with HIV. Specifically, the major concerns identified through a semistructured interview with either one or both parents encompassed the functioning of the entire immediate family. Parents emphasized social unacceptibility, the uncertainty of the child's future, the child's symptoms and pain, the mother's fatigue and physical condition, sibling response to the diagnosis, and the usual care for the affected child as major concerns. These concerns are detailed in Table 11.1. Families spoke of withholding the diagnosis from family and friends, marveling that their spouse would stand by, the "specialness" of the child and its meaning to the mother, feelings of blame for the child's illness by the mother, and the sibling's reactions to a father's prior death. Each family was unique in its experiences and coping, yet commonalities existed because of the continued stigma surrounding this disease (Cohen, Nehring et al., 1991).

The effects of pediatric HIV infection on grandparents is not well documented. In the area of developmental disabilities, grandparents have been found to fill roles of child-care assistant, caregiver, gift giver, playmate, and teacher therapist (Sonnek, 1986). In some cases, the paternal grandmother has "blamed" a daughter-in-law for the birth of a child with handicaps. An understanding of their fears and explanations of the child's condition have helped remedy this situation over time (Pieper, 1976). There is little research about grandparents' emotional response to the impending loss of both a child and a grandchild.

It is known that in many cultures the grandmother plays an important role in the upbringing of those living with her, including her grandchildren. If she is accepting of the HIV/AIDS diagnosis, often her support is tantamount to the well-being of her grandchild; therefore, grandparents should be considered in the planning of the child's care if they are viewed as an important support for the family (see Chapter 2).

Beyond the family environment are nursing issues related to the community and society. The interaction between the child and his or her family with the health-care and educational systems must be considered in any discussion of the impact of HIV infection on families. The impact of this disease on social mores and the culture of the family has already been mentioned. As noted in Table 11.1, the family's religion and feelings concerning spirituality greatly affect coping and prognosis. Members of religious communities also express their feelings regarding this disease in their words and actions. These do not always reflect sensitivity and concern and may actually convey judgment, blame and further stigmatize the child and family. On the other hand, feelings of spirituality often greatly affect coping processes in a positive manner. Finally, laws and policies that further structure how we live are mentioned in the discussions involving education and alternative living situations.

TABLE 11.1 Family Concerns and Responses to Pediatric HIV Infection/AIDS

Concern category	Adaption problems	Adaptive response	Emotional response
Social unacceptibility	Rejection of family and friends Revealing diagnosis of mother and child Fear of harm to personal possessions Loss of home Loss of personal life Isolation	Not tell father's family or friends Not trusting/Lying Overprotectiveness of child Strengthen marriage Not a normal family Play stupid	Anxiety Fear Relief "Slap in face" Sadness Anger Depression
Uncertainty of child's future	Fear of child's dying Blame Possessiveness of child Mood swings Lack of knowledge of HIV	Cherishing child World upside down Little use of babysitters Put in God's hands Take one day at a time Trying to be better parent	Hope Grief Faith in God Guilt Fear Depression Sadness
Child's symptoms and pain	Blame Future medical problems Future hospital stays and procedures	Shock Honest explanations Hope	Fear Guilt Depression
Mother's fatigue and physical condition	Change in lifestyle Loss in employment Loss of finances Child not sleeping through night Mother's mood swings Decreased socialization Loss of personal life	Hope for cure Spouse altering his work hours One day at a time Make the best of it Home health aide Support from partner, friends Continue to plan for future	Fear of future Anger Frustration Depression Denial by husband
Sibling Response to HIV	Death of father Sibs with emotional problems Financial burdens Fear of mother's death Interaction with child with HIV	Counseling for siblings Extra concern Hope for cure Treat normal except no biting No childhood compromise	Fear of death Fear of isolation Hope Confusion
Normal Care for the affected child	Social isolation Honesty in answering questions Playing with friends who don't know	Enforce no biting rules Don't leave alone	Fear of infection

Adapted from Cohen, F. L., Nehring, W. M., Malm, I. C., & Harris, D. (1991), Family relationships in pediatric HIV/AIDS and other at-risk conditions. Exploring individual family relationships, unpublished manuscript, University of Illinois, Chicago, IL.

PEDIATRIC HIV/AIDS PROGRAMS

Since the onset of AIDS in the pediatric population, medical and support programs have been created to meet needs presented by children and their families. Important factors that figure into a successful program include a family-centered approach, a multidisciplinary focus, knowledge of the demographic variables of the population served, availability of appropriate professionals, and knowledge of community resources. These points will be discussed below.

Any program established to deal with children with HIV infection must be family-centered. In addition to providing care and services for the child, programs must deal with the complex needs of the families in which these children live, whether they be natural, foster, or adoptive. Because of the complexity of the problems presented by the child infected with HIV and his or her family, a multidisciplinary approach appears to be the most effective. Members from only one discipline are simply not able to deal effectively with all of the needs presented by these children and their families.

The multidisciplinary teams set up to provide treatment and services are characterized by a basic core team, which consists minimally of a physician, a nurse, and a social worker. The composition of the multidisciplinary team is usually based on two important factors: (1) the demographic characteristics of the target population; (2) the availability of appropriate professionals and community resources, including funding.

The physician directs the medical treatment of the child. The nurse coordinates the medical and nursing plans and care. The nurse also provides health-related educational services to the child and parent and provides general information about HIV, its mode of transmission, and methods that can be used to prevent transmission. The nurse may also be a source of emotional support for the child and family. The social worker provides financial and social-service information and support. Counseling and emotional support for these families is a shared responsibility of team members, particularly of the nurse and social worker.

The demographic characteristics of the pediatric HIV population varies from area to area, and these differences directly affect membership in the multidisciplinary team. A comparison of the population at the AIDS Comprehensive Family Center at Albert Einstein College of Medicine in New York City with the population being treated in the program at Los Angeles Children's Hospital illustrates this variance in population characteristics. In the New York City program, 90% of the population is considered below the poverty level and is on public assistance. The ethnic background of the patients is predominantly Hispanic. Less than 20% of the children live with their mothers, most of whom are unmarried. Most of the children in this program became HIV-infected through perinatal transmission of HIV (Seibert, Garcia, Caplan, & Septimus, 1989).

In contrast, only 26% of the families in the Los Angeles program live below the poverty line, with 35% classified as middle income or better. The ethnic background of this group is nearly equally divided among blacks, Hispanics, and non-Hispanic whites. Over 90% of these children live with their parents, and the majority of the mothers are married. Approximately 50% of the pediatric cases were transfusion-related, and about 41% were due to perinatal transmission (Seibert et al., 1989).

The demographic differences between these two populations require different programmatic approaches. The first program must deal with a predominantly Hispanic population living in poverty. Issues of language, culture, substance abuse, and poverty are high priorities in this program. A program with this population must place a high priority on bilingual professionals, with an understanding of the cultural diversity and values of the Hispanic population groups. The poverty of this population may require a focus on such basic needs as food and housing and the provision of basic health services. In contrast, the Los Angeles program must deal with a culturally diverse population that is predominantly middle income. In this program, having a bilingual staff may not be a high priority. Since basic needs are less of a concern, team members may have to deal with the subtler issues of family adjustment and future expectations (Seibert et al., 1989).

A second issue concerns the availability of the appropriate professionals for the team. Children with HIV and their families present a wide spectrum of needs. In addition to medical and nursing care, needs related to the physical, social, and emotional development of the child as well as the supportive needs of parents or caregivers must be addressed. In situations involving parental infection, experience has shown that client needs are best met by a team of specialists such as physicians, nurses, social workers, psychologists, psychiatrists, neurologists, dieticians, speech therapists, and physical and occupational therapists. Additional specialties such as child life, pastoral care, special education, pharmacy, and others may also be represented on the team. The real constraints of the multidisciplinary team composition may be the availability of these professionals and/or funding for their services. These restraints may be the determinants of whether a professional is a permanent member of the team or utilized on a consulting basis.

Community Resources

An additional component of any comprehensive family-centered care program serving the pediatric HIV population is the linkage between families and supportive community organizations. These links give additional support to the caregivers and allow the HIV-infected child to stay in the home environment for longer periods. Hospitalizations tend to be shorter and less frequent when caregivers and children are members of service-rich supportive communities. Some of these supportive services include day care, respite care, special education services, home health nursing, hospice, visiting nurse services, counseling services, legal services, substance abuse treatment programs, and bereavement services. Some of these services focus on the child while others support the parents or caregivers. Their importance cannot be overemphasized. For instance, access to a substance abuse treatment program for the drug addicted mother is imperative if other services and agencies are to work for this family (Woodruff & Durkosterzin, 1988). When the mother is in a recovery program, she is more likely to utilize the other services available to her.

National pediatric HIV resources also exist and should be used by local programs and interested professionals and family members as appropriate. The National Pediatric HIV Resource Center (NPHRC) is funded in part by the Health Resources and Services Administration and is a project of the Children's Hospital of New Jersey. This center provides a range of services for professionals, including consultative services, technical assistance, and referrals (Centers for Disease Control, 1991). The Center can be reached by calling 1-800-362-0071 or (201) 268-8251, or by writing the National Pediatric HIV Resource Center, Children's Hospital of New Jersey, 15 South 9th St., Newark, NJ 07107.

The National Cancer Institute Pediatric Branch actively develops and carries out clinical protocols for children with HIV infection, for which any child up to 21 years of age is eligible. For additional information, contact the National Cancer Institute Pediatric Branch, Building 10, Room 13N240, Bethesda, MD 20892, or call (301) 402-0696.

The Centers for Disease Control (CDC) has also worked with various state and local education agencies to produce materials and implement effective HIV education programs. For further information, contact the Division of Adolescent and School Health, Centers for Disease Control, 1600 Clifton Rd., Mail Stop K-31, Atlanta, GA 30333, or call (404) 488-5372.

Another extremely important aspect of any comprehensive family care program is the educational component of the program. Within the program there is a need to educate parents about family planning and birth control. The possibility of transmitting HIV to sexual partners and any children born to HIV-infected mothers makes education a high priority in any program (see Chapter 4). Additionally, foster parents and other caregivers need information on how the virus is transmitted and how to incorporate universal precautions into care. Expert professionals within these programs must also assume some responsibility for community education. Professionals in these programs must become involved in the development of community education programs to stop the spread of HIV, educate the community and other health professionals about HIV, and how to care for the child with HIV infection sensitively and without fear. An urgent need exists for outreach education programs, especially for certain high-risk populations such as adolescents (see Chapter 9). Thus, the goal of any family-centered pediatric HIV program is to coordinate hospital and clinic care with community resources to serve the HIV-infected families and provide them the support they need in their own ethnic, societal, and religious context (Septimus, 1989).

EDUCATIONAL ISSUES

Early in the HIV epidemic, schools with an infected child frequently responded in ways not in the best interests of children and families. Fear and prejudice rather than scientific knowledge led some schools to isolate HIV-infected children. Legislative and legal decisions and policy development have resulted in clearer school policies and a better understanding of the disease process.

School policy recommendations have been written to address many issues (American Academy of Pediatrics, Communicable Infectious Disease Committee, 1987; Task Force on Pediatric AIDS, 1989; Centers for Disease Control, 1985). Many states have passed legislation affecting the educational rights of HIV-infected children after specific and celebrated lawsuits were filed in the cases of Ryan White (Indiana) and the Ray brothers (Florida), who all had hemophilia and contracted AIDS from transfusions. Important to these policies and laws are the concepts of significant risk, a "real and valid threat" to the school, the least restrictive environment, universal precautions, confidentiality, and screening.

Significant risk simply implies that the child cannot be refused an education based upon his or her diagnosis (Hanlon, 1991). The least restrictive environment ensures that the child is placed in a classroom that best meets the child's medical and educational needs. Such placement may require special education based upon the child's developmental learning needs and/or medical needs due to open wounds or biting behaviors. It is imperative that school personnel are well informed to avoid the social isolation and fear that can lead to social and behavioral problems in the child (Horan & Sherman, 1988). An excellent discussion of the legal history behind HIV infection and the schools is found in Hanlon (1991).

P.L. 99-142, the Education for All Handicapped Children Act, first enacted in 1975, assures every individual between 3 to 21 years a right to an education, including a due process hearing if a family feels their child's needs are not being adequately met. P.L. 99-457, Part H, of the Individuals with Disabilities Education Act (IDEA), first signed into law in 1986, discusses the right for early childhood education between the years of 3 to 5, with the option for early intervention between birth and 3 years. As part of fulfilling the criteria in Part H, an Individualized Family Service Plan must be written and periodically reviewed and updated for the child and his or her family. Therefore, the child with HIV infection should be referred to such programs as needed. These are often free, and many have available transportation. Presently, integration of children with HIV infection into these programs is slow as programs are developed and the institution of universal precautions by staff is initiated.

One such program is the Bronx Municipal Hospital Center day-care program, which was developed in 1986 in New York City. A multidisciplinary staff is present to care for two groups of children, infant-toddlers, and preschoolers infected with HIV. Besides following through on the child's educational plan and attending to any medical needs or procedures, a weekly support meeting is offered to both staff and parents (Lelyveld, 1990). It is not clear if the program follows an Individualized Family Service Plan as detailed in P.L. 99-457.

ALTERNATIVE LIVING ARRANGEMENTS

As the incidence of HIV infection in the pediatric population increases, increasing numbers of HIV-infected children are living with someone other than their biological parents. This arrangement largely stems from the inability of an infected parent to provide adequate child care. In some cases, the mother's illness has progressed to the point that she is no longer able to care for the child. In others, children have been abandoned by drug-using mothers who turn to the streets and/or prostitution to support their chemical dependence. In still other situations, the child's own illness is so severe that continued placement in the biological parents' home is impossible (Boland, Evans, Connor, & Oleske, 1988).

Initially there was little response to the growing number of those HIV-infected infants who were unwanted or abandoned. Many remained housed on pediatric units, creating an increasing number of "boarder babies" (Meintz & Lynch, 1989). Foster placement was not available to these babies at that time because of the unjustified contagion fears of potential foster families. In the New York City area where the pediatric HIV-infected population was largest, whole units were dedicated to housing and caring for these boarder babies. The Comprehensive Family Center at Albert Einstein College of Medicine found that less than 20% of the children in their program were living with their biological parents (Seibert et al., 1989). Facilities were strained to their limits.

In addition to cost-related issues, boarding these infants in specialized hospital units was counterproductive to the children's welfare since they did not need the specialized care of the hospital. Instead, these children needed the nurturing care of families and stable caregivers. As a result, intensive efforts were mounted to identify foster families for these children. Such foster families exist as either the nuclear family (one or two parents) or a group of families who share the foster parenting of children with HIV (Meintz & Lynch, 1989).

Only within the past 7 years have governmental and professional groups outlined policies related to the foster care of children with AIDS. Information on individual state policies regarding the foster care of children with HIV infection and AIDS is limited. In a recent study, only 21 states were found to have foster-care policies regarding children with HIV infection and AIDS. Licensing standards and supplementary services varied for the foster families across states (Cohen & Nehring, 1991).

In 1985, the Centers for Disease Control (CDC) issued a set of recommendations regarding the education and foster care of children with AIDS. At that time and to date, no known cases of HIV infection have been transmitted horizontally as a result of being in school, daycare, or foster care (Centers for Disease Control, 1985; Hanlon, 1991). Among the recommendations made by the CDC were the following: (1) decisions for the education and care setting for the child should be based upon behavior, neurological development, and the physical state of the child in relation to the expected type of interactions the child would be having; (2) if the infected child lacks control of bodily secretions, displays biting behaviors, and/or has oozing wounds, a more restricted environment is needed, and this environment should be reassessed regularly; (3) individuals should take routine hygienic precautions when handling secretions; and (4) HIV screening should be done prior to the child's placement in a foster home as the family has a right to know the child's HIV status (Centers for Disease Control, 1985).

In 1987, the Communicable Infectious Disease Committee of the American Academy of Pediatrics published guidelines regarding attendance of children with AIDS in daycare and foster-care settings. Their recommendations included (1) the placement of the child on an individual basis, taking into account the potential risk and need for optimal care; (2) procedures regarding the control of bodily secretions; (3) the principle that widespread screening for AIDS is not currently needed; (4) the need for physician assessment if both clinical and epidemiologic signs and symptoms of AIDS were present in a child; and (5) the child and family's right to privacy (American Academy of Pediatrics, Committee on Infectious Diseases, 1987). Another view is that parents cannot make "an informed choice" about choosing a day-care center for their child if they are not told that an HIV-infected child is present (Fenster, 1992).

In 1989, the Task Force on Pediatric AIDS of the American Academy of Pediatrics published a document on placement of children with AIDS in adoption or foster care. Considered were issues of social stigma, the fear of the spread of HIV infection among family members and the physical, and emotional burdens placed upon a family. The Task Force stressed the urgent need for additional special support services, including (1) accurate information regarding the child's health status; (2) education and counseling concerning all aspects of the child's medical care; (3) financial support, including health and psychosocial expenses; (4) respite care, including day care and babysitting; (5) psychological counseling without pay for individuals and families as a group; and (6) social and legal counseling without pay. The Task Force also concurred with the CDC recommendations (1985) that preplacement testing for HIV should be done at the request of the physician or the foster parents. If the child to be placed is not currently HIV positive, and has a risk of exposure to HIV, regular retesting should be done. Also, placement in a foster home should be done by an interdisciplinary committee.

In 1992, the Task Force on Pediatric AIDS of the American Academy of Pediatrics published guidelines for HIV-infected children and their foster families. Among their recommendations were (1) there is no reason to restrict foster care or child care to protect either the foster family members or child-care personnel, as horizontal transmission risk is negligible; (2) child-care personnel do not need to be informed of the HIV status of a child to protect either the caregiver or other children. They reiterate the necessity for universal precautions in all child-care settings and the necessity for such programs to inform all parents when an infectious disease such as chickenpox occurs in any child in the setting. They note that the parent of an HIV-positive child may choose to inform the child-care provider so that assistance for any special needs may be provided.

Initial efforts at recruiting foster families early in the AIDS epidemic were not very successful because of common misconceptions and fears. Even after educational programs were instituted to educate the public about HIV and its transmission, few foster families were recruited. At first, many families who wished to care for these children were allowed to do so without being previously licensed as foster parents (Meintz & Lynch, 1989). Experiences with these first foster families indicated that there was a need for a mechanism to screen out families that could not deal with the problems associated with an HIV-infected child. Experience also demonstrated that these foster parents needed continued emotional and financial support as well as education and guidance on care for the child and themselves. Maintenance of these foster homes required intensive medical and psychological support services (Gurdin & Anderson, 1987). Fear of the child dying, transmission of the disease to other family members, and social isolation remain major concerns in the decision to become foster parents of children with HIV (Cohen & Nehring, 1991).

Foster Care for Children with AIDS

In 1985, the first foster-care program solely for children with AIDS was founded at the Leake and Watts Children's Home in New York City. Recruitment came from personal and community networking. Criteria for foster parent selection included (1) being single or married; (2) no children living in the home below the age of 10 years to protect the child with HIV infection from potential childhood infections; (3) being well informed about the disease, expressing confidence in caring for such a child, and having little fear about the transmission of the disease. Most of the parents originally chosen had some medical background. A maximum of two children were placed in any one home (Gurdin & Anderson, 1987). Usually the selected foster parents were not employed. The major part of their income came from foster care monthly payments. In New York as in many of the states, foster care payment for children with AIDS is the highest provided by the state (Gurdin & Anderson, 1987).

Foster care is the option of choice for many children infected with HIV. In a foster home the child is able to receive the individualized care and attention needed for optimal growth and development. Unfortunately, in areas of the country where the pediatric HIV population is largest and increasing rapidly, foster care placement has not been able to keep pace with the growing need (Boland et al., 1988). In these areas, alternatives to individualized foster care are being explored. One form of alternative placement for these children is a group foster home. One model for the group home is Grandma's House in Washington, D.C., established as an alternative for HIV-infected babies remaining in the hospital. Grandma's House has four beds, with one bed reserved for emergency situations. By keeping the numbers low, the group house hopes to provide one-to-one interaction. This home provides 24-hour care for the children as well as family counseling, education, and training for volunteers. The demand for the services offered by Grandma's House has been so great that a second home is being planned that will offer daycare for children infected with HIV. Offering daycare as an option will allow some mothers to continue to work and keep their babies. It can also assist the working foster mother and offer respite for families that need some relief from care (Laxton, 1989).

Still another form of foster home is the transitional foster home, illustrated by St. Clare's Home for Children in New Jersey. This setting allows for temporary placement of children 6 years or younger with HIV infection until they can return to their biological family or an alternative placement, either foster care or adoption. A multidisciplinary staff designs each child's plan of care around his or her medical and developmental needs. Family visitation and foster parent training are also provided (Zealand, 1989). Because of a lack of foster families and the continued stigma surrounding HIV/AIDS, alternative group homes for children with or without a parent appear to be a realistic approach to providing the best medical care and maintaining a type of family environment.

In the majority of cases, the ideal situation for the child infected with HIV is to remain home with his or her biological parents. When this is no longer possible, relatives may be able to take responsibility for the care of the child. Services should remain the same when the child is cared for by relatives. When placement with relatives is not an option, a foster or adoptive home is the next best alternative. Adoption, however, is not always possible because the mother often does not wish to relinquish custody of the child. Some mothers with AIDS need to retain the final hope that at some time in the future they might be able to care for their child again.

Residential Placement

A final alternative is residential placement. Some children with AIDS who have neurological problems and developmental disabilities are placed in long-term facilities. Fear of transmission and stigma prohibit attempts at foster family placement, and the segregation of these children frequently continues until their death.

The quality of life for each child affected with HIV is the primary concern surrounding placement. Planning for the best living situation requires a team approach by the biological family and the social and health personnel. Placement, whether temporary or permanent, should be sensitively considered, and the child should be included in this decision when possible. Also, families should remain intact as much as possible, with efforts made to keep siblings together. Continued follow-up by health and social welfare professionals is vital.

THE NURSING ROLE

Nurses more than any other health workers interact with families affected by HIV in their professional and personal roles, thus encountering families in a variety of settings: homes, clinics, hospitals, religious settings, schools, and communities. Coordination of care by nurses in all arenas is important. The nurse is an advocate for the child and his or her family and must prioritize the family's needs, exercising a nonjudgmental approach at all times. Some important areas where nursing can assist the family include aiding the family in discussing the diagnosis with the affected individual and other family members, considering new treatments, using resources, identifying disease progression, and referring to respite and hospice services.

Family Reaction

Families often first have a difficult time accepting the diagnosis of HIV infection and AIDS and then find it difficult to discuss the ramifications of this illness with other family members, especially the other children. As more HIV-infected children live beyond 6 years, the diagnosis must be discussed with the child. Nurses can help parents to use age-appropriate language to communicate the information and their feelings. For the child with AIDS, parents must understand that neurological deficits require that information be shared at the child's developmental level, not for his or her chronological age.

Death is an ever-present concern of families affected by HIV infection and AIDS. Depending on the child's age and family circumstances, planning for that child's death can be very painful. If the child is older, allowing that child to express his or her feelings and plans regarding death is very helpful. Some children decide when they no longer want to continue treatment; others plan their own funerals. When parents die before the children, placement decisions must be made. If this placement is to be made with relatives, legal guardian papers must be initiated and signed. If foster or adoptive placement is desired, opportunities to meet with these families should be arranged and in some cases, placement (or at least placement planning) before the parent dies may be in the child's best interests. Today, programs are being developed to assist HIV-infected parents in identifying potential adoptive/foster home families for both their infected and uninfected children prior to the death of the parents.

When a parent has AIDS, a nurse often notices subtle changes in his or her personality or behaviors as the disease progresses. These changes may first appear as noncompliance. At this time, written rather than verbal instructions and/or information are preferred and are more apt to be comprehended and followed. Repetition of instruction or information and verbal feedback is also a confirming approach.

New treatment protocols are constantly emerging for pediatric HIV infection (see Chapter 10). These treatments create both fear of the unknown and hope for families. Nurses can help affected families to understand treatment approaches and what is needed from them to benefit from the treatment protocol. Dealing with the emotions of all family members as they consider choices can be just as important as discussing the details of the proposed treatment (see Chapter 2).

Many resources are available to assist families with children affected by HIV. Yet many families fail to fully embrace these services. Thus the nurse's role includes making the initial contact for the families and following up as needed. On the other hand, families are often able to form informal support networks from the pool of families they meet at the treatment sites. Frequently these groups are more helpful than organized groups arranged by professionals. These families may be to support one another through crises and death.

Respite, either short or long term, is important to the physical and mental well-being of the family. Respite can take the form of babysitters, daycare, in-home volunteers, or an alternative home setting. While few such respite programs exist currently, they are well worth the effort to locate and make known to the family.

Coping

A final issue for the nurse is his or her coping ability. The nurse is unable to adequately care for the families he or she sees if he or she is not well or is "burned out." The nurse must also take care of her/himself. The unexpected course of this illness in children often leaves the nurse just as emotionally involved as any family member. For example, some children may have a chronic course of illness, while another may do fine for a long period followed by an acute episode and death. Nurses too must form support groups to understand HIV infection and AIDS, to provide informed assistance to families, and to have a safe haven for sharing their feelings and concerns. Difficult issues which many nurses must face include changes in the child's illness and consequent care changes, coping with both personal and professional losses, denial in family members and other professional staff, and dealing with family members at different stages of acceptance and grief. In some cases, the health-care institution can provide such services in formal or informal ways.

CONCLUSION

In time, each person will be touched by HIV infection, either personally or professionally. The effects on families can be devastating. After the diagnosis of HIV infection, each family member's life is forever changed. Hopefully, the social stigma and isolation now still associated with HIV infection and AIDS will change, but until this happens, nurses must provide sensitive care and support to children and families in need of their expertise and strength.

REFERENCES

Abrams, E. J., & Nicholas, S. W. (1990). Pediatric HIV infection. *Pediatric Annals, 19*, 482–487.

American Academy of Pediatrics, Committee on Infectious Diseases (1987). Health guidelines for the attendance in day care and foster care settings of children infected with human immunodeficiency virus. *Pediatrics, 79*, 466–471.

Boland, M. G., Evans, P., Connor, E. M., & Oleske, J. M. (1988). Foster care needs of children with HIV infection. *AIDS and Public Policy Journal, 3*(1), 8–9.

Centers for Disease Control. (1985). Education and foster care of children infected with human T-lymphotropic virus type III/lymphadenopathy-associated virus. *Morbidity and Mortality Weekly Report, 34*(34), 517–521.

Centers for Disease Control. (1991). *HIV/AIDS prevention, July 1991* (pp. 1–19).

Cohen, F. L., & Nehring, W. M. (1991). Foster care of children with HIV/AIDS: A national study. Unpublished manuscript, University of Illinois, Chicago, IL.

Cohen, F. L., Nehring, W. M., Malm, K., & Harris, D. (1991). Family relationships in pediatric HIV/AIDS and other at-risk conditions: Exploring individual family relationships. Unpublished manuscript, University of Illinois, Chicago, IL.

Cohen, S. E., Mundy, T., Karussik, B., Lieb, L., Ludwig, D. D., & Ward, J. (1991). Neuropsychological functioning in human immunodeficiency virus type 1 seropositive children infected through neonatal blood transfusion. *Pediatrics, 88*, 58–68.

Crnic, K. A., Friedrich, W. N., & Greenberg, M. T. (1983). Adaptation of families with mentally retarded children: A model of stress, coping and family ecology. *American Journal of Mental Deficiency, 88*, 125–138.

Dailey, A. A. (1991). Terminal care for the child with AIDS. In P. A. Pizzo & C. A. Wilfert (Eds.), *Pediatric AIDS* (pp. 619–629). Baltimore: Williams & Wilkins.

Fenster, D. L. (1992). HIV and day care. *Pediatrics, 89*, 690.

Gurdin, P., & Anderson, G. R. (1987). Quality care for ill children: AIDS-specialized foster family homes. *Child Welfare, 66*(4), 291–302.

Hanlon, S. F. (1991). School and day care issues: The legal perspective. In P. A. Pizzo & C. A. Wilfert (Eds.), *Pediatric AIDS* (pp. 693–703). Baltimore: Williams & Wilkins.

Horan, P. F., & Sherman, R. A. (1988). School psychologists and the AIDS epidemic. *Professional School Psychology*, *3*(1), 33–49.

Laxton, C. E. (1989). Grandma's house. *Caring, 14*, 37–39.

Lelyveld, C. (1990). Caring for children with AIDS in a day care setting. In G. Anderson (Ed.), *Courage to care* (pp. 53–64). Washington, DC: Child Welfare League of America.

Longo, M. B., Spross, J. A., & Locke, A. M. (1990). Identifying major concerns of persons with acquired immunodeficiency syndrome: A replication. *Clinical Nurse Specialist*, *4*, 21–26.

Luginbill, M., & Spiegler, A. (1989). Specialized foster family care. *Children Today*, *18*(1), 5–9.

Meintz, S., & Lynch, R. D. (1989). The human right of bonding for warehoused "AIDS babies." *Community Health*, *12*(2), 60–64.

Meyers, A., & Weitzman, M. (1991). Pediatric HIV disease: The newest chronic illness of childhood. *Pediatric Clinics of North America*, *58*, 169–194.

Pieper, E. (1976). Grandparents can help. *The Exceptional Parent*, *6*, 7–10.

Schmitt, B., Seeger, J., Kieciz, W., Enenhel, S., & Jacobi, G. (1991). CNS involvement of children with HIV infection. *Developmental Medicine and Child Neurology*, *33*, 535–540.

Seibert, J., Garcia, A., Caplan, M., & Septimus, A. (1989). Three model pediatric AIDS programs: Meeting the needs of children, families and communities. In J. M. Seibert & R. A. Olson (Eds.), *Children, adolescents & AIDS* (pp. 25–57). Lincoln, NE: University of Nebraska Press.

Septimus, A. (1989). Psychosocial aspects of caring for families of infants infected with human immuno-deficiency virus. *Seminars in Perinatology*, *13*, 49–54.

Sonnek, I. M. (1986). Grandparents and the extended family of handicapped children. In R. R. Fewell & P. F. Vadasy (Eds.), *Families of handicapped children: Needs and supports across the life span* (pp. 99–120). Bellevue, WA: Edmark.

Task Force on Pediatric AIDS (1989). Infants and children with acquired immuno-deficiency syndrome: Placement in adoption and foster care. *Pediatrics*, *83*, 609–612.

Task Force on Pediatric AIDS. (1992). Guidelines for human immunodeficiency virus (HIV)-infected children and their foster families. *Pediatrics*, *89*, 681–683.

Waterbury, M. (1991, February 9–11). *Identifying and addressing the needs of non-infected siblings of children with HIV infection*. Paper presented at the 5th Annual Pediatric HIV/AIDS Conference, Washington, DC.

Woodruff, G., & Durkotsterzin, E. (1988). The transagency approach: A model for serving persons with HIV infection and their children. *Children Today*, *17*(4), 9–14.

Zealand, T. P. (1989). St. Clare's home for children: A transitional foster home for children with AIDS. *Quality Review Bulletin*, *15*, 17–20.

12

HIV-Infected Women and Children: Social and Ethical Perspectives

John Douard and Jerry D. Durham

The HIV/AIDS epidemic has highlighted a broad range of ethical concerns, widely discussed in the literature since the mid-1980s. Ethical concerns unique to HIV-infected women and children, however, have received less attention. These unique concerns stem partially from several realities:

• Women and children generally hold less power in interpersonal relationships than men in most cultures;
• Women and children are disenfranchised in public policy-making arenas;
• Women and children are economically disadvantaged in comparison to men;
• HIV/AIDS affects minority women and children disproportionately;
• Women and children, because of their social and economic circumstances, frequently do not receive adequate health care and the benefits of cutting-edge research;
• Women, because of their caregiver roles, often subjugate their needs to those of their partners and children;
• Infected women have been viewed as vectors of disease, resulting in their stigmatization;
• Women and children have until relatively recently been invisible in the HIV/AIDS epidemic.
• Women at highest risk of infection (sex workers, injecting drug users [IDUs], partners of IDUs) have few resources in the traditional health-care community or the AIDS-care networks to assist them (Anastos & Marte, 1989; Bayer, 1989; Campbell, 1990; Diaz, 1990–1991; Hankins, 1990; Mitchell, 1988; Levine, 1990; Powers, 1990; Smeltzer & Whipple, 1991a, 1991b).

As a result of these realities, issues related to distributive justice and duties and rights (moral and legal) are central concerns in any discussion of ethical issues connected to the lives of women and children who are HIV-infected. Any consideration of such issues must occur within the social and economic contexts that shape women's and children's lives. Because of space limitations, only major issues salient for nurses and other health-care workers who care for HIV-infected women and children will be addressed in this chapter.

Many of the ethical issues in health care have their source in a tension between two ideals: respect for persons as autonomous agents and the altruistic ethic of service and care. Both ideals are important in sustaining human sociality, but both can be distorted by the pressure of circumstances or the substitution of mechanically applied rules for good judgment. If good judgment is lacking, respect for persons can lead to withdrawal of care and concern. And in the absence of good judgment, the ethic of service and care can become an unjustifiable paternalism. This tension will become apparent throughout this chapter.

AIDS AND STIGMA

According to Goffman (1962), "In an important sense, there is only one complete, unblushing male in America; a young, married, white, urban, Northerner, heterosexual Protestant father of college education, fully employed, of good complexion, weight, height, and a recent record in sports" (p. 7). Those who are "shamefully different," or stigmatized, *know* that they are different. Strategies used to "fit in" or "pass" are often fraught with anxiety, and even people considered normal by a society are aware not only of the ways stigmatized persons are different but also that those who are different are aware that "normals" are aware of the differences. This "infinite regress of mutual consideration" sets such awkward interactions adrift and results in a "spoiled identity," or a lack of a secure sense of place in the social order in the stigmatized. People who are stigmatized, then, must adjust their public behavior to appear to satisfy social norms or accept their status as social outcasts. Both gays and injecting drug users have been, and continue to be, stigmatized. They have been placed in socially constructed categories of deviance and are therefore particularly vulnerable to various forms of discrimination.

Initially in the HIV epidemic, AIDS was considered a gay man's disease since it first affected men in the gay community. Hence, AIDS became widely associated in the public's mind with male homosexuality and sexual "promiscuity," even after it was discovered to be transmitted by routes clearly independent of a gay lifestyle. While several years of education have somewhat altered that association, stigma still accompanies AIDS because it continues to be prevalent among gay males.

Injecting drug users (IDUs), also stigmatized as engaging in socially unacceptable behavior, make up the second largest demographic category of people who contract HIV infection (Cohen, 1991). Again, the possibility of discrimination against people with AIDS is heightened by its association with a group labelled as deviant. IDUs are particularly vulnerable to discrimination because they are a less cohesive, less well organized group than gays. The latter have been organized, at least in large cities, into support and political-action organizations for about 15 years. Injecting drug users, on the other hand, remain fragmented and isolated.

Another morally relevant social fact about AIDS is that employers, insurance companies, and people with HIV/AIDS all express fears about the costs of treating people with AIDS. It is difficult (and can be misleading) to estimate the costs of AIDS treatment, but it is important to note that the health care system in the United States does not provide a consistent and reliable method of financing health care. In general, the system does not provide fair access to health care, and people with AIDS in particular have to contend with the anxiety and financial problems associated with uncertainty about health-care costs (Bartlett, 1990).

For all of these reasons, health workers need to be sensitive to the interest people infected with HIV have in maintaining their confidentiality. The interest is strong enough to warrant the claim that HIV-infected persons have a right to confidentiality, a right that can be overridden only by a justifiable claim on the part of others to have an even more serious right. The limits on a right to confidentiality, however, cannot be determined in abstraction from legal and social structures, and people who are vulnerable to discrimination if a "secret" about them is divulged can argue reasonably that their right to confidentiality is violable only under the most extreme circumstances. Society thus has a duty to protect its most vulnerable members, especially when society is responsible for some of its citizens' vulnerability by virtue of its role in constructing categories of deviance.

SOCIAL CONCERNS

HIV-infected women and children suffer from an additional burden: Until a few years ago, they were relatively invisible. This invisibility resulted partially from a focus on gay men prior to 1986, but it is also the result, at least in the United States, of the low social status of women in general. Most women with AIDS have been diagnosed since 1986 (see Chapter 3). For much of medical history, women's health issues have been marginalized in the context of the male-dominated medical profession and the patriarchal nature of social life. Rosser (1989) argues, for example, that "considerable resources and attention are devoted to women's health issues when these issues are directly related to women's interest in controlling production of children." She concludes that "AIDS represents a prime example of a disease in which androcentricism has placed women at a disadvantage for diagnosis, treatment and care" (1991, p. 231).

Black and Hispanic women have been even further marginalized by the racism endemic to American culture. Most of the HIV-infected women in the United States are members of racial and ethnic minorities, and the majority are IDUs, or sexual partners of IDUs, as discussed in Chapter 3. HIV infection exacerbates the systemic social problems created by institutionalized racism and class discrimination.

The injustices produced by a social structure that is racist, sustains stigmatization and deviance labeling, and has kept women in a subordinate social role must be taken into account by health workers. Nurses in particular are in a unique position to play the role Gadow (1980, p. 97) called "existential advocate." She summarized advocacy nursing as "the participation with the patient in determining the *personal meaning* which the experience of illness, suffering, or dying is to have for that individual." But to play this role well in caring for women with AIDS, nurses (and ideally other health workers) need to have an adequate grasp of the meaning of *social experience* and the illness for people who have been marginalized by a dominant white middle-class male culture.

Existential advocacy, it is important to note, is possible only if health workers are equipped to understand the full range of women's social experiences. Experience is culture-specific, and Western societies, not to mention the international context, contain a plurality of cultures. In the United States, social stratification is often masked by homogenizing cultural mechanisms such as mass media and political rhetoric, but health workers have an obligation to recognize the *differences* among people with AIDS to the extent that good practice requires such recognition.

CHILDREN WITH AIDS: PERINATAL TRANSMISSION

The decision of an HIV-infected pregnant woman to carry her child to term is often based on estimates of risk that are at least fallible if not contestable. Perinatal transmission raises several ethical dilemmas that arise from a clash between women's reproductive rights and the preventive perspective on health care. On the one hand, preventive measures are the most effective intervention in the AIDS epidemic. Treatments for people with symptomatic HIV infection are still relatively limited, even for adults, and for children, the treatment choices are even more limited. The range of preventive measures available to pregnant women are, first, HIV-antibody testing; education about routes of transmission, risk of perinatal transmission, and methods for preventing HIV infection; and for HIV-infected women, counseling and pregnancy termination. However, trials testing the efficacy of zidovudine during pregnancy may offer additional options (see Chapter 6).

At present, throughout most of the United States, involuntary HIV testing is generally illegal and probably not effective since it might drive people away from the health-care system to avoid discrimination and social isolation (exceptions include mandatory testing of sex workers and prison inmates in some states). Hence, prenatal care, even when it is available, might not be utilized by pregnant women if they were afraid it would involve HIV-antibody testing. Indeed, the ethnic minority women whom AIDS has affected most may be least likely to run the risk of further discrimination if HIV testing was routinely coupled with prenatal care.

What of women who fall into a high-risk category? Some policymakers have argued that women at highest risk of HIV infection be persuaded (even required) to be tested for HIV. There are two difficulties with this proposal. First, the notion of a "high-risk category" is misleading. It is a statistical property attributable to a group on the basis of past documented cases. The notion is useful for demographic purposes but not for the purpose of counseling individuals. No assumptions can be made about an *individual's* risk solely on the basis of such qualities as race or gender. Second, the distinctions between persuasion and coercion, and between information and persuasion, are flexible. Whether a piece of advice counts as coercion depends on the context in which it is given, the relations of dominance and submission between advisor and advisee, and the social experience of the parties.

Counseling that is coercive is immoral, even if it is believed to be in the client's best interest (i.e., is paternalistic), because people have a right to choose their own medical treatment unless their choice can be expected to cause others unnecessary and unreasonable harm. This point, however, results in a serious dilemma: If prevention of HIV infection is the only effective strategy for protecting the public's health, it may be argued, some coercion is morally required from a public health perspective. The dilemma is exacerbated in the case of counseling HIV-infected pregnant women about whether they ought to abort their fetuses.

By the 1980s, a legal and moral tradition had developed in which women were considered to have a right to privacy over their own bodies. The landmark *Roe v. Wade* abortion decision embodied that moral right in the common law, and until recently, state statutes followed suit. Although the right to privacy was claimed primarily to defend the right to choose an abortion, this might also extend to the situation in which an HIV-infected woman may be required or persuaded to have an abortion she might not choose on her own (Bayer, 1990).

Health workers who counsel HIV-infected pregnant women should avoid persuasive rhetoric in favor of the language of empathy and support. Women with AIDS, particularly poor black and Hispanic women, may very well consider the chance of perinatal transmission worth taking. As Bayer (1990) points out, "From the perspective of an infected woman whose own life prospects are not good and for whom the grim reality of an impoverished existence limits options of every kind, the . . . chance of having a healthy baby might seem worth the risks entailed" (pp. 69–70). One cannot, therefore, conclude that this choice is an irrational one. But even if it were, a client's irrational preferences do not ordinarily warrant coercive interference on that ground alone.

END-OF-LIFE DECISIONS

Among the decisions people with AIDS have to make are decisions about termination of treatment. The rule of thumb (and law) is that competent individuals have the right to make such decisions. If a patient loses respiratory function, for example, a decision to resuscitate has to be made. The dilemma in such situations is that obviously the patient cannot then make the decision. People with AIDS in the late stages of their disease have a right to know before it is too late whether resuscitation after respiratory failure is expected to have any medical benefits. There is increasing concurrence that patient's with AIDS have a right to have "Do Not Resuscitate" orders in their charts if they choose. The recent implementation of advance directives in health-care facilities have underscored that right for all patients.

Similarly, patients have a right to refuse heroic measures of other sorts, such as total parenteral nutrition (TPN). TPN is an invasive procedure that can save some peoples' lives, but it can also be used to prolong death. Ventilators can also be used to prolong death, especially if a patient has no cerebral brain function left. But in emergency situations, patients aren't always able to make their preferences known. Hence, it is important for them to let family members and physicians and nurses know in advance whether they want such measures taken. Alternatively, in some states, a patient can legally authorize a family member or friend to make her medical decisions even if she is not capable of deciding for herself. This is known as a *durable power of attorney*, to distinguish it from the power of attorney that authorizes a person to make someone else's decisions *unless* that someone is incapable (Winslade, 1990).

End-of-life decisions can be particularly difficult for women with AIDS, especially those who are heads of households for whom it may be difficult to acknowledge that they will no longer be able to protect and care for their families. Nurses and other health workers must be responsive to this difficulty and at the same time provide enough information to women for them to make maximally autonomous decisions. Empathy and respect for patients as autonomous agents are both key components of ethical health care, and both involve the capacity to make good judgments.

An attitude that interferes with empathy and respect is paternalism, demonstrated on the part of some health workers with an inability to share decision making in care issues. Paternalism is deeply embedded in the historical traditions from which modern medicine emerged, and health workers are often so deeply committed to caring for patients that paternalism frequently interferes with clients' rights to autonomy. However, it is important for nurses and other health workers to avoid a paternalistic posture toward patients if they are to act as existential advocates. Sick people are in some ways always dependent on their caregivers. Women, children, and the poor are often further dependent because of their social status. In a sense, health care should aim at restoring as much autonomy to patients as possible. Paternalism conflicts with, while the practice ideal of existential advocacy is compatible with, this ideal. Indeed, one can view health care as a form of politics that tries to help people to realize their *own* conception of a good life, including the way that life will end.

PROFESSIONAL DUTIES AND RIGHTS

Nurses who are occupationally exposed to HIV while treating infected persons run a very small risk of infection. Since AIDS is a life-threatening condition, the possibility of occupational transmission raises the question whether health workers have an obligation to treat HIV-infected patients and whether they have a right to know the HIV status of all their patients.

On the other side of the ledger, the question has recently been raised whether HIV-infected health workers have an obligation to inform their patients about *their* HIV status. Recently documented cases of individuals who became HIV-infected as the result of dental treatment (Ciesielski et al., 1992) have created fear in the public about the adequacy of universal precautions and a flurry of legislative activity at both state and federal levels.

HIV-Infected Patients

The health-care worker is subject overall to a small risk of occupational transmission per exposure after percutaneous injury, estimated at less than 1 percent (0.56%, according to one authoritative study, Henderson et al., 1990). This risk is roughly comparable to the occupationally related risk of death of a fire fighter in a large city and is generally considered reasonable. In 1988, the American Medical Association's Council on Ethical and Judicial Affairs (p. 1360) asserted:

> A physician may not ethically refuse to treat a patient whose condition is within the physician's current realm of competence solely because the patient is seropositive. . . .
> A physician who is not able to provide the services required by persons with AIDS should make an appropriate referral to those physicians or facilities that are equipped to provide such services.

Health workers in general have a limited obligation to treat people with AIDS. The justification for attributing this obligation is that under certain conditions, health workers give their *consent* (tacit or explicit) to providing treatment by virtue of entering a health-care profession. Among these conditions are the following (Douard, 1991)

- The attribution of a duty is sensitive to a reasonable level of risk.
- Society implements a workable plan to distribute risks fairly.
- Hospitals implement policies that require physicians to treat AIDS patients in ways it is reasonable to expect will benefit them.

Even when condition (1) is satisfied, conditions (2) and (3) are often contestable. It isn't obvious that society as a whole or hospitals have fair and explicit policies regarding the obligation to treat. Even so, once health workers have engaged a patient in a treatment regimen or in an emergency situation, health care workers have a moral and legal obligation not to abandon their patients, which often amounts to an obligation to treat.

The ethical requirements of an obligation to treat, however, may be more stringent in the case of HIV-infected women and children than in the usual case. First, women and children with AIDS have been neglected until recently; hence, society has failed to provide information and treatment that might have reduced the number of women and children who contract HIV and may have reduced the severity of symptoms with which they present at hospitals and clinics. Second, many of the women with AIDS are from marginalized groups, as previously noted. Hence, they are less likely than men to have had access to adequate health care throughout their lives. They are less likely than men to have insurance coverage when they become infected, and therefore they have fewer resources for treatment. Moreover, children who are infected perinatally may be orphaned by the time they are symptomatic. They are dependent on the state for care. Nurses and other health workers in these situations should be aware of their special responsibilities to treat particularly vulnerable people with a very narrow range of options.

Nurses can play a special role in caring for women and children with AIDS. Children often need advocates in the health-care system to protect their rights, and if an HIV-infected child's mother is also infected, the responsibility to care can fall directly on nurses. Nurses can also play an important counseling role for mothers who feel guilty about bringing their children to term and can provide accurate information about children's HIV status and prognosis. Given these special roles, nurses must be well informed about the minimal risk involved in treating people with AIDS. They cannot refuse to assist in providing care without also abdicating their advocacy role.

HIV-Infected Health Care Workers

Questions surrounding whether health workers ought to be tested for HIV and, if infected, ought to be prevented from practicing are currently being contested in the media, Congress, and professional organizations. It is reasonable to believe that at least five people were infected by the same dentist. The exact routes of transmission are unknown: the dentist may not have followed universal precautions, or he may have transmitted the virus even if he did follow Centers for Disease Control (CDC) guidelines (Ciesielski et al., 1992). No well-designed studies have been completed to determine risk of iatrogenic infection, but the CDC has recommended that health workers at known risk of infection be voluntarily tested, that workers who perform or assist in performing certain invasive procedures either stop doing such procedures or inform their patients of their HIV status (Centers for Disease Control, 1991).

These recommendations are clearly unworkable in many emergency situations. They also have been proposed in a context in which HIV-infected health workers do not have job, malpractice, and health insurance protection. HIV-infected health workers are, or can expect to be, patients and therefore have a right to confidentiality. While this issue cannot be resolved here, one can persuasively argue that presently health workers who do not perform invasive procedures do not have a moral obligation to inform their patients of their HIV status. Moreover, several major professional health organizations maintain that because of the low risk, HIV-infected health workers do not have an obligation to inform their patients even when performing invasive procedures, except in very circumscribed situations.

The moral dilemma raised by the possibility of iatrogenic transmission is this: Good nursing practice rests on trust between health workers and patients. If health workers do not inform their patients of their HIV status, trust may be undermined. Yet it seems unreasonable to require anyone, patient or health worker, to divulge her HIV status without well-designed studies that support the claim that there are unavoidable and unreasonable occupational or iatrogenic risks of infection. The vulnerability of people with AIDS to social discrimination creates a context in which secrecy about one's HIV status is the only protection available.

EXCLUSION OF WOMEN AND CHILDREN FROM RESEARCH

For nearly three decades, women and children have been underrepresented in clinical research protocols. This has led to research that does not take into account the possibility that women and children may respond differently to a variable being tested in men. Much less is known about the natural course of HIV infection and the effects of experimental drugs in women and children than in men, probably because historically women and children have not been recruited as research subjects (Rosser, 1989).

The Food and Drug Administration (FDA) and the Department of Health and Human Services (DHHS) have ethical requirements relative to government-funded research that set conditions for human subjects of research. These requirements stem primarily from the shocking abuse of women and children in research prior to 1970. Violations and fundamental ethical standards were revealed in the 1960s: institutionalized children were subjects in one experiment without consent from their guardians; poorly educated Hispanic women were sterilized without their consent; and radical mastectomies were performed without providing adequate information to women about less invasive or noninvasive technologies (Katy, 1972). However, it is difficult to justify the degree to which women and children have been excluded from clinical research. This exclusion has been recognized as a serious problem in AIDS research. Since women and children with AIDS have been diagnosed in larger numbers only relatively recently, most of the early experiments (e.g., on zidovudine) have included primarily male subjects.

A confluence of forces has resulted in increasing recognition of the injustice of excluding women and children. First, feminist critics of research strategy have pointed out that in a male-dominated scientific establishment, men have chosen the research problems and methods, subject populations, goals of research, and ethics of research. This research bias has led, according to these critics, to a partial and biased scientific practice that has excluded not just women but their point of view. A similar point can also be made about racial and class bias in scientific research.

Second, AIDS activists such as the AIDS Coalition to Unleash Power (ACT-UP) have challenged the FDA and DHHS regulations as being woefully slow to produce approved therapies and biased in the choice of experimental therapies. Among the results of these criticisms has been an effort to rethink these regulations, an indirect benefit of which is reevaluation of the stringency of requirements on the inclusion of women and children as research subjects.

Third, the interests of the pharmaceutical companies are on the side of widening the population that can be recruited as subjects since these companies desire a potentially large market for drugs approved for use by women and children.

The rights of clinical research subjects must be protected. Nonetheless, there are strong arguments to support the views expressed by feminists and AIDS activists that women and children have been unfairly excluded from research and that people with AIDS have been unfairly prevented from receiving the best available treatment because the scientific establishment serves the narrow interests of the scientists themselves. Clinical research, in short, is highly contested terrain. Here too, nurses have a responsibility to act as advocates representing the interests and rights of women and children with AIDS during the debates about AIDS research.

AIDS AND HEALTH CARE

As drugs became available for treating HIV infection and the associated opportunistic infections that affect people with AIDS, it is tempting to think of AIDS as a chronic illness. Chronic illnesses require medical and supportive home care, self-care, empathy, prevention. These are features of a health-care system that is not centered in tertiary-care settings, and many people with AIDS, like people with chronic illnesses, need help learning to cope during periods of relative stability. Family members, friends, and home-care nurses are essential participants in such nonhospital-based care (Strauss & Corbin, 1988).

Nonetheless, in the United States, the health-care system has been hospital-centered and not home-centered. Economic resources, for better or worse, are allocated to expensive technologies located in hospitals. Furthermore, many of the people with AIDS are poor, black, or Hispanic and IDUs. In many cases, they have no stable home or community lives, and public hospitals are the only place they can get relief and referral to scarce nursing homes. Politically, as Gostin (1990, p. 4) points out, the temptation to view AIDS as a chronic illness should be resisted:

> If AIDS is viewed as a chronic disease, it could sink to the mediocre level of health policy, research, and financing to which other chronic diseases have been relegated. Indeed, the demographics of AIDS virtually ensure that it will lose desperately needed resources. As the burden of the disease moves disproportionately to African-Americans and Hispanics, to the urban poor and to drug-dependent populations, it will surely lose political clout.

It is true, however, that hospital-based AIDS programs can and will discharge people with AIDS back to their communities whenever possible. Nurses and other health workers who help people with AIDS at home to care for themselves will increasingly have to be prepared to be health educators as well as advocates, skilled and empathic counselors as well as technicians. Women with AIDS are often the heads of households, and the time they can afford to spend in the hospital may be very limited. Hence, they need the best help they can get to learn to care for themselves while organizing their households. This responsibility will fall primarily on home-care nurses.

SOCIAL RESPONSIBILITIES

In a recent book, *The AIDS Disaster*, Perrow and Guillen (1990, p. 4) argue that "AIDS is unique among epidemics in the United States in its ability to disable organizational and community defenses and in its interaction with the pervasive social problems of poverty and discrimination." They consider the scope of the epidemic to have been widened by organizational failure. Among the organizations that failed are public health departments, hospitals, and professional health care associations.

The best response to this failure on the part of health workers is to engage actively in the societywide debates about how the AIDS epidemic can be addressed at this point. Perhaps the most effective place to engage in these debates is in health-care associations. The American Nurses Association and the American Medical Association, to name only two, can play an effective role in pressuring federal and state agencies, Congress, and the White House to allocate adequate funds to AIDS research and treatment, to design a health-care system based on democratic principles of justice, to focus attention on preventive measures, and to eliminate discrimination, at least at an institutional level, against women, blacks, Hispanics, and people who are drug-dependent. In other words, nurses and other health workers must have a political perspective and engage in political activities if they are to enact ethical health care. And good health care is ethical health care.

REFERENCES

American Medical Association Council on Ethical and Judicial Affairs. (1988). Ethical issues involved in the growing AIDS crisis. *Journal of the American Medical Association, 259*, 1360–1361.

Anastos, K., & Marte, C. (1989). Women—the missing persons in the AIDS epidemic. *Health Policy Advisory Center Bulletin, 19*, 6–13.

Bartlett, L. (1990). Financing health care for persons with AIDS. Balancing public and private responsibilities. In L. Gostin (Ed.), *AIDS and the health care system* (pp. 211–220). New Haven: Yale University Press.

Bayer, R. (1989). Perinatal transmission of HIV infection: The ethics of prevention. *Clinical Obstetrics and Gynecology, 32*(3), 497–505.

Bayer, R. (1990). Perinatal transmission of HIV infection: The ethics of prevention. In L. Gostin (Ed.), *AIDS and the health care system.* New Haven: Yale University Press.

Boland, M. G. (1991). The child with HIV infection. In J. Durham and F. Cohen (Eds.), *The person with AIDS* (2nd ed., pp. 316–347). New York: Springer.

Campbell, C. (1990). Women and AIDS. *Social Science in Medicine, 30*(4), 407–415.

Centers for Disease Control. (1991). Recommendations for preventing transmission of human immunodeficiency virus and hepatitis B virus to patients during exposure-prone invasive procedures. *Morbidity and Mortality Weekly Report, 40*(RR-8), 1–9.

Ciesielski, C., Marianos, D., Ou, C-Y, Dumbaugh, R., Witte, J., Berkelman, R., et al. (1992). Transmission of human immunodeficiency virus in a dental practice. *Annals of Internal Medicine, 116*, 798–805.

Cohen, F. L. (1991). The etiology and epidemiology of HIV infection and AIDS. In J. Durham and F. Cohen (Eds.), *The person with AIDS* (2nd ed., pp. 1–59). New York: Springer.

Diaz, E. (1990–1991). Public policy, women, and HIV disease. *SEICUS Report, 19*, 4–5.

Douard, J. (1991, February). Do physicians have an obligation to treat people with AIDS? Medical Humanities Rounds. Institute for the Medical Humanities, UTMB.

Gadow, S. (1980). Existential advocacy: philosophical foundation of nursing. In S. Spicker and S. Gadow (Eds.), *Nursing: Images and ideals* (pp. 62–73). New York: Springer.

Goffman, E. (1962). *Stigma: Notes on the management of spoiled identity.* New York: Simon & Schuster.

Gostin, L. (1990). Preface: Hospitals, health care professionals, and persons with AIDS. In L. Gostin (Ed.), *AIDS and the health care system* (pp. 3–12). New Haven: Yale University Press.

Hankins, C. (1990). Issues involving women, children, and AIDS primarily in the developed world. *Journal of Acquired Imune Deficiency Syndromes, 3*, 443–448.

Henderson, D. K., Fahey, B. J., Willy, M., Schmitt, J. M., Carey, K., Koziol, D. E., Lane, H. C., Fedio, J., & Saah, A. (1990). Risks for occupational transmission of human immunodeficiency virus type 1 associated with clinical exposures. *Annals of Internal Medicine, 113*, 740–746.

Katy, J. (1972). *Experimentation with human beings.* New York: Russell Sage Foundation.

Levine, C. (1990). Women and HIV/AIDS research: The barriers to equity. *Evaluation Review, 14*(5), 447–463.

Mitchell, J. (1988). Women, AIDS, and public policy. *AIDS and Public Policy Journal,* *3,* 50–51.

Perrow, C., & Guillen, M. (1990). The AIDS disaster. New Haven: Yale University Press.

Powers, M. (1990). Ethical considerations in HIV screening for infected women and children. *AIDS Patient Care, 4,* 40–41.

Rosser, S. (1989, Summer). Re-visioning clinical research: Gender and the ethics of experimental design. *Hypatia, 4*(2), 125–139.

Rosser, S. (1991). AIDS and women. *AIDS Education and Prevention, 3*(3), 230–240.

Smeltzer, S., & Whipple, B. (1991a). Women and HIV infection: The unrecognized population. *Health Values, 15,* 41–45.

Smeltzer, S., & Whipple, B. (1991b). Women and HIV infection. *Image, 23*(4), 249–256.

Strauss, A., & Corbin, J. M. (1988). *Shaping a new health care system.* San Francisco: Jossey-Bass.

Winslade, W. (1990, Summer). Whose will prevails? *Biomedical Inquiry, 2*(2), 24.

13

Psychosocial and Economic Concerns of Women Affected by HIV Infection

Carol Ren Kneisl

In almost all cultures, women maintain and support the family network, do the mothering and nurturing, and care for the sick. When HIV enters the picture, either because the woman herself is infected with the virus or a family member or friend is infected, these tasks become even more difficult, and the psychosocial needs more complex. AIDS has a profound and lasting influence on the nature, structure, and functions of families (Levine, 1990). An HIV-related illness may serve as the final insult to disrupt nuclear and extended families which are already fragile (Staples, 1990).

In addition, women affected by HIV have to a large extent been isolated and alienated from the larger society. Whereas many homosexual males are involved in community organizations that support gay lifestyles, women affected by HIV are more often heterosexuals without strong identification with a group or community organization (McGough, 1990). This chapter discusses the psychosocial needs of women affected by HIV and suggests guidelines for nursing involvement.

PSYCHOSOCIAL CONCERNS

Sociocultural Hostility and Discrimination

Most women with HIV infection are members of groups whose skin color, ethnic background, or lifestyle may be viewed negatively by mainstream Americans. Most women with HIV infection are either injecting drug users (IDUs) themselves, or sexual partners of IDUs. Most are people of color. Some are prostitutes. Some are the sexual partners of bisexual men. Durham (1991) suggests that persons with HIV infection are doubly stigmatized because most are already members of these stigmatized groups. Stigma and discrimination are intensified for HIV-infected women (Weiner, 1991). Many women's lives are further complicated by the fact that they are single heads of households with young children who may also be ill. The illness, poverty, oppression, invisibility, and lack of community support often experienced by HIV-positive women severely test their ability to cope with an already difficult situation.

Moral indignation is a frequent response to both gay and bisexual people, IDUs, and prostitutes. Many people consider homosexuality, bisexuality, prostitution, and substance use evidence of lack of character, criminal behavior, or a sinful lifestyle. Families of origin may be unaware of, or may reject, the individuals's lifestyle and thus be unable or unwilling to provide support.

In *Illness as Metaphor* (1977), Susan Sontag suggests that people with illnesses that evoke feelings of apprehension and vulnerability in others become objects of that dread. This is especially true of HIV and AIDS. Those who are well fear contamination by an illness for which there is no known cure. Sometimes hostility is generated by this fear.

Sexuality

The HIV epidemic has intruded into the sexual lives of women. Women who have been exposed to risk-reduction education have heard that they should practice safer sex and that they are responsible for ensuring that safer sex practices are followed. However, many women find it difficult if not unrealistic to follow this advice. There are a variety of sexual, economic, political, legal, cultural, and religious issues that influence a woman's sexual behavior (see Chapter 4). For example, in a study of poor black and Latina women (Flaskerud & Nyamathi, 1989), only 23% used condoms. Resistance to condom use may come from both men and women. In some cultures, only prostitutes use condoms, and in some religions, sex has reproduction, not recreation, as its purpose. If attractiveness is associated with sexual purity and sex without reproduction is associated with immorality or sin, then it is unlikely that the woman will encourage the use of condoms.

It is also unlikely that the new Reality condom for women will alter these attitudes. It requires the woman to manipulate her genitals, something that some women may be uncomfortable doing. And even if she was willing, men in many cultures, especially black and Hispanic men, have negative attitudes toward using condoms. In these cultures the balance of power in sexual decision making is weighted heavily toward the man. It may be considered improper for women to be aware of what kinds of barrier protection are available and how they are used. Such concerns about the sexual act may be interpreted by the woman's partner as improper and impure. Shared responsibility for safer sex practices, pregnancy termination options and choices, and health teaching for women are discussed in Chapters 5 and 6. Barrier protection for women who have sex with women may be subject to the same or similar sexual, economic, cultural, and religious issues.

Economic Issues

HIV disease disproportionately affects persons already at the economic edge. For women, HIV disease often means an even more unstable financial situation. The woman or her partner, if her partner is HIV-infected, may lose days or months from work because of illness. Jobs may be completely lost because of discrimination on the basis of race, lifestyle, or HIV diagnosis. New jobs may be difficult if not impossible to find. Many black and Hispanic women either lose their insurance benefits or have no insurance protection to draw on in time of illness. Family and friends may be unable or unwilling to help out financially. Seeking public assistance such as Medicaid requires time, energy, and assertiveness—all of which can be in short supply when one is coping with HIV infection. Unfortunately, many women fail to receive early diagnosis and early intervention because of these financial barriers.

In most large- and medium-size cities, volunteer programs often provide lifelines for persons with HIV infection. While these volunteer programs are usually well known in the gay community, women, especially black and Hispanic women, are less likely to know what is available or to feel comfortable asking for assistance. As the epidemic continues, however, greater numbers of programs and more outreach efforts are targeted toward HIV-infected women and minorities (see Chapter 14). Assisting women with AIDS, at least from a public policy perspective, requires intervention to combat drug use, teenage and unwanted pregnancies, poverty, discrimination against people of color, and lack of education (Shayne & Kaplan, 1991).

A growing and critical problem associated with economic constraints is the lack of decent, appropriate housing for the growing number of persons with HIV disease. HIV disease is disproportionately high in persons who are targets of discrimination in housing and medical care. Shelters for the homeless may not be the answer, since many shelters refuse to accept persons with, or at risk for, HIV infection. A homeless woman with HIV infection may find herself and her family members barred from shelters.

Caregiving

Family caregivers grapple with diverse issues that revolve around traditional versus nontraditional definitions of family, ineffective family coping, altered family processes, grieving, and survivorship. In many instances, women are the core of the family support system. Being the support system for a person with HIV infection is a challenge that requires special emotional stamina. Being HIV-positive and the core of the support system of others—husband, lover, children, father, brother, mother, sister, friend—is more than a challenge. Imagine what it must be like to assume these heavy responsibilities while attempting to cope with one's own fears. A diagnosis of AIDS presents a tremendous challenge to many women to maintain roles which bolster their self-esteem. Loss of health, drug addiction, lack of social and economic support, lack of information about AIDS, and inadequate health care can further erode these women's sense of control and ability to fulfill their social roles (Nyamathi, 1989).

Stress

The degree and kind of stress experienced by the HIV-infected woman goes beyond the routine and essential stress of everyday life. The ability of HIV-infected women to cope with stress may differ from that of infected men who often have more economic resources and social support than infected women do. Men may have fewer role responsibilities (e.g., caretaker). Indeed, these women encounter undesirable or excess stress that threatens their well-being and may even be life-threatening.

Selye's general adaptation syndrome, a framework for understanding stress, is based upon the belief that stress affects the whole person, and therefore the whole person must adjust to the changes brought about by stress. Selye's third stage of the general adaptation syndrome is the stage of exhaustion that occurs if stress continues over a prolonged period of time. It also occurs when multiple stressors are active simultaneously, or when a person undergoes repeated or overwhelming stress, such as occurs with HIV infection. Adaptive energy is exhausted, and the body surrenders to stress. Prolonged or multiple stress have both biological and psychological consequences. The adrenal glands enlarge and become depleted, and the lymph nodes enlarge. These changes lower the person's overall resistance and cause disturbances in interpersonal relationships. For example, persons under prolonged stress may show such behavioral changes as increased irritability, hypersensitivity or overreaction to minor stimuli, sleep disturbances, and recurrent nightmares. The highest incidence of illness and death occur in persons who experience stress after infection with HIV.

An exciting new field of research—psychoneuroimmunology, the study of the communication between the mind, the brain, the endocrine system, and the immune system—attempts to explain the relationships between mind and body and the role of attitudes and emotions in combating a serious illness like AIDS. For example, a common characteristic of long-term survivors is their refusal to accept the diagnosis of HIV disease as a death sentence. While they accept the diagnosis, they defy the fatal outcome that is supposed to be connected to it. Long-term survivors are extremely goal-oriented and social. They treat their symptoms as if they were minor impediments; they are determined to prevail. Their immune systems seem to function better. They have higher T-cell counts, and in many cases other immune system components compensate for the ravaged T-cells.

Anxiety

Anxiety is an inevitable result of the attempt to maintain equilibrium in a changing world. Because the world of the woman with HIV disease is constantly changing, she often experiences frequent and prolonged anxiety. Emotional distress has been found to accompany negative immune function factors in HIV-infected persons. The general causes of anxiety have been classified into two major threats:

1. threats to biologic integrity: actual or impending interference with basic human needs, such as the needs for food, drink, or warmth; and
2. threats to the security of the self:
   a. unmet expectations important to self-integrity
   b. unmet needs for status and prestige
   c. anticipated disapproval by significant others
   d. inability to gain or reinforce self-respect or to gain recognition from others
   e. guilt, or discrepancies between self-view and actual behavior

Threats to biological integrity are a general cause of anxiety. As the other chapters in this book document, threats to biological integrity are frequent and common to persons with HIV disease. Threats to the security of the self however, are not as easily categorized. In some instances they are obvious; in others, they are more obscure because each person's sense of self is unique. To one woman, continued career growth may be essential to the security of the self. To another, keeping her family happy, healthy, and well cared for may be essential. HIV disease often threatens one's ability to perform these tasks or fulfill roles related to essential values. When these unmet needs or expectations are coupled with the anticipated or actual disapproval of others who are important, anxiety is generated. It is important to understand that either actual or impending interference may cause anxiety (actual interference with a biologic or psychosocial need is not a necessary condition). All that is necessary is the anticipation of one of these major threats.

Depression

The concept of loss is central to an understanding of the psychological impact of HIV and the depression and suicidal ideation that often accompany it. Depression is often a situational reaction to loss of one or more of the following (Kneisl & Pheifer, 1992):

- energy, appetite, strength, and physical stamina
- control of body functions such as elimination, mobility, speech, sight, hearing, and tactile sensations
- control of body appearance because of dramatic weight loss, oozing wounds, skin breakdown, hair loss, skin lesions, and so on
- self-worth
- mental clarity and cognitive ability

- privacy
- self-sufficiency and self-determination
- employment, health insurance, salary
- personal competence
- physical intimacy, including sexual expression
- friends and lovers to earlier deaths from AIDS
- social support
- hope
- peace of mind and spirit
- life itself

Feeling sad and occasionally depressed because one has HIV disease is certainly not abnormal. Some people's feelings of sadness may extend beyond occasional depression to the psychiatric disorder of depression. Such persons may have a variety of symptoms in addition to obvious feelings of sadness. For example, some gain weight during a depressive episode, while others lose weight. Many feel so tired that they could sleep all day, while others take brief naps but never feel rested. As depression progresses, symptoms like difficulty in concentrating, difficulty in making decisions, slowed movements, slowed thinking, apathy, withdrawal, and constipation emerge.

The clinical problem becomes one of determining whether the symptoms signal psychiatric depression or are characteristic of HIV dementia or other HIV sequelae. For example, weight loss and fatigue are common in HIV disease. Problems in cognition such as loss of concentration, slowness of thought, and difficulty in making decisions can also be symptoms of HIV dementia. Slowed movements are not unusual in fatigued persons or those who have motor deficiencies because of HIV dementia.

Research regarding the risks of suicide among persons with AIDS, conducted primarily with male subjects, suggests this risk is higher than among persons with other illnesses (Marzuk, Tierney, Tardiff, Gross, Morgan, Hsu et al., 1988; McKegney & O'Dowd, 1992). Still other studies (Holland & Tross, 1985; O'Dowd & McKegney, 1990) have reported lower suicide rates among persons with AIDS when compared to uninfected individuals. These discrepancies may reflect differences in risk groups studied, stage of HIV-related illnesses, socioeconomic factors, and other sampling biases (McKegney & O'Dowd, 1992). Limited research has suggested that HIV-infected women, when compared with infected men, rarely demonstrate suicidal tendencies. The reasons for these differences are unclear; however, many HIV-infected men are homosexual or bisexual, states which have been suggested as risk factors for suicide (Brown & Rundell, 1989). A key to the prevention of suicide is accurate and early assessment of persons with AIDS for depression and careful evaluation for suicide risk (Marzuk et al., 1988). Saunders and Buckingham (1988) suggest the following approaches in assessing suicide risk in persons with AIDS: (1) Explore their situations; (2) identify their intentions; (3) find out if they have a plan and evaluate its lethality; (4) find out if they have a means to carry out the plan; and (5) evaluate their risk factors and resources. In dealing with suicide, these authors recommend that health care workers: listen but not overreact; understand their legal/ethical obligations; be able to identify crises resources (e.g., AIDS hotlines); develop professional relationships within populations at risk of AIDS; and stay in touch with their own feelings.

Resolution of ethical quandries related to the right of persons with AIDS to end their own lives is further complicated when quality of life issues are considered. Quality of life for persons with AIDS, like that for persons with other serious illnesses, usually deteriorates as the disease progresses and living becomes more difficult. Psychological wellbeing is a particularly important factor in the wellbeing of persons with AIDS (Ragsdale & Morrow, 1990). Other factors affecting quality of life (and thus psychological wellbeing) in persons with AIDS include ability to work, physical symptoms, hospitalization, pain, and perception of health (Wachtel, Piette, Mor, Stein, Fleishman & Carpenter, 1992). As quality of life deteriorates, reflecting changes in physical, mental, social and role functions, persons with AIDS may be at higher risk for depression and suicide. In HIV-infected women, the loss of role may be particularly pronounced, and, in the absence of adequate social support, may engender alterations in mood.

Other common psychiatric disorders seen in people with HIV and AIDS are anxiety disorders, panic attacks, adjustment disorders with depressed mood, and major depression. These problems have been widely discussed in the psychiatric and mental health literature (Wallack, Snyder, Bialer, Gilfand, & Poisson, 1991), although few are specific to psychiatric/mental health concerns of HIV-infected women.

Bereavement

Family caregivers may feel it necessary to mask the cause of illness because of the stigma associated with HIV infection. They may experience little or no support from others in coping with illness, mourning losses, or expressing feelings associated with bereavement.

A relationship with a partner may have been strained before diagnosis or before death because of lifestyle choices. Some women are unaware that their partners inject drugs or that they are sexually active outside the relationship. Anger and guilt related to bereavement may arise and block progress in grieving for a partner's illness or death. Some partners may also be feeling guilt if they think they may have transmitted HIV to their loved one; others may feel fear or anger at having been exposed to a probable fatal illness. Still other HIV-infected women may have to deal with the illness and death of an infected child or children, fully aware of their own role in unintentionally transmitting the virus. For such women, many of whom are struggling with their own illness and the need to grieve for their own losses, the toll can be inexorable. Under these circumstances of grief and bereavement, women may find themselves unable to reach out for social support to maintain the fabric of their lives.

The women must also cope with the untimely nature of death—her own or her partner's, friend's, or family member's (see Chapter 2). HIV disease requires people to face issues of mortality much sooner than they normally might, since it is generally young people who have HIV-related illnesses or die of AIDS. For some, there is inadequate time to prepare to accept illness, life changes, or death.

PSYCHOSOCIAL NURSING INTERVENTIONS

Research suggests that nurses should initiate psychosocial interventions with newly-diagnosed HIV-infected persons before symptoms of AIDS become apparent. The nature of these interventions will depend upon such factors as the age and developmental level of the client; the nature of the presenting problems; the therapeutic context; the types and availability of resources; the amenability of the client to intervention; and the knowledge, attitudes, and skills of the nurse. These interventions include individual, group, and family therapeutic approaches to assist clients and their significant others to deal with such common problems as loss and grief; guilt; prejudice and discrimination; isolation; uncertainty; and fear of abandonment. HIV-infected women need emotional support and look to nurses to provide such support or to link them to supportive resources. Nurses should also focus on or incorporate crisis intervention and psychoeducational methodologies and pay particular attention to women of color. Women are key figures in educating others in their family and community.

Because the research describing psychoneuroimmunology is investigational, and has not been controlled for several factors such as mutational changes in the HIV, the amount of HIV in the body, and so on, one cannot assume that HIV-infected persons are in total control of the disease process and the state of their health, or that the mind can cure AIDS. However, nurses can and should teach self-care behaviors that long-term survivors are using to maintain their health.

Nurses should also assess the level of stress, quality of social support, and mood, factors that influence the quality and quantity of life of persons with HIV disease. Psychosocial nursing interventions to help clients enhance neurological, immunological, and cognitive functioning should focus on stress reduction, social support, and adequate sleep-wake patterns.

Nurses also play key roles in providing AIDS education to HIVinfected women or those at risk of such infection. Such counseling can take place in both individual and group contexts and should be culturally sensitive (Flaskerud & Nyamathi, 1989; Nyamathi, Shuler & Porche, 1990). Such sites as sexually transmitted disease clinics; drug treatment sites; WIC clinics; high schools and colleges; psychiatric units and jails may offer nurses unique opportunities for educational intervention to prevent HIV infection among women (Aruffo, Coverdale, Chacko & Dworkin, 1990). Such topics as reproductive decision-making, assertiveness training, and communication skills are particularly important if women are to achieve balanced relationships with their sexual partners (Levine & Dubler, 1990; Arras, 1990).

Case management of women caught in stressful family, financial, or emotional situations should be directed toward supportive problem solving. The early creation of psychosocial support groups is indicated because newly-infected individuals experience greater alienation. Bereavement support is critical throughout in order to help the woman cope with losses throughout the illness phase up until her death or the death of friends or family.

CONCLUSION

Women affected by HIV suffer from many of the same psychosocial and economic issues that are also confronted by men. However, they also suffer some unique problems related to their less-powerful place in society, their caretaking roles, and to reproductive issues. It is only recently that education and support services especially for women have begun to appear. Health care givers need to recognize some of the unique problems of women posed by the AIDS epidemic and actively participate in finding solutions.

REFERENCES

Arras, J. (1990). AIDS and reproductive decisions: Having children in fear and trembling. *Milbank Quarterly, 68*, 353–382.

Aruffo, J., Coverdale, J., Chacko, R., Dworkin, R. (1990). Knowledge about AIDS among women psychiatric outpatients. *Hospital and Community Psychiatry, 41*, 326–328.

Brown, G., & Rundell, J. (1989). Suicidal tendencies in women with human immunodeficiency virus infection. *American Journal of Psychiatry, 146*, 556–557.

Durham, J., (1991). The HIV epidemic: Ethical and legal dimensions. In J. Durham and F. Cohen (Eds.), *The person with AIDS: Nursing perspectives.* (2nd ed.). pp. 261–367. New York: Springer.

Flaskerud, J., & Nyamathi, A. (1989). Black and Latina women's AIDS knowledge, attitudes and practice. *Research in Nursing and Health, 12*, 339–346.

Holland, J. & Tross, S. (1985). The psychosocial and neuropsychiatric sequelae of acquired immunodeficiency syndrome and related disorders. *Annals of Internal Medicine, 103*, 760–764.

Kneisl, C. R., & Pheifer, W. G. HIV/AIDS: A mental health challenge. In H. S. Wilson and C. R. Kneisl (Eds), *Psychiatric nursing* (4th ed.), 585–611. Redwood City, California: Addison-Wesley.

Levine, C. (1990). AIDS and changing concepts of family. *Milbank Quarterly, 14*, 61–68.

Levine, C., & Dubler, N. (1990). Uncertain risks and bitter realities: The reproductive choices of HIV-infected women. *Milbank Quarterly, 68,* 321–351.

Marzuk, P., Tierney, H., Tardiff, K., Gross, R., Morgan, E., Hsu, M., & Mann, J. (1988). Increased risk of suicide in persons with AIDS. *Journal of the American Medical Association, 259,* 1333–1337.

McGough, K. (1990). Assessing social support of people with AIDS. *Oncology Nursing Forum, 17*(1), 31–35.

McKegney, F., & O'Dowd, M. (1992). Suicide and HIV status. *American Journal of Psychiatry, 149,* 396–398.

Nyamathi, A. (1989). Impact of poverty, homelessness and drugs on Hispanic women at risk for HIV infection. *Hispanic Journal of Behavioral Sciences, 11,* 299–314.

Nyamathi, A., Shuler, P. & Porsche, M. (1990). AIDS educational program for minority women at risk. *Family and Community Health, 13*(2), 54–64.

O'Dowd, M., & McKegney, F. (1990). AIDS patients compared with others seen in psychiatric consultation. *General Hospital Psychiatry, 12,* 50–55.

Ragsdale, D. & Morrow, J. (1990). Quality of life as a function of HIV classification. *Nursing Research, 39,* 355–359.

Saunders, J. & Buckingham, S. (1988, July). When the depression turns deadly. *Nursing 88,* 59–64.

Selye, H. (1976). *The stress of life.* New York: McGraw-Hill.

Shayne, V. & Kaplan, B. (1991). Double victims: Poor women and AIDS. *Women and Health, 17,* 21–37.

Sontag, S. (1977). *Illness as metaphor.* New York: Farrar, Straus, Giroux.

Staples, R. (1990). Substance abuse and the black family crisis: An overview. *Western Journal of Black Studies, 14*(4), 196–204.

Wachtel, T., Piette, J., Mor, V., Stein, M., Fleishman, J., & Carpenter, C. (1992). Quality of life with human immunodeficiency virus infection: Measure by the Medical Outcomes Study Instrument. *Annals of Internal Medicine, 116,* 129–137.

Wallack, J., Snyder, J., Bialer, P., Gilfand, J., & Poisson, E. (1991). An AIDS bibliography for the general psychiatrist. *Psychosomatics, 32,* 243–254.

Wiener, L. (1991). Women and immunodeficiency virus: A historical and personal perspective. *Social Work, 36,* 375–378.

14

The Community: Mobilizing and Accessing Resources and Services

Risa Denenberg

MAKING WOMEN VISIBLE IN THE EPIDEMIC

The AIDS epidemic is aptly portrayed as an iceberg. Those diagnosed with AIDS, people now living with AIDS, and those who have died from AIDS represent the visible cap. The Centers for Disease Control (CDC) counts their numbers and publishes monthly reports, stratified by race, gender, and exposure category. At the murky level of the iceberg beneath the surface where the true picture is less discernible are people who have tested as HIV positive. If and when they will develop AIDS is uncertain, and there is no general medical or governmental agency responsible for collection and distribution of information regarding their numbers.

The largest, most unexposed portion of the AIDS iceberg, however, contains the unknown numbers of people who are infected with HIV but don't know it. They may be able to guess that they are "at risk" from public information about the risk of injecting drug use or certain kinds of "high-risk" sex. At the base of the iceberg, invisible to everyone, are those who have no idea that they are at risk for contracting HIV through their sexual activities. Many of these are women. This group may include a married woman whose husband has been her only lifetime sexual partner. It may include a lesbian woman who is unaware of her current lover's former injecting drug use. Or it might include a college student who experienced date rape but has never been sexually active.

Women comprise the fastest-growing group of Americans currently being diagnosed with AIDS, even though the definition of AIDS used by the CDC does not yet adequately reflect the spectrum of disease seen in women. One review of HIV-related deaths in women found that 65% died without fitting the official government definition for AIDS (Chu, Buehler, & Berkelman, 1990). Because of this unclear epidemiologic picture of women with HIV/AIDS, the true numbers of women who are HIV-infected is likely to be underestimated.

Estimating HIV seroprevalence in women is further complicated by a lack of research, attention, and understanding of the presentation and progression of HIV-related illness in women.

To examine how women have accessed and utilized available resources as people living with HIV disease, one must first look at the early years of the AIDS epidemic to learn how women became visible. Pediatric HIV programs and research preceded active detection and treatment of HIV illness in women, although the link between perinatally infected infants and their mothers was an obvious one. As mothers of sick children and often partners of men living with the disease as well, most HIV-infected women were overwhelmed. If no programs existed for them, it was just as well since they had no time to take care of themselves anyway. Of course, many children diagnosed with AIDS were separated from their parents by circumstances of death, drug abuse, and poverty. The mothers of these children were simply invisible to the system.

As it became clearer to clinicians and policymakers that each infant with AIDS probably represented an HIV-positive woman, the issue of perinatal transmission became a topic for research. Several states undertook blind HIV seroprevalence studies of newborns (Hoff et al., 1988). Each HIV-positive newborn reflected an HIV-infected mother. Still, programs to enter these women into care and support them with resources available in the community were largely nonexistent when these HIV seroprevalence studies were first undertaken. Women were thus first defined in the epidemic as mere vessels for HIV-positive babies, who were portrayed dramatically in the media as "innocent victims."

Next, women were tangentially defined in the epidemic as vectors of the virus through prostitution—passing HIV to their male clients, who then transmitted HIV to their "innocent" wives and children. This purported route of transmission has proven unsubstantial in the actual number of cases of HIV transmission, yet it concretizes some basic public perceptions about women—as vectors of disease (Alexander, 1988). This portrait, reminiscent of earlier decades when prostitutes were quarantined as a strategy to slow the spread of sexually transmitted diseases, resurfaced in the early 1980s with virulence. The stereotyping of female sex workers is inaccurate in several respects. Sex workers generally use condoms with male clients and promote safe sex when possible. Sex workers who are also drug addicts are more likely to practice unsafe sex to procure drugs. The representation of HIV positive women as "AIDS carriers," junkies, and prostitutes has obstructed public education campaigns about HIV transmission and has served as a barrier to the message that AIDS should be everyone's concern. Because of this view of HIV-infected women, those with HIV infection and women at risk of infection have naturally responded with grave fear of testing and disclosure of HIV status to family, community, and medical providers.

Even if AIDS had been recognized and studied in women early in the epidemic, there might still be a lack of resources and services specifically to address their needs in the present decade. The majority of women with HIV infection are urban dwellers, poor women from ethnic minority groups (see Chapter 3). These women's health-care needs have traditionally been neglected in areas such as infant mortality, alcohol and drug rehabilitation, primary care (meaning, among other things, access to regular Papanicolaou [Pap] smears, mammograms, hypertension screening, cancer screening, etc.), and health education. Undereducation, poverty, discrimination, the status of women, and lack of access to health care have combined to insure that most HIV-infected women and those at risk of infection will fare the worst in this epidemic.

The epidemic was first defined in gay men in 1981. Current retrospective analyses suggest that IDUs, including female IDUs, probably had an AIDS-like syndrome as early as, or before, the illness was recognized in gay men. There is now a recognition of an increase in the rate of pneumonia deaths in women that parallels the identification of *Pneumocystis carinii* pneumonia (PCP) in men (Norwood, 1988). AIDS was referred to at the time as Gay Related Immune Disorder (GRID). It was not until 1986, after antibody screening tests for HIV were available, that women were consistently identified with HIV infection and AIDS.

Why was it so difficult to see that the disease had appeared in IDUs and women? Mainly because most of the affected gay men were basically healthy, were often seen in the private sector, and often were resourceful in their ability to procure needed health-care services. Many were seen by their peers—gay physicians who were accustomed to treating sexually transmitted infections in gay male clients. These physicians who observed a unique syndrome of illness in previously healthy clients were more likely to pay attention and provide follow-up care for their patients than physicians seeing poor clients in crowded settings such as public health clinics, methadone programs, and emergency rooms, clients who were and are traditionally viewed as likely to be ill.

The gay community, already a cohesive group in many parts of the country, mobilized in a number of ways in the early 1980s to reduce their risk of HIV infection. Prevention efforts were combined with a positive attitude toward sexuality, and the resulting concept of "safe sex" was promoted by forums, educational campaigns, posters, videos, classes, and seminars, and by making condoms available in clinics, bars, and community meeting places. As men began to see their friends and lovers become ill and die, they combined resources and developed buddy programs, food programs, and other services. Some programs grew into thriving organizations such as the Gay Men's Health Crisis in New York and the Shanti Project in San Francisco. Further, gay men started to meet and develop strategies for demanding more funding and research into treatments for AIDS, founding such groups as ACT UP (AIDS Coalition to Unleash Power).

These same strategies were not available to women, who face special barriers in recognizing themselves as at risk for HIV illness. This is particularly true of women most at risk of infection. Just as the health-care system, social-service system and the government failed to recognize early on that women were affected, women themselves found difficulty in being visible in the epidemic.

WHAT ARE WOMEN'S HIV ISSUES?

Until very recently, women have not been perceived as part of the HIV community. It is difficult for women to see themselves as at risk, and HIV infection often causes medical distress in women long before it is actually identified and diagnosed. Even women who are considered to be at risk—IDUs, for example— have a different set of concerns than their male counterparts. Women IDUs are more likely to exchange sex for drugs and to encounter sexual assault. Some studies show that female IDUs are more likely to share needles with other drug users (Villalobos, 1989) and have more medical problems than men. Drug treatment may be harder for women to procure, especially if they are pregnant or have children to care for.

Women in prison represent still another group with special concerns. Much of the research on HIV in prison populations has focused on male prisoners. Most women who end up in the prison system are there because of drug use and related economic "crime." The federal prison system and some state prison systems test prisoners routinely, and many segregate on the basis of positive-HIV status. Peer support groups are sorely needed in the prison system as well as an effective method of drug treatment and rehabilitation.

Prostitutes have been scapegoated as vectors of HIV infection and recently have been subjected to laws that mandate HIV testing if they are arrested. While sex workers are discriminated against, their customers are not. Women who work the streets are more likely to spend time in jail, to be drug addicts, and are less likely to require that their "johns" use condoms. Since sex workers are at high risk of HIV infection from drug use and unsafe sex, they are a special population that requires services and support.

Lesbians also have particular needs for appropriate and sensitive services and educational materials. Lesbians may be at risk for HIV infection through IDU, sex work, or sex with men at risk. Yet these same women may feel uncomfortable discussing their relationships and sex lives with providers who are insensitive to their sexual preference. A female partner may be excluded when family interventions are planned simply because the system renders this partner invisible. Children may also be ignored in lesbian families due to misconceptions about lesbian lifestyles.

Women who have contracted HIV infection from male sexual partners are often overwhelmed and unable to reach out for the help they need. Their partner and children may be enrolled in appropriate services long before they are.

Condom campaigns targeted to women may be a cruel joke to women who experience domestic violence. These women are often unable to find networks of support, support groups, and feelings of camaraderie with other patients enrolled in HIV clinics. They often feel shame and embarrassment at their predicament, rendering them less able to seek and procure services for themselves.

WHAT DO WOMEN NEED?

Many women affected by HIV illness, as well as women at risk of contracting the virus, do not have a sense of belonging to any specific community. While many are poor women of color, they belong to many different cultural and ethnic groups. "Black" women may be African-American, Afro-Caribbean, or Latina; "Hispanic" women may be Puerto Rican, Dominican, Mexican, Central American; "Asian" woman may be Chinese, Japanese, Filipino, and so on. In immigrant families, young women with children are often the last to have opportunities to be in public settings or study English. Language is often a barrier to prevention and educational campaigns, yet even when pamphlets and videos are translated into appropriate languages, cultural barriers may limit the usefulness of such resources. To reach women, neighborhood programs must be available, offered by accepted community leaders who can provide relevant information in appropriate languages. These types of programs need funding and technical assistance to be effective.

Many urban centers such as New York, Chicago, Miami, or San Francisco have programs for treating people with HIV infection and AIDS. Yet these programs often do not reach women living in the communities they serve. Women may feel uncomfortable sitting in a waiting room, often for hours, with a clientele that is predominately male. Or they may feel that it is not a suitable setting to bring their children into, but they have nowhere to leave them. Women may feel stigmatized and embarrassed, especially if they are not already connected to other sources of support regarding their HIV status. In less urban areas, HIV patients may be managed in more general medical settings, yet transportation may be a problem because of a lack of money, a lack of experience in using the public transportation system, or difficulty in negotiating transportation for themselves and young children.

Women need the same kinds of health services that men need when they have HIV infection, but they also need the full range of obstetrical and gynecological services. Most women are accustomed to entering the health-care system to deliver a baby, to receive prenatal care, to obtain family planning services, or to find care for their children. To require that women receive HIV-related health services in settings entirely different from those with which they are familiar is a prescription for failure. The responsibilities of caring for home, children, partners, and elderly family members are often more than women can handle without neglecting their own needs routinely. Women need comprehensive primary-care programs where they can be seen along with their children, where they can get a Pap smear as well as a T-cell count, and where tuberculosis testing and routine immunizations can be provided to the entire family.

In addition to these centralized services, women also need on-site child care, assistance with transportation, social services, nutritional services (including WIC programs), and the opportunity to relate to peers in support groups. For some women, having female providers for obstetrical and gynecological services is crucial to accepting such services. Because women with HIV infection frequently have gynecological complaints such as recurrent vaginal candidiasis and high rates of cervical dysplasias, it is particularly useful if gynecological services, including colposcopy, are routinely available on site.

Women have also faced special obstacles in accessing the drug trial system which provides experimental treatments for AIDS and HIV illness. Women have been excluded from drug trials explicitly and implicitly. Often they have been required to give proof of contraception or sterilization to enroll, and they are tested for pregnancy during enrollment (Long, 1991). Trial sites do not generally consider women's special needs for child care, appropriate transportation, and appointments that match their needs for caring for children and other family members. The percentage of women enrolled in formal drug trials through the AIDS Clinical Trial Groups (ACTG), sponsored by the National Institute of Allergy and Infectious Diseases (NIAID), or in the Community Program for Clinical Research in AIDS is far below the percentage of women these programs serve. These enrollment figures suggest that women have had limited access to promising therapies, raising troubling ethical concerns about equity.

RESPONDING TO WOMEN'S NEEDS

Governmental Response

In December 1990, several governmental agencies, including the Centers for Disease Control (CDC), the National Institutes of Health (NIH), and the National Institute of Allergy and Infectious Diseases (NIAID), sponsored a conference titled the National Women and HIV Conference in Washington, D.C. More than 1,000 women attended, including many women living with HIV-AIDS. The meeting was punctuated by the frustrations of women with HIV, health-care providers who serve them, and an activist community that advocates for them. In a compelling scene, at one point during the day-long conference, the schedule had to be adjusted as woman after woman lined up at the microphone to address the audience. Stories of discrimination, lack of services, denial of benefits, recurrent gynecological problems, inadequate information about treatments, and inability to access drug trials were told. Providers expressed frustration at the systemic denial that women have experienced; the lack of appropriate resources, funding, and services; and the inadequate research into the natural history of HIV infection in women.

Another recent governmental response to women has been the establishment of an Office of Research on Women's Health in the NIH. Congressional hearings in 1990 revealed that the NIH had never accomplished its mandate to study any disease (or its treatment) in women in the same manner as these are studied in men. A Women's Health Committee now exists in the AIDS Division of NIAID to recommend research needed to understand HIV infection in women.

Medical Community Response

Among the first to notice women with HIV illness were health-care providers, often female nurses or physicians, who saw women in their clinics or in emergency departments and felt that they were the sole witnesses to the horrors of this disease in women patients. Pat Kloser, a physician who is the clinical director of AIDS services at the University of Medicine and Dentistry of New Jersey Hospital in Newark, New Jersey, where the HIV seroprevalance in women is the highest in the nation, was an early witness. Her response was to establish the first women's HIV clinic, where complete primary care, including obstetrical and gynecological services, are provided to women by women in weekly clinic sessions. Her research revealed the greatly shortened survival of women in her community who died of AIDS, yet established the improved survival for similar women who were enrolled in the clinic. Care, as usual, does make a difference. She comments:

> As an internist, I have spent a great deal of my time with patients who have incurable diseases. Most of these diseases, however, do not kill people in the 20–40 year old age group. My particular interest in this disease has become that of women with AIDS. I think that this group is much without advocacy.

Other female physicians and nurse practitioners have been instrumental in setting up programs for women and children, such as the Women and Children AIDS Project at Cook County Hospital in Chicago, the Heterosexual Transmission Study at Kings County Hospital in Brooklyn, Family and Gynecological Clinic Sessions at Bronx-Lebanon Hospital in the Bronx, and others. However, the need for women's programming exists in all facilities where women with HIV infection are seen.

The medical and scientific community have also played a role in describing and researching specific women's issues. Dr. Constance Wofsy, Codirector of AIDS Activities at San Francisco General Hospital, has spearheaded important epidemiological research for women. Dr. Howard Minkoff and colleagues at Kings County Hospital in Brooklyn, Carola Marte at Beth Israel Hospital in Manhattan, Machelle Allen at Bellevue Hospital in Manhattan, and others have studied and described standards for care of HIV-positive women.

COMMUNITY-BASED ORGANIZATIONS

Community-based organizations have sprung up throughout the country to address issues faced by women with HIV illness. Some of these are the projects of broader-issue groups (e.g., the women's support groups in such AIDS service organizations as the Shanti Project in San Francisco). However, many of the services provided to women are those found in small grass-roots projects that too often are underfunded and understaffed. The hope of such organizations, which work to link services for women in various communities, is to build a solid network that can match services to women's needs and to create strategies for their own survival through the crisis. Cynthia Acevedo, of the Women and AIDS Resource Network (WARN) in Brooklyn, describes the work as

> . . . always an uphill battle. We work without money, or have to accept money with strings attached to it, which decreases our effectiveness. We're often forced to exclude women who do not match the profile our funding sources want us to serve. Yet most of the time we manage to be creative, to be effective, to create language-appropriate materials, to really serve the women who turn to us.

Such grass-roots projects often provide peer counseling, run support groups, teach safer sex, provide support and technical assistance to health-care providers and service workers, hold conferences and meetings, and serve specific community groups. Several such projects are described below.

SisterLove Women and AIDS Project in Atlanta is a partner of the Black Women's Health Project. It provides support and services to women affected with HIV infection and their families. It has a peer program to run safe sex parties for women in homes, churches, and schools.

The California Prostitutes Education Project (CAL-PEP) has produced materials to assist sex workers to promote a safer working environment and address the specific needs of these women in negotiating with customers to use condoms.

Women in Need provides housing, childcare, and drug counseling to HIV-positive women in New York City.

The South Carolina AIDS Education Project runs out of the beauty parlor of its director, Diana Diana. The project provides women clients of the business with safe-sex education and safe-sex kits. It does outreach to teens, runs a drama group, and produces educational materials for women, teenagers, and people with low reading skills.

The Native American Women's Health Education Resource Center (Lake Andes, South Dakota), the Haitian Women's Program (New York City), the Caribbean Women's Health Association (Brooklyn, New York), Project Aware (San Francisco), and the Women's AIDS Project (Los Angeles) all represent women's AIDS projects struggling to provide direct service and advocacy to affected women in their communities.

AIDS Counseling and Education (ACE) is a peer support group at Bedford Hills Correctional Facility, a maximum-security women's prison in New York. Women prisoners created the group and worked with the prison administration to make it work. They provide AIDS education to new inmates, HIV-antibody test counseling, peer support, and a buddy system for women with AIDS in the prison infirmary. This inspiring but fragile organization has had a tremendously positive impact on the lives of women in this prison.

The New Jersey Women and AIDS Network produced a booklet entitled *Me First! Medical Manifestations of HIV in Women* as an alert to physicians and health-care providers who care for women but may not be aware of the gynecological manifestation of HIV illness in women.

ACTIVISTS

Activists who advocate for women with AIDS exist within all of the spheres already mentioned—the medical community, governmental organizations, and community-based projects. In addition, activist groups exist solely to exert pressure for needed changes, more funding, better services, research into women-specific issues, and better access to drug trials and drug treatment services relevant to women.

ACT UP, with chapters around the country, has spearheaded a campaign to create a treatment and research agenda for women with HIV infection. The ACT UP Book Group of ACT UP, New York, published *Women, AIDS, and Activism* (1990), and a number of national demonstrations have been organized by this group on issues pertaining to women and AIDS. Women activists have a unique perspective on these issues and demonstrate a persistent urgency to see change that will benefit women affected by the epidemic. As Ruth Rodriguez (founding board member of the Hispanic AIDS Forum in New York City) puts it,

What does the presence of a deadly, presently incurable disease, that can be prevented but that is fraught with superstition, fear and social stigma, mean in the Hispanic community? It means a woman hiding in her apartment, if she's lucky enough to have housing, taking care of her sick son, who may be gay . . . but these same women are not taking any measures to protect themselves from the real risks they face.

Gail Harris (formerly of the Center for Women's Policy Studies in Washington, D.C.) adds,

Women are at risk for HIV and AIDS because they don't recognize themselves in standard prevention and education campaigns. A major obstacle to education is sexism—dealing with women as a preconceived group—with no attempt to focus on women as individuals, without understanding how women live. . . . What I'm talking about is no less than a whole revolution in our way to seeing this crisis and in the way women are perceived.

Perhaps it is the women living with AIDS, or who have died of it, who can address women's needs most articulately. Iris De La Cruz, who died in May 1991, spoke eloquently of the role that support plays in the lives of women living with HIV illness:

> I started attending a group for women with HIV. I felt like I was the only woman in the world with AIDS. It was all gay white men. This group changed that. All of a sudden I discovered other women with the virus. There were black women, white women, Latinas, rich women, and poor women. There were addicts and transfusion women. They were mothers and sisters and lovers and daughters and grandmothers. Some were militant lesbians and others were Republicans (imagine that! even Republicans get AIDS). And we were all connected by the virus. Outside differences became trivial; feelings and survival were everyone's main concern.

Iris De La Cruz's comments underscore the importance of community support groups in providing women with the knowledge, the strength, and the love they must share to survive the AIDS epidemic. Through a network of community support, women can join together to address their needs and influence the direction of their lives as they struggle with the oppressive effects of prejudice, poverty, and indifference. Women must look to themselves to find the strength to live with AIDS.

REFERENCES

ACT UP/New York Women and AIDS Book Group. (1990). *Women, AIDS & Activism*. Boston: South End Press.

Alexander, P. (1988) *Prostitutes prevent AIDS: A manual for health educators* (available from CAL-PEP, P.O. Box 6297, San Francisco, CA 94101).

Allen, M. H. (1990). Primary care of women infected with the human immunodeficiency virus. *Obstetrics and Gynecology Clinics of North America, 17*(3), 557–569.

Carpenter, C. C. J., Mayer, K. H., Stein, M. D., Leibman, B. D., Fisher, A., & Fiore, T. C. (1991). Human immunodeficiency virus infection in North American women: Experience with 200 cases and a review of the literature. *Medicine, 70,* 307–325.

Chu, S. Y., Buehler, J. W., & Berkelman, R. L. (1990). Impact of the human immunodeficiency virus epidemic on mortality in women of reproductive age, United States. *Journal of the American Medical Association, 264,* 225–229.

Hoff, R., Berardi, V. P., Weiblen, B. J., et al. (1988). Seroprevalence of human immunodeficiency virus among childbearing women. *New England Journal of Medicine, 318,* 525–530.

Long, I. (1991). *Women's AIDS treatment issues: 1991 Update* (available from Iris Long, Ph.D., c/o ACT UP New York, 496 Hudson Street, Suite 4G, New York, NY 10014).

Marte, C., & Allen, M. (1992). *Gynecological protocol for HIV-infected women* (available from Carola Marte, MD, Beth Israel Hospital Methadone Program, 245 East 17th Street, New York, NY 10003; unpaginated).

Me first! Medical manifestations of HIV in women. (1990). New Brunswick, NJ: New Jersey Women and AIDS Network (available from NJWAN, 5 Elm Row, Suite 112, New Brunswick, NJ 08901).

Minkoff, H. L., & DeHovitz, J. A. (1991). Care of women infected with the human immunodeficiency virus. *Journal of the American Medical Association, 266,* 2253–2258.

Norwood, C. (1988, July). Alarming rise in deaths: Are women showing new AIDS symptoms? *MS Magazine,* 65–67.

Villalobos, A. (1989, November 26). Women twice as likely to continue sharing needles. *Gay Community News.*

RESOURCES

Programs for Women and Children

Boston Women's AIDS Information Project
c/o Fenway Community Health Center
7 Haviland Street
Boston, MA 02115
(617) 267-0900 or (617) 267-0159

Brooklyn AIDS Task Force-Women's
  Initiative and the Haitian Women's
  Program
465 Dean St.
Brooklyn, NY 11217
(718) 783-0883

Women and AIDS Resource Network
  (WARN)
30 Third Ave., Suite 212
Brooklyn, NY 11217
(718) 596-6007

Women in Crisis
133 West 21st St., 11th floor
New York, NY 10011
(212) 242-4880

Women in Need—AIDS Project
323 W. 39th St.
New York, NY 10018
(212) 695-4758

AIDS Counseling and Education (ACE)
Bedford Hills Correctional Facility
247 Harris Road
Bedford Hills, NY 10507
(914) 241-3100, ext. 275

New Jersey Women and AIDS Network
5 Elm Row, Suite 112
New Brunswick, NJ 08901
(908) 846-4462

National Black Women's Health Project
1237 Ralph David Abernathy Blvd., SW
Atlanta, GA 30310
(404) 758-9590

SisterLove Inc.
1237 Ralph D. Abernathy Blvd., SW
Atlanta, GA 30310
(404) 753-7733

AID Atlanta
1438 W. Peachtree St., NW, Suite 100
Atlanta, GA 30309
(404) 872-0600

South Carolina AIDS Education Network
2768 Decker Boulevard, Suite 98
Columbia, SC 29206
(803) 736-1171

Kupona Network-Women's Project
4611 South Ellis Ave.
Chicago, IL 60653
(312) 536-3000

Native American Women's Health
Education Resource Center
P.O. Box 572
Lake Andes, SD 57356
(605) 487-7072

Project Aware
3180 18th St.
Suite 205
San Francisco, CA 94110
(415) 476-4091

Women and AIDS Risk Network
Project L.A.
900 North Alvarado
Los Angeles, CA 94110
(213) 650-1508

Women's AIDS Network
P.O. Box 426182
San Francisco, CA 94142
(415) 864-5855 ext. 2007

Wholistic Health for Women—
    The Women's AIDS Project
8235 Santa Monica Boulevard, Suite 308
West Hollywood, CA 90046
(213) 650-1508

California Prostitutes Education Project
    (CAL-PEP)
P. O. Box 23855
Oakland, CA 94623-0055
(510) 874-7850

15

The Threat of AIDS for Women in Developing Countries

Kathleen Norr, Sheila Tlou, and James Norr

The AIDS pandemic seriously threatens women in developing countries. The direct and indirect negative consequences of AIDS in developing countries reviewed below make AIDS prevention important for all women, regardless of their age, social status, or personal risk of contracting AIDS. The many economic, political, social, and cultural factors that affect discrimination against women in other aspects of their lives also present barriers to the recognition of women's special needs related to AIDS and the allocation of resources to meet those needs. Women in developing countries suffer more inequality and lack opportunities relative to both men and women in industrialized countries. The effects of AIDS for women and their children in developing countries are devastating and require more programs responsive to women's specific needs.

This chapter identifies key factors affecting women in all developing countries, with attention to the most important regional variations. A review of ongoing prevention efforts and treatment programs in developing countries reveals that such programs have not been adequately responsive to the unique needs of women, although the number of programs for women and their sensitivity to women's issues is increasing. Awareness of the social position of women can facilitate development of prevention and treatment programs that will minimize the negative impact of AIDS on women in developing countries.

THE THREAT OF AIDS FOR WOMEN IN DEVELOPING COUNTRIES

Three-quarters of all women live in developing countries. For a variety of reasons, women in developing countries are also at much greater risk of contracting AIDS than women in developed countries. One-third of the world's HIV-positive individuals are women, and the proportion of HIV-positive women worldwide with AIDS is expected to climb to 50% by the year 2000 (Petros-Barvazian & Merson, 1990). The World Health Organization (WHO) estimates that there are about 3 million HIV-positive women in the world today, and 2.5 million of them live in sub-Saharan Africa (Chin, 1990). Latin America and the Caribbean have the second greatest number of HIV-positive women. While the incidence of AIDS was relatively low in Asia throughout the early 1980s, since 1985, there has been a rapid rise in the rate of transmission (Palca, 1991). There are now at least 200,000 HIV-positive women in Asia, mainly in Thailand, India, and China, and this region has the potential for rapid spread of HIV in the 1990s (Chin, 1990). The only developing countries where the rate of infection remains low for both women and men are in North Africa and the Middle East.

Sexual contact is the most important route of transmission for women in developing countries, although the importance of other routes differs by region. In sub-Saharan Africa, heterosexual transmission predominates for both men and women. In Latin America, sexual transmission is both homosexual and heterosexual, with transmission from bisexual males an important source of HIV infection for women. This is especially well documented in Mexico (Garcia, Valdespino, Salcedo, Magis, & Sepulveda, 1991). In Latin America, the Caribbean, and parts of Asia, injecting drug use (IDU) is also an important route of transmission. However, IDU is a much less important transmission route for women than for men due to lower rates of injecting drug use, as documented by recent studies of IDUs in Brazil (81% male) and Thailand (95% male) (Lima, Bastos, & Friedman, 1991; Vanichseni et al., 1991). In these regions, female partners of IDUs and bisexuals are at high risk for HIV infection through sexual contact. Blood contact from transfusions or other procedures has also been a significant source of infection for women, especially in more prosperous developing countries like Mexico and Brazil (Basanez, Izazola, Valdespino, & Sepulveda, 1991; Sanches, Matida, & Sole-Pla, 1991) where transfusions are more available. However, since most countries have now instituted regular testing of blood donors, this route of infection should continue to decline in importance.

In nearly all developing countries, the AIDS epidemic began in urban areas, and the number of persons with AIDS and HIV infection in urban areas remains considerably higher than in rural areas. The infection eventually spreads to the much larger rural population as infected individuals return to their partners and families. However, even in Uganda, one of the first developing countries where AIDS became widespread, urban areas, market centers, and towns continue to have higher prevalence rates than rural areas (Ankrah, Sekeeboobo, Asingwire, & Kengeya-Kayondo, 1991).

Where heterosexual transmission is the main route of infection, nearly equal numbers of women and men have AIDS and HIV infection. However, women become infected at younger ages. This means that the long-run social and economic consequences of AIDS deaths will be even greater for women than for men because earlier deaths mean a greater loss of years of childbearing and economic productivity (Decosas, 1991).

Mortality from the AIDS pandemic may be so large that the fastest-growing populations among developing countries may decelerate to zero growth, but at an unbearable cost. AIDS strikes hardest the age group any society can least afford to lose—economically active young men and women. The loss of young adults and their future contributions imposes a serious burden on economic and social systems and will severely diminish the prospects for economic growth in developing countries. In sub-Saharan Africa, even subsistence food production will be seriously threatened.

HIV and AIDS exert important indirect effects on women in developing countries. HIV-positive women face the physical and emotional burden of bearing potentially infected infants or limiting their fertility. This is especially difficult because in most developing countries, women's status and future financial security depend on their capacity to produce healthy sons. In their almost universal roles as providers of family health care, women assume much of the caregiving burden for AIDS sufferers. Caregiving is made more difficult in developing countries by the inability of the overburdened health-care system to provide adequate supportive services. Women's lower earning capacities and economic dependency on men means that women who lose their partners, sons, and other family members to AIDS are often impoverished as well as burdened with the care of AIDS orphans. In most developing countries, the AIDS pandemic will also decrease the financial and human resources available to address women's other urgent health and welfare needs, such as those addressed by maternal mortality and child survival programs (Petros-Barvazian & Merson, 1990).

While effects of AIDS are not unique only to women in developing countries, their generally lower status and their greater poverty make these effects far more devastating. In the allocation of human and material resources for the fight against AIDS, women in developing countries are all too often at the end of the line.

CONDITIONS IN DEVELOPING COUNTRIES AFFECTING WOMEN AND AIDS

Economic Factors

In all developing countries, lower levels of production and incomes mean that individuals, their families, communities, health-delivery organizations, and government agencies all have fewer resources for the AIDS pandemic. Developing countries can be divided into two groups: (1) the poorest countries that comprise most of sub-Saharan Africa and South Asia all have a per capita gross national product (GNP) lower than $600 per year compared to the average GNP per capita of $12,000 for the industrialized countries; (2) the middle-income developing countries that predominate in Latin America, the Middle East, North Africa, and the Pacific, which have average GNPs of less than $2,000 (UND Programme, 1991). Compared to industrial countries, the nonfarming resources of developing countries are more concentrated geographically, leading to greater urban-rural and regional inequalities and potential conflicts over the use of scarce resources. Most developing countries rely on only a few raw materials for international trade, making their economies more volatile and more dependent on the larger industrial economies of Japan, Germany, Great Britain, France, and the United States. When industrialized nations suffer recession, developing countries are affected by decreased exports and decreased aid from foreign donors. Greater economic volatility hampers effective planning for and efficient implementation of AIDS programs.

Discrimination against women in income and in access to economic resources is even greater in developing than in developed countries. Most available work is in either agriculture or services. Women are especially concentrated in these low-paying economic activities. Women are also more likely to work in the underground economy of informal exchange and barter, outside government controls to protect workers. They are dispersed geographically and more difficult to reach in their workplaces with information or behavioral-change programs.

The lack of economic resources in developing countries means that people suffer from health problems due to malnutrition, unsafe water and waste disposal, lack of health facilities and essential drugs, and serious shortages of trained health professionals. The average life expectancies of around 65 years in middle-income developing countries are a full decade less than the 75 years found in industrialized countries. Life expectancy in the poorer countries of sub-Saharan Africa and South Asia is more than two decades less, around 55 years or less (UNDP, 1991). Infant mortality frequently exceeds 100 per 1,000 in the poorer countries and is around 50 per 1,000 in the middle-income developing countries, compared to less than 10 per 1,000 in high-income industrialized countries (UNDP, 1991). Lack of treatment facilities for sexually transmitted diseases (STDs) is especially serious. STDs that cause genital lesions have been associated with HIV infection and may increase the risk of sexual transmission of AIDS. Developing countries spent an average of only $11 per capita in public expenditures on all health care in 1986, compared to $521 per capita in developed countries (Sivard, Brauer & Roemer, 1991). In some of the poorest countries like Bangladesh and Zaire, per capita expenditures are only $1 per capita. A health system so inadequately funded faces very stark choices in dealing with the costs of AIDS prevention and treatment programs for the population as a whole, much less the special needs of women.

The degree to which women have access to economic resources independent of men is one factor that differs greatly by region and country. In the Muslim

Middle East and North Africa, women are severely limited in their participation in wage labor (participation rates generally less 10%), although they participate heavily in subsistence agriculture and family-based crafts. Women in most of Latin America are also limited in their independent economic activities (participation rates averaging 25%), while in Africa, non-Muslim Asia, and the Caribbean, women more often have independent economic activities (labor-force participation around 50%) (Sivard et al., 1991). Women who lack independent access to economic resources will suffer more severely from the AIDS pandemic. Economic dependency makes negotiation with partners to adopt safer sex practices more difficult and increases the burden on women from the loss of partners, fathers, and other male relatives to AIDS. Lack of economic alternatives may also force some women into the commercial sex industry, further increasing their risk of HIV infection.

Even in regions like the Middle East, North Africa, and Latin America, where women have generally low labor-force participation rates, women still are critical for subsistence agriculture and household production. This means that the economies of entire countries will suffer if large proportions of rural women and their children have AIDS or must reduce their economically productive work to care for relatives who are AIDS sufferers. In sub-Saharan Africa especially, women provide most of the labor in subsistence agriculture, and the AIDS epidemic may seriously threaten food production and family income, particularly for female headed households (Norse, 1991).

In some developing countries, economic growth has fostered wholesale migration of young men, with devastating effects on family structure and on subsistence agriculture. Brown (1989) provides an excellent description of the impact of male migration to South African mines on women and families in Botswana from 1890 to the present. Similar patterns also occur in cities where work opportunities are restricted to men, in some types of plantation agriculture, in trucking and other transportation routes, and in the armed services. The existence of a high concentration of young males who are unmarried or separated from their partners often leads to the development of a local commercial sex industry. This economic pattern has had a direct effect on the AIDS pandemic by increasing sexual transmission both in the areas of male concentration and in the rural areas where the men return periodically. Hunt (1989) has shown how the spread of HIV infection in sub-Saharan Africa follows the Pan-African trucking route.

Political Factors

Political dependence on more powerful neighbors, industrial countries, and foreign donors limits developing countries in designing and implementing their own programs of response to meet their country's AIDS-related needs. In most developing countries, differences in power among classes, regions, ethnic groups, genders, and communities are greater than in industrial societies, and these differences frequently become sources of political conflict and competition. Cleavages and competition then become obstacles to an effective response to a crisis such as the AIDS pandemic. In some countries, the ability to mount an adequate response to social problems is also hampered by the general lack of effective organizations and bureaucratic personnel outside the army and large multinational corporations. The stability, representativeness, and responsiveness of the government vary considerably by region and country. Less stable governments and those less responsive to citizen needs are less likely to recognize AIDS-related needs and to develop effective AIDS programs. AIDS can easily become a political issue. Some politicians, for example, have promoted the claim that AIDS is a foreign invasion from neighboring countries or the decadent West.

The legal status and political activism of women in developing countries vary tremendously. Many developing countries restrict women's legal rights, criticism of government policy, and political protest even when other aspects of legal equality have been adopted. In Botswana, for example, the overall legal code recognizes equal rights for all races and religions, yet married women's property and child custody rights are restricted (Tlou, 1990). Women's more limited access to resources and traditional lack of political participation make political organization by women difficult. The more limited women's legal rights and ability to mobilize are, the less responsive the government and society will be to the needs and concerns of women related to AIDS and other issues.

Perhaps the most direct effect of the political structure is in the way health care is delivered and financed. Most developing countries have a national health service and support the WHO primary-health-care model emphasizing accessibility in rural as well as urban areas, affordability, preventive care, and community input. However, in some countries, more affluent citizens use private health-care facilities, resulting in a two-tiered health system. The effectiveness of health-care planning and implementation also varies greatly. Where the health system is patterned after the primary-health model, it can more effectively function and respond to the threat of AIDS for women.

Social Factors

The rural character of most developing countries means that much of the population lives in small communities with relatively little access to the economic, political, educational, and health resources of urban centers. Most of the population in developing countries, and especially most women, live in rural areas, yet most AIDS prevention and treatment programs are urban even in countries where AIDS has already spread to rural areas.

Relatively high levels of fertility and a very high value on childbearing that makes motherhood important to a woman's status are common social patterns affecting women in nearly all developing countries. Condom use, perhaps the most effective way to prevent heterosexual AIDS transmission, is problematic when couples desire more children. In addition, higher fertility means that perinatal transmission from HlV-infected women will be much higher than in developed countries, further increasing the burden of AIDS on the society.

A potential advantage in coping with the AIDS pandemic is a social pattern common to most developing countries: cooperation within the extended family unit and other social groups within communities. Given the lack of economic and health-care resources in many developing countries, this cooperation and support at the familial and community levels are among the few factors that can minimize somewhat the tremendous social disruption of the AIDS pandemic. However, it is women who usually do most of the work of cooperation, especially in caring for the sick and orphaned children, and this burden increases as the pandemic worsens. Planners must also remember that traditional support structures may not exist for marginalized groups of men and women such as commercial sex workers or migrant workers far from home, many of whom are also at especially high risk of AIDS.

In nearly all developing countries, the lives of women are highly integrated into the family, and the family usually is much larger, more cohesive, and more important than in developed countries. All societies distinguish between socially recognized marriages and informal unions or casual sexual encounters. Cultural norms and values always place some restrictions on the sexuality of men and women outside marriage, and women usually have less sexual freedom than men and suffer more serious consequences for violating cultural restrictions.

There are also wide variations in the size and nature of family and social regulation of male and female sexuality. Variations in the formation and disso- lution of sexual-partner bonds within and outside legal unions are especially critical to AIDS prevention. Developing societies differ greatly in whether polygamy is allowed, and if so, how common it is. Polygamy is not practiced at all and is illegal in Latin America and the Caribbean. In Buddhist and Hindu Asia, polygamy is not illegal, but it is extremely uncommon. All of the Moslem world and most of sub-Saharan Africa permit polygamy for men. However, in some countries like Botswana, it has always been quite rare, while in other countries it is a fairly common occurrence. A survey in Unganda found that 30% of married women were in polygamous unions (McCombie, Bukombi, & Dupree, 1991).

In some societies as in most of South Asia, social norms restrict sexual activ- ity to marriage, marriage is monogamous, and the marriage bond is very diffi- cult to break for both wives and husbands. These norms are seldom fully fol- lowed in practice, and violations by men are tolerated far more than violations by women. A variant of this pattern, widespread in the Middle East, North Af- rica, and Latin America, and parts of Southest Asia, restricts sexual activity and divorce for women but tolerates extramarital sex and easy divorce or separation for men. Where women's sexuality is very restricted, most women are at rela- tively low risk of HIV infection from their own behavior, but they are at risk of contracting AIDS from their regular partners. Two studies of wives of workers in Southern India found almost no extramarital sexual activity among the women (Kandaswami et al., 1991; Ravinathan et al., 1991). However, one of these studies looked at STDs and found that 100 women out of 573 were infected, presumably due to their husband's behavior (Ravinathan et al., 1991). In Thailand, a large survey of Buddhist Thais found that 17% of married men, but only 0.9% of married women, reported having sex outside marriage (Sittitrai, Brown, Phanuphak, Barry, & Sabaiying, 1991). Confronting the problem of AIDS and devoting resources to AIDS prevention is difficult in societies with these behavior patterns. The spread of AIDS reveals the actual, as opposed to the ideal, patterns of behavior, and it is often easier to stigmatize persons with AIDS than to recognize these realities. Because wives cannot easily challenge husbands, married women are especially vulnerable to infection due to their husbands' behavior.

A different pattern occurs in the Caribbean and most of sub-Saharan Africa. Many men and women go through a series of easily broken unions, usually not in formal marriage, before eventually "settling down." The woman often assumes the major burden of support for her children, frequently with help from her kin. Female-headed households, births outside marriage, the presence of children in the same families with different fathers, extramarital affairs, and divorce are all common. This pattern is often associated with migratory or plantation labor that makes it difficult for men to support or to stay with a family. Men and women with more economic and other resources usually have earlier and more stable unions in the same society, creating substantial differences in union patterns by social class. Surveys in five African countries find that men have more casual and commercial sex than women and that currently married persons have less casual sex than the never married or formerly married (Carael, Carballo, Ferry, Mehryar, & Slutkin, 1991). In Uganda, a comparison of HIV-positive and HIV-negative women attending a pediatric clinic found that HIV-positive women had more partners (2.5 versus 1.95 in the last five years), lower income, and more often agreed that women have boyfriends for economic reasons (Rwabukwali et al., 1991). In Rwanda, women not legally married and those with more partners were more likely to be HIV positive (Chao et al., 1991). A study of low-risk women in Kenya concluded that while the women's number of lifetime sexual partners was related to HIV status, this factor only partially explained their HIV status, and concluded that many women were at greater risk from their partners' behaviors than their own (Reyes, Oberle, Leoro, Rubio, & Kreiss, 1991). These studies document that more frequent union formation and dissolution favor the relatively rapid heterosexual transmission of AIDS. Both women and men are likely to have multiple lifetime partners and to be without a regular partner periodically (and thus vulnerable to casual sexual encounters), increasing women's risk of AIDS from their own and their partners' behaviors. Women in these societies can more readily recognize that they are at risk than women in societies with more rigid union patterns, but this does not mean it is easy for them to change these behaviors. Even women in a more stable relationship may not want to question their partners because of concern for breaking the more fragile bonds of the relationship.

In virtually all developing societies, a group of women are commercial sex workers full-time or part-time, but the size of the commercial sex industry and the degree to which it is tolerated, or regulated, vary greatly. Most of these women are young and poor, highly stigmatized by the rest of society, and are at the most immediate risk of HIV infection. They are often blamed as the source of infection for their clients rather than viewed as people with a personal need for protection. Among the poor, in addition to commercial sex workers there is often a much larger group of women who have multiple partners in their search for economic and emotional security and perhaps occasional presents. These women have economic motives for sexual relations but are not commercial sex workers. This is especially common where a large number of women are not in legal marriages.

Cultural Factors

While all cultures have values and beliefs that legitimate the lower status of women, there are also differences in the nature and strength of these values and beliefs. Generally, there is high congruence between women's economic independence, role in families, and cultural values. The greater the culturally defined inferiority of women, the more difficulty women will have in initiating safer sex. Values and beliefs about sexuality also differ greatly, from near total repression of female sexuality in many Middle Eastern cultures to recognition and legitimization of the sexuality of women common in most of sub-Saharan Africa. Ambivalence about female sexuality is present to some degree in most cultures and is pronounced in Latin American cultures where women are dichotomized into "good" mothers and "bad" promiscuous women. The degree to which sexuality can be discussed greatly affects the ease of AIDS education, especially for young people.

The rate of AIDS transmission is also affected by specific cultural practices. In some African countries such as Zaire, the use of vaginal irritants to enhance the sexual experience creates vaginal lesions and increases the likelihood of heterosexual transmission for women (Brown & Brown, 1991). In Sierra Leone, 95% of adults have participated in ceremonies involving bloodletting for ritual scarification, male and female circumcision, and traditional healing (Makiu, Kosia, & Mansaray, 1991).

Traditional health beliefs and practices also have a direct impact on AIDS. Unfortunately, this area has not been well researched. In Botswana, AIDS was initially identified with boswagadi, a life-threatening condition caused by violation of the taboos against sexual intercourse after widowhood (Ingstaadt, 1990). While these taboos apply to both men and women, in practice it is only women who are accused. Obviously, this interpretation of AIDS blames the woman. Traditional healers today differ about whether AIDS is boswagadi, and therefore curable, or a new disease from Europeans that cannot be cured by traditional methods. Traditional beliefs are often ignored by the "official" health system, but a recognition and incorporation of these beliefs is more likely to lead to successful prevention and treatment approaches. In Botswana, for example, a meeting with traditional healers discussed how the condom could prevent the "mixing" of fluids that is the reason for sexual taboos, thus preventing both boswagadi and HIV infection (Ingstaadt, 1990).

AIDS PROGRAMS FOR WOMEN IN DEVELOPING COUNTRIES

The lack of resources in developing countries has meant a considerable lag between the international recognition of women's needs and development of research and interventions to address these needs. At the 1991 International Conference on AIDS, only 33 of over 200 presentations in the areas of epidemiology and social and behavioral factors related to AIDS were about women, and only 20 presentations (less than 10%) focused on women in developing countries.

Mass Media

Widespread mass media campaigns in developing countries have increased knowledge about AIDS, but there is little evidence that these efforts have led to behavioral changes or that knowledge about AIDS relates to preventive behaviors (Schopper, 1990). The accomplishments of mass media campaigns in increasing public awareness and correct knowledge of AIDS are an essential first step in the process of behavioral change. However, changes in sexual behaviors will require more personally relevant messages and support for change. While both women and men have benefited from mass-media campaigns, messages for the public in general are likely to be messages designed from the perspective of men. Now that the basic AIDS-prevention messages have been disseminated, messages that address women's lack of power to control their level of risk due to their partners' behaviors should be disseminated. A second difficulty is that mass media do not reach many women in developing countries. Hailegnaw (1991) has pointed out that in the poorest developing nations, many people lack access to the mass media of radio and television, especially in rural areas. Lower literacy levels, less urban migration, and greater seclusion of women in some cultures makes reaching women through mass media more difficult than reaching men, as documented in Cote d'Ivoire (Messou, 1991). Combining mass media with other strategies can increase the effectiveness of educational intervention. In Sierra Leone, street theater rather than radio is used for mass campaigns as a way to overcome low literacy levels (Mansaray, Kosia, Bangura,

Nicolls, & Makiu, 1991). In Zaire, linking mass media with personal contacts such as listening groups has increased the impact of media campaigns in rural areas (Convisser, Kyungu, Kambamba, & Eiger, 1991). AIDS programs in developing countries need to assess carefully how well their mass-media campaigns reach women, especially rural and low-status women.

Targeting Sexual Transmission

Most AIDS-prevention and research programs in developing countries have focused on heterosexual activities, the most common route of transmission. Unlike the United States, where most women with AIDS are economically disadvantaged and women of color, epidemiologic studies show that in developing countries AIDS can threaten women at all social levels. In Malawi and Rwanda, women of higher social status (for example, defined as married to a man with more than eight years of education) are more likely to be HIV positive (Chao et al., 1991; McCombie, Rwakagiri, Bukombi, & Cohn, 1991). On the other hand, a study in rural Uganda found higher economic level associated with lower rates of HIV infection for both male and female-headed households (Seeley, Malamba, Nunn, & Mulder, 1991).

Despite evidence of risk throughout the social spectrum, few programs in developing countries focus on reducing heterosexual transmission in general populations. In Uganda, community health workers succeeded in increasing condom knowledge in the areas they served, but they did not succeed in reducing risky behaviors (Ssembatya, Kelley, Nduhura, & Wawer, 1991). A program in Cote d'Ivoire has integrated AIDS prevention into its primary-health-care mobile teams serving rural villages. There has been good acceptance by the villagers, but no data on impact have yet been reported (Poinsignon, Lavreys, & Boni Mel, 1991).

Condoms are an important part of programs aimed at preventing sexual transmission of HIV for both the general public and high-risk groups like commercial sex workers. Condom use in the eastern Caribbean and workplaces in Uganda is not associated with AIDS awareness, knowledge, or perceived risk, but is related to the belief that peers use condoms and discussion about condoms with peers and partners (McCombie, Bukombi, et al., 1991; Middlestadt, Zucker, Ramah, & Eustace, 1991). The social marketing of condoms has proven an effective way to reach a large number of persons in both Zaire (high prevalence) and Cameroon (low prevalence) (Hassig, Price, Earle, & Spilsbury, 1991). Promotion of condoms emphasizing positive and relational values rather than AIDS prevention, health, or family planning has been successful in the eastern Caribbean (Ostfield, Fevrier, Jagdeo, Coles, & France, 1991). In the Caribbean, skill with condoms was related to more frequent use (Uribe et al., 1991), and in Santo Domingo breakage rates for older condoms were much higher than for new ones (Guerrero, Zacarias, Jordan, & Rosario, 1991). Among Mexican sex workers, condoms were rejected due to vaginal irritation by those with three or more clients per day (Uribe, et al., 1991). For women, condoms are difficult because they are a male method of protection. The development of a female condom will be an important breakthrough for women, especially since this new product will start out with fewer negative stereotypes. Commercial sex workers in Thailand have used an experimental female condom and liked it (Sakondhavat et al., 1991).

Since women in developing countries contract HIV infection at younger ages than men, promotion of safer sex for teens is especially important for women. Even in countries with the highest rates of HIV infection, young teenagers are largely free of infection, so protecting them from future infection is extremely important. Studies in several different regions document that lack of knowledge and early sexual activity put many adolescents at risk (Bagarukayo, 1991; Duale, Vangu, Bange, Duale, & Munkatu, 1991; Sanchez, Vega, Alvarez, & Gotuzzo, 1991; Uwakwe, 1991).

Unfortunately, in many developing countries programs aimed at teens are hampered by cultural restrictions on sex education and denial of teen sexual activity. These barriers must be broken down through intensive work with parents, teachers, health workers, and teens before programs for teens can achieve success. In Zaire, the local chapter of the Society for Women and AIDS in Africa (SWAA) brings trained SWAA members into secondary schools to conduct weekly classes on AIDS prevention with pupils over two months (Bishagara et al., 1991). Education of teachers is another approach that has been used successfully in five Latin American countries (Erbstein, Schenker, & Greenblatt, 1991) and in Botswana (de Wildt et al., 1991). A program in Benin uses students participating in an educational program in school as a way to also reach their parents (Verbeke & Fransen, 1991). All of these programs explicitly address cultural barriers to frank discussion about sexuality with teens. The SWAA program also explicitly recognizes the special needs of women and younger girls.

Programs aimed at helping young women remain free of AIDS need to consider the different social situations of adolescent females and males. In many developing countries, cultural reticence about discussing sexuality remains, but the traditional social patterns that regulated sexual behaviors of adolescents (such as sequestering or limiting movement of young women, presence of adults in the home most of the time, absence of private meeting places for the young, etc.) have disappeared, especially in urban areas. Young women need to be given the social skills to handle these new situations. More long-term approaches to protection for young people should also focus on greater education and economic opportunity for women that will increase women's ability to insist on safer sex practices and decrease pressures for early marriage and childbearing.

The largest number of programs to reduce heterosexual transmission in developing countries has focused on groups at highest risk, predominately commercial sex workers. Higher levels of seropositivity for commercial sex workers in many developing countries are well documented, and computer simulation identifies this group as an important route of transmission to the general population (Schopper, 1990). The pioneering project of Ngugi and her associates uses a peer education and empowerment model that has increased condom use and slowed the seroconversion rates of commercial sex workers in Nairobi, Kenya (Ngugi et al., 1988; Ngugi et al., 1991). This project is important because it works collaboratively with the community of women affected rather than being imposed by more powerful people, mostly male, from above. Another successful program in Zaire provides HIV testing, STD treatment, and condom promotion and distribution for commercial sex workers at an STD clinic. In 22 months, the rate of HIV seroconversion decreased from 18% to 2.2%, and regular condom use with clients increased from 4% to 55%. However, this project and one in Zimbabwe also found a persistant lack of condom use in the sex workers' noncommercial relationships (Tuliza et al., 1991; Wilson et al., 1991).

A recent review by WHO and the AIDS prevention division of Family Health International (known as AIDSTECH) identified 45 peer education programs for commercial sex workers in developing countries (Ferencic, Alexander, Slutkin, & Lamptey, 1991). Almost all of these programs have had a positive impact, increasing condom use some or all of the time by as much as 81%. However, client resistance, lack of power of sex workers to negotiate with clients, lack of support by brothel managers, and inadequate condom access remain important barriers to consistent condom use by commercial sex workers. Equally important is the small scale of most projects and major organizational and funding difficulties that hamper expansion and sustainability.

Programs in several countries are beginning to address some of the barriers to safer sex for commercial sex workers. Several projects have found that nongovernmental organizations have greater flexibility in program development that permits them to be more responsive to the specific life situations and needs of marginalized groups (Crane, Filgueiras, Row Kavi, & Swaminathan, 1991). A project in Thailand, for example, is working directly with brothel managers to institute mandatory condom use policies (Sakondhavat, Werawatakul, & Bennett, 1991). In Nigeria, a prevention program developed solidarity among prostitutes, so they succeeded in insisting upon condom use and raising their prices, thus maintaining income with fewer partners (Williams, Lamson, Lamptery, 1991). A pilot study with commercial sex workers in India found that clients' social power is so much greater than the commercial sex workers' that condom promotion must focus on or at least include the client (Swaminathan & Kumaresan, 1991). Several projects are addressing male clients in Kenya, Tanzania, and Zimbabwe through outreach and condom promotion to truckers, a group especially likely to use commercial sex workers and engage in other casual sex (Mwizarubi, 1991; Omari Mohamed, 1991; Wilson, Lamson, Nyathi, Sibanda, & Sibanda, 1991). The Tanzania project has found that the truckers' partners are motivated to practice safer sex but have less power to implement changes in the sexual relationship (Mwizarubi et al., 1991). A major criticism of all these programs from a woman's perspective is their lack of attention to the social and economic structures that permit the sexual exploitation of women and give women little control over partner behaviors.

Perinatal Transmission

Because motherhood is often critical for women's status and long-term security, childbearing is a high priority for most women. The plight of the HIV-positive woman is especially tragic if she is childless or pregnant. A counseling program for HIV-positive pregnant women in Zaire found that despite counseling about the risk to their infants, 68% did not want to make any change in their current pregnancy or future fertility plans (Batter et al., 1991). Recent studies have found perinatal transmission rates of 30% in Rwanda (Lepage et al., 1991) and 39–45% in Kenya (Datta, Embree, Ndinya-Achola, Kreiss, & Plumer, 1991). Several recent studies have documented lower birth weights and higher infant mortality and morbidity for infants born to HIV-positive mothers (Adjorlolo et al., 1991; Guay et al., 1991; Lepage et al., 1991; Miotti et al., 1991), and even for infants who remain HIV negative (Datta et al., 1991). In Rwanda, there has been documented postnatal transmission for infants of 9 out of 16 mothers, most often in the first trimester (van de Perre et al., 1991).

Perinatally acquired AIDS raises many serious public-policy and ethical issues regarding widespread screening of pregnant women, counseling, therapeutic abortion, breast-feeding recommendations for HIV-positive and HIV-negative mothers in high-prevalence areas, and surveillance and treatment for infants. These issues must be resolved in the cultural context and epidemic pattern of specific countries. Research findings will help in these decisions but cannot resolve them. However these issues are resolved, it is extremely important that the rights and dignity of women be respected. Where decisions affect a woman's body directly, the woman should have the most important input into that decision. In particular, public policy and practices by health-care professionals must ensure that the more powerful male partners do not make unilateral decisions about what happens to women.

Direct Contact with Blood

Blood transfusion or procedures involving direct contact with blood such as scarification, circumcision, or traditional healing ceremonies have also been the focus of prevention efforts in developing countries. Women are more affected by the safety of the blood supply than men because blood transfusion is often used for childbirth-related bleeding. WHO has successfully initiated a worldwide program of technical assistance and financial support to provide safe blood in 22 countries (Watson, Fournel, Sondag, & Fransen, 1991). A program in the Dominican Republic has succeeded in reducing the proportion of AIDS cases attributable to blood transfusion from 20% in 1985 to under 5%, even though not all the blood supply is screened (Pena, De Moya, Garris, & Gomez, 1991). They point out that half the transfusions are for dubious reasons and that a decrease in unnecessary transfusions is also important in reducing transmission. Reduction of HIV transmission due to traditional practices can be promoted by helping traditional healers to adopt safety measures like the use of a new razor blade for each client.

Protection of health-care workers exposed to HIV infection through needle-stick injuries and other accidents is also important. In developing countries as well as industrial countries, the majority of health-care workers are women. Unfortunately, a review of practices in developing countries and specific studies in the Caribbean, Brazil, and Uganda all document a lack of adequate knowledge, training, and resources such as disposable equipment, gloves, and sterilization equipment that result in inadequate safety precautions for health workers (Bailey, 1991; Byahuka, Naamara, Byangire, Duggan, & Rushota, 1991; Lauria et al., 1991; Wilson, Mooteeram, Gayle, & Hull, 1991). Health workers also suffer great psychological stress as a result of the AIDS pandemic, and few developing countries have programs to address these needs. Women in the health professions need to initiate activities for mutual support and self-protection from occupational exposure to HIV.

The initiation of widespread screening of blood has led to the need for counseling of those found to be HIV-positive. However, such programs require substantial resources to train medical personnel or others to act as effective counselors. Setting up and maintaining counseling programs has been difficult for health personnel in both northern Thailand (Taywaditep, Mandel, Vithayasai, Leelamanit, & Kearst, 1991) and the Congo (M'Pele, Lallemant LaCoeur, Lallemant, & Samba, 1991). Posttest counseling raises many issues since many HIV-positive persons are reluctant to inform their partners out of fear of rejection, and it is important that programs involve the couple and not just the seropositive individual. The importance of posttest counseling, especially where one partner is seronegative, is documented by findings in Cote d'Ivoire and Kenya that the seronegative partner is very likely to become HIV-positive (Moss et al., 1991; N'Gbichi et al., 1991). A counseling program in Kenya for discordant couples (one partner HIV-positive and one HIV-negative) has been successful in increasing condom use, but seroconversion remained high (Moss et al., 1991) In Uganda, a model testing center provides long-term support for those who are HIV-negative to help them remain negative, and also provides support to HIV-positive persons and their partners (Barugahare, Byaruhanga, & Muller, 1991).

Caring for Persons with AIDS

Programs for persons with AIDS highlight the many differences between industrialized and developing nations. In developing countries, HIV-positive persons generally progress to AIDS symptoms more quickly and die sooner after AIDS develops. Twenty-five per cent of asymptomatic blood donors in Zaire who were HIV-positive died within 12 months (Luo, Mwendafilumba, & Chipoka, 1991). Developing countries cannot afford the costly preventive drugs or the aggressive treatment of opportunistic infections now commonly used in industrialized countries. Persons with AIDS in developing countries usually do not experience rejection by the family but often fear rejection by neighbors, as found by a study in urban Uganda (McGrath, Ankrah, Schumann, Lubega, & Nkumbi, 1991). The families of persons with AIDS also suffer many negative consequences. In Zaire, poverty, family breakup, and early end to education for children are all documented negative consequences of AIDS for families (Haworth et al., 1991). Programs of home care by the Chikankata Hospital (Campbell, Bodwell, & Rader, 1991) and the Society of Women Against Aids in Africa (Mwadi et al., 1991) in Zaire provide a model now being considered for replication in industrialized countries. Regular visits provide education and support to the caregiving family and medical treatments to alleviate suffering. This program allows persons with AIDS to die with dignity in the comfort of their homes without undue burden on caregiving families or the health-care system and helps destigmatize AIDS and dispel myths about persons with AIDS in the community as a whole. Such programs are especially important for women in developing countries who bear the primary burden of caring for persons with AIDS.

IMPLICATIONS FOR FUTURE PROGRAMS

This review of programs directed at AIDS prevention for women in developing countries shows that women need greater equity in the proportion of resources devoted to their AIDS-related needs, that AIDS prevention programs need to explicitly address discriminatory barriers that affect women, and that improving women's overall position is an important component of AIDS prevention.

The share of resources devoted to women is substantially below the proportion of women who are HIV-infected and should be increased to at least half of all programs. Women in rural areas and women who are not commercial sex workers are especially underserved, and these women are the substantial majority in all developing countries. Most existing programs explicitly for women focus on commercial sex workers and pregnant women. While there are often good epidemiological reasons for this approach, unfortunately this allocation of resources conveys the messages that women only matter as potential sources of infection to men and children and that AIDS is a concern only for a small subgroup of women. The lack of equity for women can be addressed through programs that serve both men and women, but such programs need to recognize the special needs of women.

In nearly all developing countries—indeed in all countries—women's relative lack of status, power, and economic resources make them dependent on men and limit their ability to convince partners to practice safer sex. Programs focused on heterosexual transmission need to help women learn partner-negotiating skills and ways to support each other in AIDS prevention. Methods of AIDS prevention that give more control to women, such as female condoms, need to have more emphasis. Efforts to reduce perinatal transmission should consider the impact of pregnancy on the health of the HIV-positive woman as well as her infant and formulate public-policy responsive to the needs of women as well as children. Programs focused on commercial sex need to expand their focus to male clients and the social and economic conditions that maintain the commercial sex industry. Women in their roles as health professionals and as home caregivers need the knowledge and resources to protect themselves from HIV infection and the economic and psychological support for their difficult tasks.

Helping women to adopt risk-reducing behaviors requires the legal, economic, political, social, and psychological empowerment of women, not just increasing AIDS-prevention knowledge. Education for women is an extremely important long-run component of AIDS prevention for women because of its overall impact on economic opportunity, greater awareness, self-esteem, and other critical factors. Another serious issue is the provision of alternative sources of economic and social security for men and women that will help to reduce the pressure on women to have children regardless of the HIV status of both partners. These changes are all politically and culturally controversial and will not be accomplished overnight. Most also require a substantial economic investment, but others, such as providing women with legal rights, can be afforded by even the poorest developing nations. While these efforts may not have immediate effects on the AIDS pandemic, there will be many economic and social benefits from these changes that will affect overall development and health as well as AIDS prevention.

REFERENCES

Adjorlolo, G., Gayle, H., Ekpini, E., Sibailly, T., Brattegaard, K., & DeCock, K. M. (1991). Prospective study of HIV-1 and HIV-2 mother-to-child transmission in Abidjan, Cote D'Ivoire. (Abstract M.C. 3053). In *VII International Conference on AIDS Abstract Book* (Vol. 1, p. 311). Florence, Italy.

Ankrah, M., Ssekeboobo, A., Asingwire, N., & Kengeya-Kayondo, J. (1991). The environment, HIV testing and Ugandan women (Abstract M.D.4246). In *VII International Conference on AIDS Abstract Book* (Vol. 1, p. 451). Florence, Italy.

Bagarukayo, H. (1991). KAP study on AIDS among school pupils in Kabale District, Uganda (Abstract W.D.4222). In *VII International Conference on AIDS Abstract Book* (Vol. 2, p. 443). Florence, Italy.

Bailey, M. (1991). Assessment of risk in developing country health work (Abstract W.D.4176). In *VII International Conference on AIDS Abstract Book* (Vol. 2, p. 432). Florence, Italy.

Barugahare, L., Byaruhanga, T., & Muller, O. (1991). The POSTTEST club—project of the AIDS information center in Kampala/Uganda (Abstract M.D.4215). In *VII International Conference on AIDS Abstract Book* (Vol. 1, p. 443). Florence, Italy.

Basanez, R. A., Izazola, J. A., Valdespino, J. L., & Sepulveda, J. (1991). Risk perception, sexual practices and AIDS related health service use among women in Mexico (Abstract M.D.4228). In *VII International Conference on AIDS Abstract Book* (Vol. 2, p. 447). Florence, Italy.

Batter, V., Malulu, M., Mbuyi, K., Mbu, L., Kamenga, M., & St. Louis, M. (1991). HIV seronotification and counselling of childbearing women in Kinshasa, Zaire (Abstract M.D.4013). In *VII International Conference on AIDS Abstract Book* (Vol. 1, p. 393). Florence, Italy.

Bishagara, K., Kasali, M., Tuliza, M., Mulanga, K., Grandpierre, J., & Piri Piri, L. (1991). Mobilization of women in the struggle against AIDS in urban areas: Action among young people (Abstract TU.D.111). In *VII International Conference on AIDS Abstract Book* (Vol. 1, p. 86). Florence, Italy.

Brown, B. B. (1989). Women in Botswana. In J. L. Parpart, (Ed.), *Women and Development in Africa*. Lanham, VA.: University Press of America.

Brown, R. C., & Brown, J. E. (1991). The use of intra-vaginal irritants as a risk factor for the transmission of HIV infection among Zairian prostitutes (Abstract M.C.3006). In *VII International Conference on AIDS Abstract Book* (Vol. 1, p. 299). Florence, Italy.

Byahuka, E., Naamara, W., Byangire, M., Duggan, M., & Rushota, R. (1991). AIDS: a challenge to the nursing profession (Abstract W.D.4167). In *VII International Conference on AIDS Abstract Book* (Vol. 2, p. 429). Florence, Italy.

Campbell, I. D., Bodwell, S., & Rader, A. (1991). Transferable concepts in AIDS programme development—a South/North Exchange (Abstract M.D.4297). In *VII International Conference on AIDS Abstract Book* (Vol. 1, p. 464). Florence, Italy.

Carael, M., Carballo, M., Ferry, B., Mehryar, A, & Slutkin, G. (1991). Prevalence of high risk sexual behaviors in some African countries: Evidence from recent surveys (Abstract M.D.4109). In *VII International Conference on AIDS Abstract Book* (Vol. 1, p. 417). Florence, Italy.

Chao, A., Bulterys, M., Musanganire, F., Mukafaranswa, B., Nawrocki, P., Dushimiana, S., Hoover, D., & Saah, A. (1991). Risk factors for HIV-1 Seropositivity among pregnant women in Rwanda (Abstract M.C.3097). In *VII International Conference on AIDS Abstract Book* (Vol. 1, p. 332). Florence, Italy.

Chin, J. (1990, November & December). Challenge of the nineties. *World Health*.

Clerici-Schoeller, M., Plebani, A., Bardare, M., Zehender, G., Capelli, C., & Zanetti, A. R. (1991). Mother to child transmission of HIV infection (Abstract W.C.3267). In *VII International Conference on AIDS Abstract Book* (Vol. 2, p. 362). Florence, Italy.

Convisser, J., Kyungu, M., Kambamba, S. A., & Eiger, R. (1991). AIDS communication programs in the African context: integrating mass media and interpersonal approaches in Zaire (Abstract W.D.4267). In *VII International Conference on AIDS Abstract Book* (Vol. 2, p. 454). Florence, Italy.

Crane, S. F., Filgueiras, A., Row Kavi, A., & Swaminathan, S. (1991). Reaching marginalized groups through local non-governmental organizations (Abstract W.D.56). In *VII International Conference on AIDS Abstract Book* (Vol. 2, p. 37). Florence, Italy.

Datta, P., Embree, J., Ndinya-Achola, J. O., Kreiss, J., & Plumer, F. A. (1991). Perinatal HIV-1 transmission in Nairobi, Kenya: 5 year follow-up (Abstract M.C.3). In *VII International Conference on AIDS Abstract Book* (Vol. 1, p. 20). Florence, Italy.

Decosas, J. (1991). The demographic AIDS trap for women in Africa—Implications for health promotion strategies. (Abstract W.D. 6). In *VII International Conference on AIDS Abstract Book* (Vol. 2, p. 21). Florence, Italy.

de Wildt, G. R., Frenken, H., Makgonedi, F., Molosiwa, K., Seeletso, L., & Stronkhornst, R. (1991). AIDS and the science curriculum in Botswana (Abstract W.D.110). In *VII International Conference on AIDS Abstract Book* (Vol. 2, p. 51). Florence, Italy.

Duale, S., Vangu, N., Bange, N., Duale, L., & Munkatu, M. (1991). Knowledge and beliefs about AIDS among high school students in two health zones in the Ubangi area of Zaire (Abstract W.D.4230). In *VII International Conference on AIDS Abstract Book* (Vol. 2, p. 445). Florence, Italy.

Erbstein, S., Schenker, I., & Greenblatt, C. (1991). Training teachers in AIDS education: evaluation of the first 12 courses in Latin America (Abstract W.D.4220). In *VII International Conference on AIDS Abstract Book* (Vol. 2, p. 443). Florence, Italy.

Ferencic, N., Alexander, P., Slutkin, G., & Lamptey, P. (1991). Study to review effectiveness and coverage of current sex-work interventions in developing countries (Abstract TU.C.56). In *VII International Conference on AIDS Abstract Book* (Vol. 1, p. 70). Florence, Italy.

Garcia, M. L., Valdespino, J. L., Salcedo, R. A., Magis, C., & Sepulveda, J. (1991). Impact of bisexuality on AIDS cases in Mexico (Abstract M.C.3310). In *VII International Conference on AIDS Abstract Book* (Vol. 1, p. 375). Florence, Italy.

Guay, L., Ball, P., Ndugwa, C., Kenya-Mugisha, Hom, D., Kataaha, P., Goldfarb, J., Vjecha, M., Mmiro, F., & Olness, K. (1991). Preliminary results of the natural history of HIV infection in Ugandan infants (Abstract M.C.96). In *VII International Conference on AIDS Abstract Book* (Vol. 1, p. 47). Florence, Italy.

Guerrero, E., Zacarias, F., Jordan, J., & Rosario, S. (1991). Use and breakage of condoms with and without Nonoxinol in Santo Domingo, Dominican Republic (Abstract M.C.3346). In *VII International Conference on AIDS Abstract Book* (Vol. 1, p. 384). Florence, Italy.

Hailegnaw, W. (1991). Factors affecting the dissemination of information on AIDS in Ethiopia (Abstract TH.D.115). In *VII International Conference on AIDS Abstract Book* (Vol. 2, p. 85). Florence, Italy.

Hassig, S. E., Price, J., Earle, D., & Spilsbury, J. (1991). A tale of two programs—Social marketing in Zaire and Cameroon (Abstract W.D.4011). In *VII International Conference on AIDS Abstract Book* (Vol. 2, p. 390). Florence, Italy.

Haworth, A., Kalumba, K., Kwapa, P., Hamavhwa, C., Van Praag, E., & Nyirenda, J. (1991). Social consequences of AIDS in 49 Zambian Families (Abstract M.D.4264). In *VII International Conference on AIDS Abstract Book* (Vol. 1, p. 456). Florence, Italy.

Hunt, C. H. (1989). Migrant labor and sexually transmitted disease: AIDS in Africa. *Journal of Health and Social Behavior, 30*(4), 345–352.

Ingstaad, B. (1990). The cultural construction of AIDS and its consequences for prevention in Botswana. *Medical Anthropology Quarterly, 4*(1), 145.

Kandaswami, J., Ravinathan, R., Padmarajan, S., Sethuraman, Venkataram, M. K., Ganesh, R., & Jayakumar, W. (1991). Sero-epidemiological study of HIV infection in two major centres of South India (Abstract M.C.3302). In *VII International Conference on AIDS Abstract Book* (Vol. 1, p. 373). Florence, Italy.

Lauria, L. M., Vieira, M., Werneck, E., Janini, M., Carvalho, C., Oliveira, J., Carreira, M., Marques, M., Lucarevschi, B., Kritski, A., Barroso, P., & Hearst, N. (1991). Knowledge, attitudes and practices (KAP) about HIV infection and AIDS among health care workers in Rio de Janeiro, Brasil (Abstract W.D.4158). In *VII International Conference on AIDS Abstract Book* (Vol. 2, p. 427). Florence, Italy.

Lepage, P., Van de Perre, P., Msellati, P., Hitimana, D. G., Van Goethem, C., Bazubagira, A., Stevens, A. M., Mukamabano, B., Simonon, A., & Dabis, F. (1991). Natural history of HIV-1 infection in children in Rwanda: A prospective cohort study (Abstract W.C.46). In *VII International Conference on AIDS Abstract Book* (Vol. 2, p. 34). Florence, Italy.

Lima, E., Bastos, F., & Friedman, S. (1991). HIV-1 epidemiology among IVDU's in Rio de Janeiro, Brazil (Abstract W.C.3287). In *VII International Conference on AIDS Abstract Book* (Vol. 2, p. 367). Florence, Italy.

Luo, N. P., Mwendafilumba, D., & Chipoka, L. (1991). Development of AIDS in asymptomatic, HIV positive, non-remunerated blood donors (Abstract M.C.3139). In *VII International Conference on AIDS Abstract Book* (Vol. 1, p. 332). Florence, Italy.

MacCallum, L. R., Johnstone, F. D., Brettle, R. P., Hamilton, B. A., Peutherer, J., Burns, S. M., & Gore, S. (1991). Population based, controlled study: Effect of HIV infection on infectious complications during pregnancy (Abstract W.C.3238). In *VII International Conference on AIDS Abstract Book* (Vol. 2, p. 355). Florence, Italy.

Makiu, E., Kosia, A., & Mansaray, N. (1991). Socio-cultural beliefs and practices—possible impediments to AIDS control efforts in Sierra Leone (Abstract W.D.4118). In *VII International Conference on AIDS Abstract Book* (Vol. 2, p. 417). Florence, Italy.

Mansaray, N., Kosia, A., Bangura, I. H., Nicolls, A., & Makiu, E. (1991). Community theatre performance—a model of AIDS health promotion activity in Sierra Leone (Abstract W.D.4018). In *VII International Conference on AIDS Abstract Book* (Vol. 2, p. 392). Florence, Italy.

McCombie, S., Bukombi, S., & Dupree, J. D. (1991). Changes in condom use among women in Uganda (Abstract W.D.4104). In *VII International Conference on AIDS Abstract Book* (Vol. 1, p. 414). Florence, Italy.

McCombie, S., Rwakagiri, F., Bukombi, S., & Cohn, P. (1991). Sociodemographic predictors of AIDS related knowledge and practice in Uganda (Abstract M.D.107). In *VII International Conference on AIDS Abstract Book* (Vol. 1, p. 50). Florence, Italy.

McGrath, J. W., Ankrah, E. M., Schumann, D. A., Lubega, M., & Nkumbi, S. (1991). The psychosocial impact of AIDS in urban Ugandan families (Abstract M.D.4261). In *VII International Conference on AIDS Abstract Book* (Vol. 1, p. 455). Florence, Italy.

Messou, E. (1991). Information sources about AIDS in the Ivory coast (Abstract W.D.4249). In *VII International Conference on AIDS Abstract Book* (Vol. 2, p. 460). Florence, Italy.

Middlestadt, S. E., Zucker, D., Ramah, M., & Eustace, M. A. (1991). Using KABP data to develop communication interventions to increase condom use among heterosexuals in the eastern Caribbean (Abstract M.D.4036). In *VII International Conference on AIDS Abstract Book* (Vol. 1, p. 399). Florence, Italy.

Miotti, P., Liomba, G., Odaka, N., Dallabetta, G., Chiphangwi, J., Wangel, A. M., Hoover, D., & Saah, A. (1991). Timing of excess mortality in children of HIV-infected African mothers (Abstract M.C.3144). In *VII International Conference on AIDS Abstract Book* (Vol. 1, p. 334). Florence, Italy.

Moss, G., Clemetson, D., D'Costa, L. J., Maitha, G. M., Reilly, M., Ndinya-Achola, J. O., Plummer, F. A., & Kreiss, J. K. (1991). Despite safer sex practices after counselling, seroconversion is high among HIV serodiscordant couples in Nairobi, Kenya (Abstract W.C.3119). In *VII International Conference on AIDS Abstract Book* (Vol. 2, p. 325). Florence, Italy

M'Pele, P., Lallemant LaCoeur, S., Lallemant, M., & Samba, L. (1991). Screening for HIV-1 infection in Africa: A problem within a problem (Abstract M.D. 4154). In *VII International Conference on AIDS Abstract Book* (Vol. 1, p. 428). Florence, Italy.

Mwadi, K., Manoka, Shamavu, Kakanda, Grandpierre, J., & Nkisi, M. (1991). Women's role in managing the impact of AIDS: patients care taking (Abstract M.D.4252). In *VII International Conference on AIDS Abstract Book* (Vol. 1, p. 453). Florence, Italy.

Mwizarubi, B., Laukamm-Josten, U., Maijonga, C., Lwihula, G., Outwater, A., & Nyamwaya, D. (1991). HIV/AIDS education and condom promotion for truck drivers, their assistants and sex partners in Tanzania (Abstract M.C.3344). In *VII International Conference on AIDS Abstract Book* (Vol. 1, p. 384). Florence, Italy.

N'Gbichi, J. M., Yebouet, K., Ackah, A. N., Zadi, M. F., Diallo, M., & De Cock, K. M. (1991). Comparisons of heterosexual transmission of HIV-1 and HIV-2 infections in Abidjan, Cote d'Ivoire (Abstract M.C.3025). In *VII International Conference on AIDS Abstract Book* (Vol. 1, p. 304). Florence, Italy.

Ngugi, E. N., Plummer, F. A., Simonsen, J. N., et al. (1988). Prevention of transmission of human immunodeficiency virus in Africa: Effectiveness of condom promotion and health education among prostitutes. *Lancet, 2*, 887–890.

Ngugi, E. N., Njeru, E. K., Kariuki, A., Plummer, F. Q., Muchunga, E. D., & Moses, S. (1991). A model for behavioral change and the promotion of condom use among women working as prostitutes in Kenya (Abstract W.D.4107). In *VII International Conference on AIDS Abstract Book* (Vol. 2, p. 414). Florence, Italy.

Norse, D. (1991). Socio-economic impact of AIDS on food production in East Africa (Abstract TU.D.57). In *VII International Conference on AIDS Abstract Book* (Vol. 1, p. 70). Florence, Italy.

Nzila Nzilamba, Laga, M., Brown, C., Jingu, M., Kivuvu, M., & St. Louis, M. (1991). Does pregnancy in HIV(+) women accelerate progression to AIDS? (Abstract M.C.3149). In *VII International Conference on AIDS Abstract Book* (Vol. 1, p. 335). Florence, Italy.

Omari Mohamed, A., Bwayo, J. J., Mutere, A. N., Kreiss, J. K., Moses, S., & Plummer, F. A. (1991). Changes in behavior and the incidence of HIV and other sexually transmitted diseases in truck drivers from East Africa (Abstract W.C.3118). In *VII International Conference on AIDS Abstract Book* (Vol. 2, p. 325). Florence, Italy.

Ostfield, M., Fevrier, W., Jagdeo, T., Cole, L., & France, B. (1991). "Condoms . . . because you care"—a lifestyle approach to condom promotion in the eastern Caribbean (Abstract W.D.4003). In *VII International Conference on AIDS Abstract Book* (Vol. 2, p. 388). Florence, Italy.

Palca, J. (1991). The sobering geography of AIDS. *Science, 252*, 372–373.

Pena, C., De Moya, E. A., Garris, I., & Gomez, E. (1991). Epidemiologic surveillance of HIV infections in blood-donors and blood-related AIDS cases in the Dominican Republic, 1983–1990 (Abstract M.D.4173). In *VII International Conference on AIDS Abstract Book* (Vol. 1, p. 433). Florence, Italy.

Petros-Barvazian, A., & Merson, M. H. (1990, November–December). Women and AIDS: A challenge for humanity. *World Health.*

Poinsignon, Y., Lavreys, L., & Boni Mel, J. (1991). AIDS prevention in a West African rural environment: Integration into a primary health care program (Abstract W.D.4005). In *VII International Conference on AIDS Abstract Book* (Vol. 2, p. 389). Florence, Italy.

Ravinathan, A., Ravinathan, R., Meeran, M. M., Sivarajan, N., Rosy Vanilla, B., Raghu Raman, R., & Premila, M. (1991). Oral contraception, IUD, condom use and man to woman heterosexual transmission of STD/HIV infection (Abstract M.D.4232). In *VII International Conference on AIDS Abstract Book* (Vol. 1, p. 448). Florence, Italy.

Reyes, O., Oberle, M., Leoro, G., Rubio, V., & Kreiss, J. (1991). HIV-1 seroprevalence and sexual behavior in Quito's prostitutes (Abstract M.D.4240). In *VII International Conference on AIDS Abstract Book* (Vol. 1, p. 450). Florence, Italy.

Rwabukwali, C., McGrath, J. W., Schumann, D. A., Mukasa, R., Nakayiwa, S., Nakyobe, L., Namande, B., & Carroll-Pankhurst, C. (1991). Socioeconomic determinants of sexual risk behavior among Baganda women in Kampala, Uganda (Abstract M.D.4226), In _VII International Conference on AIDS Abstract Book_ (Vol. 1, p. 446). Florence, Italy.

Sakondhavat, C., Metanawin, T., Tanbanjong, A., Wacharamporn, R., Kraus, S., & Bennett, T. (1991). Acceptability trial of Femidon the female condom among sexually active Thai women at high risk of contracting HIV (Abstract M.C.3086). In _VII International Conference on AIDS Abstract Book_ (Vol. 1, p. 319). Florence, Italy.

Sakondhavat, C., Werawatakul, Y., & Bennett, A. (1991). Promoting condom-only brothels through solidarity and support for brothel managers (Abstract W.D.53). In _VII International Conference on AIDS Abstract Book_ (Vol. 2, p. 36). Florence, Italy.

Sanches, K., Matida, A., & Sole-Pla, M. (1991). AIDS and women in the state of Rio de Janeiro (Abstract M.D.4238). In _VII International Conference on AIDS Abstract Book_ (Vol. 1, p. 449). Florence, Italy.

Sanchez, J., Vega, O., Alvarez, H., & Gotuzzo, E. (1991). Knowledge, attitudes and practices related to AIDS and STD among high school students of low socioeconomic status in Lima (Abstract M.D.4102). In _VII International Conference on AIDS Abstract Book_ (Vol. 1, p. 393). Florence, Italy.

Schopper, D. (1990). Research on AIDS interventions in developing countries: State of the art. _Social Science and Medicine, 30_, 1265–1272.

Seeley, J. A., Malamba, S. S., Nunn, A. J., & Mulder, D. W. (1991). Socio-economic status and vulnerability to HIV infection in a rural community in south-west Uganda (Abstract M.D.4030). In _VII International Conference on AIDS Abstract Book_ (Vol. 1, p. 397). Florence, Italy.

Sittitrai, W., Brown, T., Phanuphak, P., Barry, J., & Sabaiying, M. (1991). The survey of partner relations and risk of HIV infection in Thailand (Abstract M.D. 4113). In _VII International Conference on AIDS Abstract Book_ (Vol. 1, p. 418). Florence, Italy.

Sivard, R., Brauer, A., & Roemer, M. (1991). _World military and social expenditures, 1989._ Washington, D.C.: World Priorities.

Ssembatya, J., Kelley, R., Nduhura, D., & Wawer, M. J. (1991). An evaluation of community health workers to promote low risk behavior in Rakai district (Abstract W.D.4031). In _VII International Conference on AIDS Abstract Book_ (Vol. 2, p. 395). Florence, Italy.

Swaminathan, S., & Kumaresan, G. (1991). Shifting focus: Prostitute intervention to client intervention (Abstract W.D.58). In _VII International Conference on AIDS Abstract Book_ (Vol. 2, p. 37). Florence, Italy.

Taywaditep, K., Mandel, J., Vithayasai, V., Leelamanit, V., & Kearst, N. (1991). Barriers to the development of HIV counseling services in Northern Thailand (Abstract M.C.3329). In _VII International Conference on AIDS Abstract Book_ (Vol. 1, p. 380). Florence, Italy.

Tlou, S. (1990). Perimenopausal experiences of menopausal Botswana women. Doctoral Dissertation, University of Illinois at Chicago.

Tuliza, M., Manoka, A. T., Nzila, N., Way Way, St. Louis, M., Piot, P., & Laga, M. (1991). The impact of STD control and condom promotion on the incidence of HIV in Kinshasa prostitutes (Abstract M.C.2). In _VII International Conference on AIDS Abstract Book_ (Vol. 1, p. 20). Florence, Italy.

UND Programme. (1991). _Human development report._ New York: Oxford University Press.

Uribe, P., Hernandez, M., DeZalduondo, B., Lamas, M., Hernandez, G., Chavez Peon, F., & Sepulveda, J. (1991). HIV spreading and prevention strategies among female prostitutes (Abstract W.C.3135). In _VII International Conference on AIDS Abstract Book_ (Vol. 2, p. 329). Florence, Italy.

Uwakwe, C. B. (1991). Trends in Nigerian students' heterosexual behaviors: counseling implications in the age of AIDS (Abstract M.D.4002). In *VII International Conference on AIDS Abstract Book* (Vol. 1, p. 390). Florence, Italy.

van de Perre, P., Simonon, A., Msellati, P., Hitimana, D. G., Vaira, D., Bazubagira, A., Van Goethem, C., Mukamabano, B., Karita, E., Sondag-Thull, D., Dabis, F., & Lepage, P. (1991). Mother-to-infant postnatal transmission of HIV1: A cohort study (Abstract W.C.33). In *VII International Conference on AIDS Abstract Book* (Vol. 2, p. 31). Florence, Italy.

Vanichseni, S., Choopanya, K., Plangsringarm, K., Sonchai, W., Carballo, M., & Des Jarlais, D. C. (1991). HIV testing and sexual behavior among drug injectors in Bangkok, Thailand (Abstract M.C.3332). In *VII International Conference on AIDS Abstract Book* (Vol. 1, p. 381). Florence, Italy.

Verbeke, R., & Fransen, L. (1991). Reaching family environment through schoolchildren. Characteristics and impact of a strategy applied in Benin (Abstract W.D.4231). In *VII International Conference on AIDS Abstract Book* (Vol. 2, p. 445). Florence, Italy.

Watson, W., Fournel, J., Sondag, D., & Fransen, L. (1991). Safe blood programmes policies and strategies in view of controlling AIDS in developing countries (Abstract W.D.4066). In *VII International Conference on AIDS Abstract Book* (Vol. 2, p. 404). Florence, Italy.

Williams, E., Lamson, N., & Lampety, P. (1991). Nigeria: empowering commercial sex workers for HIV prevention (Abstract W.D.4041). In *VII International Conference on AIDS Abstract Book* (Vol. 2, p. 398). Florence, Italy.

Wilson, D., Lamson, N., Nyathi, B., Sibanda, A., & Sibanda, T. (1991). Ethnographic and quantitative research to design an intervention for truckers in Zimbabwe (Abstract M.C.104). In *VII International Conference on AIDS Abstract Book* (Vol. 2, p. 49). Florence, Italy.

Wilson, V., Mooteeram, L., Gayle, C., & Hull, B. (1991). Knowledge, attitudes and practices among Caribbean laboratory workers with reference to prevention of laboratory acquired HIV infection (Abstract W.D.4161). In *VII International Conference on AIDS Abstract Book* (Vol. 2, p. 428). Florence, Italy.

Wilson, D., Lavelle, S., Hood, R., Mavesere, D., Simunyu, E., & Zenda, A. (1991). Behavioral research to develop intervention strategies among prostitutes and clients in urban and rural Zimbabwe (Abstract W.C.3083). In *VII International Conference on AIDS Abstract Book* (Vol. 2, p. 316). Florence, Italy.

16

The Challenge of AIDS for Health Care Workers

Jerry D. Durham and John Douard

Since it first was recognized, health-care workers have been affected by the AIDS epidemic, both professionally and personally. Professional issues for health-care workers in regard to HIV have included the provision of quality care for HIV-infected persons; workplace transmission including issues of patient-to-provider transmission; and practice issues for the HIV-infected health-care worker. Women comprise the majority of health-care workers. Furthermore, in the United States, professional nurses are the largest group of health-care workers.

Nurses have played pivotal roles in providing quality care for HIV-infected persons since the epidemic began to unfold in 1981 (Selby, 1989). The key nursing activities which have defined nurses' leadership in the epidemic have included direct patient care, coordination of care, client education and advocacy, professional education, and research (American Nurses Association, 1988). The HIV epidemic presents nurses with both an opportunity and a challenge ". . . to develop and effect appropriate societal responses to the HIV epidemic and to counter those that are inappropriate, both among our professional colleagues and among the lay public" (American Nurses Association, 1988, p. 20). Moreover, nurses' scientific knowledge base, historical advocacy for justice in health care, understanding of ethical dimensions of the nursing roles in care delivery, and their family and community-centered focus mandate that they assume leadership roles in the present epidemic. For nurses to do less is tantamount to abandonment not only of persons most in need of their professional services but also of nursing's mandate to care—an imperative increasingly viewed as the "cornerstone and quintessence of their profession" (Fox, Aiken, & Messikomer, 1990, p. 226).

Caring, an increasingly important concept for nursing theory, research, practice, and education, takes on special meaning within the context of the HIV/AIDS epidemic (Morse, Bottorff, Neander, & Solberg, 1991). The epidemic has provided nurses with both an opportunity and a challenge to engage in creative professional caregiving of the highest order—often "against extraordinary odds of limited resources, difficulties in organizing care, and limited knowledge about the epidemic" (Gebbie, 1990, p. 21). Expert professional nursing care, provided for HIV-infected persons "in the midst of health, pain, loss, fear, disfigurement, death, grieving, challenge, growth, birth, and transition on an intimate front-line basis" is the "privileged place of nursing" in the HIV/AIDS epidemic (Benner & Wrubel, 1989, p. xi). This "privileged place," however, can also have a limiting effect on the larger influence which nurses might otherwise exert on the course of the epidemic:

> One obstacle is that nurses in this field are invisible. You hear physicians being interviewed about the crisis and even about patient care issues. But do reporters interview nurses? . . . [nurse] clinicians are so busy that they don't have the time to go out and be heard. Our energies at the end of the day are in going home and healing our wounds . . . . (Bennett, 1987, pp. 1151–1152)

One unintentional outcome of nursing's emphasis on individual caring has been nurses' lessened influence in HIV research and public policy, both of which shape nursing practice at the population level. While nurses have risen to the call to care for and to care about HIV-infected persons, the end result of this emphasis on individuals may be that nurses have unwittingly set themselves up to be forgotten and unrecognized for their contributions through what has been called the "historical forgetting process" (Fox et al., 1990, p. 252). Nurses, however, have an opportunity to interrupt this process by demonstrating their leadership and expert professional caregiving not only through individual care but also through such activities as research; development of inpatient, outpatient, and community care models; development of cost-effective treatments; and provision of support for professional caregivers.

CHALLENGES TO NURSING AND OTHER HEALTH WORKERS

The "privileged place" of nursing in the present epidemic presents many challenges forged by complex social, ethical, political, economic, legal, and professional factors. These factors not only shape the epidemic itself, but also influence solutions to the many problems associated with the epidemic. Nonmedical factors which have profoundly influenced the course of the epidemic include such phenomena as poverty, discrimination, stigma, prejudice, injustice, inequality, sexophobia (fear of sex), homophobia, sexism, and lack of access to adequate health care.

Historically in the United States, women and persons from ethnic minority groups, populations increasingly vulnerable to HIV infection and AIDS, have been most adversely affected by these phenomena. Nurses, 97% of whom are women, are challenged by these social phenomena both in their personal and professional lives. If nurses are to provide effective and compassionate care for persons with HIV/AIDS, they must understand the dynamics of these phenomena in American culture, in health care, and in their own lives.

Professional practice involving persons with HIV/AIDS (and their significant others) requires practitioners to be knowledgeable not only about HIV/AIDS but also sensitive to cultures and subcultures, human behavior, and family dynamics. While the literature on the concerns of nurses working in this area has focused largely upon disease transmission issues, many other concerns also provide challenges to practitioners (Baer & Longo, 1989; Grady, 1989).

Work with HIV-infected persons causes considerable discomfort in some health-care professionals because they must confront their attitudes and feelings about sexuality, childbearing, gay people, drug use, and death. In the second decade of the epidemic, new challenges are faced as the number of HIV-infected women seeking care increases, possibly triggering counter-transference[1] reactions in the female health-care worker regarding childbearing; sexual partner infidelity; current and past sexual experiences; and powerlessness in relationships. While men health care workers, particularly those who are gay, who have worked with large numbers of HIV-infected persons over the course of the epidemic may have already confronted many of their own counter-transference issues, women may not have confronted such a broad range of concerns since, until recently, the number of HIV-infected women in the United States has been relatively small (see Chapter 3). Health-care workers who overidentify with clients, their needs, and their problems risk engaging in counterproductive behaviors, failing to set limits for themselves and their clients, blending personal and professional obligations, and experiencing a sense of hopelessness.

Attitudes, Knowledge, and Concerns

Since the beginning of the epidemic, health care workers have expressed a mixture of attitudes and concerns about HIV/AIDS (Breault & Polifroni, 1991; Gerbert, 1987; Kelly, St. Lawrence, Smith, Hood, & Cook, 1987; Scherer, Haughey, & Wu, 1989; Larson, 1988; Smyser, Bryce, & Joseph, 1990; Somogyi, Watson-Abady, & Mandel, 1990; Swanson, Chenitz, Zalar, & Stoll, 1990). Attitudes and concerns of nurses, also present in varying degrees among both the general public and other health care workers, have shifted somewhat over the course of the epidemic as knowledge about the causes, prevention, and treatment of HIV/AIDS has improved. However, gaps in nurses' knowledge of HIV/AIDS have been identified through numerous surveys, including disease

---

[1]Counter-transference may be defined as the conscious or unconscious emotional response of the health care worker to a patient as a result of the health care worker's unresolved past conflicts with other persons and/or situations.

symptomatology, means of transmission, infection control procedures, and information about means of protection in the work setting (Swanson et al., 1990).

Since the beginning of the epidemic, fear of HIV transmission has been a paramount concern of health-care workers (Bachner, 1990; Gerbert, 1987; Schneiderman and Kaplan, 1992; Smyser, Bryce, & Joseph, 1990; Wallack, 1989; Wormser & Joline, 1989). These fears appear to stem from several causes: (1) Fear of contagion/illness/disability/death; (2) the lack of vaccines or effective treatments for HIV/AIDS; and (3) lack of knowledge about and/or disapproval of alternate lifestyles initially associated with the epidemic. In the last category, disapproval has also been associated with anger toward persons with AIDS, possibly as a result of patient behaviors and some nurses' perceptions that some persons with HIV/AIDS lack social responsibility (Breault & Polifroni, 1992). Other factors that contribute to health-care workers' attitudes toward persons with AIDS include a sense of helplessness associated with the fatal outcome of AIDS; fatigue; and a sense of lack of support (Breault & Polifroni, 1992). These factors can produce in caregivers a stress response characterized by "avoidance, extreme precautions, and verbal expressions of fear regarding the disease" (Bachner, 1990, p. 31; Jemmott, Freleicher, & Jemmott, 1992).

In their review of research conducted over the first several years of the epidemic, Swanson and colleagues (1990) concluded that:

1. fear of AIDS transmission is persistent despite the use of universal precautions;
2. nurses spend less time with AIDS patients than with other patients;
3. some nurses believe they have the right to refuse to care for persons with AIDS;
4. nurses' significant others have concerns about nurses' care of persons with AIDS;
5. a minority of nurses favor patient testing, isolation in hospital rooms, and limitations in school attendance;
6. a small proportion of nurses believe that persons with AIDS deserve their plight;
7. if their caseload of persons with AIDS increases, some nurses may begin to question their career;
8. negative attitudes toward homosexuals is associated with negative attitudes toward caring for persons with AIDS; and
9. a decrease in negative attitudes and fears is associated with accurate knowledge, experience in caring for persons with AIDS, and personally knowing someone with AIDS.

While increased knowledge about HIV/AIDS is associated with fear reduction (Gordin, Willoughby, Levine, Gurel, & Neill, 1987), common concerns expressed by some caregivers apparently stem from irrational causes (Wormser & Joline,

1989), suggesting that factual approaches alone are insufficient to reduce HIV-related anxiety and to change attitudes and behaviors among caregivers. Flaskerud (1991) has proposed a psychoeducational model in order to change nurses' AIDS knowledge, attitudes and practices. Strategies for attitude change in this model include provision of information; exploration of feelings in small groups; use of knowledgeable group leaders whose social and cultural backgrounds are similar to those of group participants; and inclusion of gay men, drug users, persons with AIDS, clergy, ethicists, and attorneys in discussion groups.

Since health-care workers who follow universal precautions are at minimal risk of acquiring HIV infection occupationally, one can reasonably conclude that the basis for some health-care workers' reluctance to provide care is not rooted in fear of contagion but rather in other intrapersonal and cultural dynamics. In the culture of caring associated with nursing, a culture which places a premium on serving all those needing care, such dynamics must be recognized at both a personal and organizational level. Because the HIV/AIDS epidemic has now spread to every corner of America, all caregivers in clinical practice now encounter persons who are HIV infected; thus it is no longer possible (and it was never appropriate) to delegate the care of persons with HIV/AIDS to "AIDS nurses" and health-care workers with "special knowledge" or with a preference to treat such clients. All health-care workers are now directly affected by the epidemic in their professional activities (and all too often their personal lives). All, therefore, bear a responsibility to recognize their own fears relative to HIV/AIDS, to grapple with these fears, and to overcome them in order to fulfill society's expectations for safe, effective, and compassionate care.

Safety in the Workplace

Health-care workers have become increasingly aware that their work exposes them to occupational hazards, including infectious diseases. This awareness can result in more fully informed professional practice, but can also produce, in the face of inadequate or incorrect information, unnecessary or exaggerated anxieties. (Interestingly, one result of this increased concern is the availability of insurance policies to cover occupationally acquired HIV infections and the emergence of HIV protection language in nursing union contracts (Boston RNs, 1992). Less information has been published regarding other occupational hazards related to care of persons with HIV/AIDS, including risks to providers delivering standard and experimental drug treatments (e.g., see Ganciclovir, 1992; and Nokes, 1992).

Occupational Risk Related to HIV Acquisition. The HIV/AIDS epidemic has had the unintended effect of reminding health-care workers that their work may expose them to harm (Bosk and Frader, 1990). However, wide discussion of transmission risk in the literature (Gerberding et al., 1987; Marcus & CDC,

1988; McKinney & Young, 1990; Centers for Disease Control, 1991a) underscores the low risk to health providers of acquiring an HIV infection from an accidental parenteral exposure to HIV-infected blood. That risk is currently estimated at less than 1% (and perhaps as low as 0.25%, depending on a variety of patient, caregiver, viral and exposure factors). Of the health-care workers who have been identified with AIDS, 95% of these cases have been attributed to established risk behaviors (Fahrner & Gerberding, 1991). The risk of infection following accidental exposure to the hepatitis B virus (HBV), however, is much higher, in the range of 25%–30%, but with only about 5% of those infected eventually dying from fulminant or chronic disease (Centers for Disease Control, 1985, 1989a; Schneiderman & Kaplan, 1992). Federal regulations (discussed below) mandating that employers provide HBV vaccination (available since 1982) to health-care workers at risk of exposure to bloodborne pathogens is certain to reduce even further the risk of occupationally acquired HBV. However, the certainty of serious illness and eventual death associated with HIV infection may explain much of the exaggerated fear of HIV infection in occupational settings despite the low risk (Burtis & Evangelisti, 1992).

By early 1992, the Centers for Disease Control (CDC) had documented 29 cases worldwide of occupationally acquired HIV infection among health-care workers, with another 70 cases under investigation but lacking substantive data (Occupational risk, 1992). Of these 29 cases, 11 (38%) were among nurses and another 11 among laboratory workers. Ten of the 11 nurses were women and all but one of the nurses suffered a percutaneous injury, most often in the hand. Seven nurses were infected while performing a phlebotomy. Ongoing studies by the CDC will undoubtedly verify additional occupationally acquired HIV infections in future years. In view of the large number of persons with HIV/AIDS and their significant use of healthcare services, however, the present number is remarkably small and provides clear evidence of the low risk of occupationally acquired HIV infection, particularly when universal precautions and safe techniques are consistently observed by health-care workers (McNabb & Keller, 1991). (See also Durham & Cohen, 1991, for a discussion of universal precautions). In some health care facilities, some techniques, equipment and procedures have been altered to make health-care worker exposure and injury less likely (Cohen, Ferrans, & Dudas, 1992).

The administration of a course of zidovudine therapy following exposure to blood or body fluids potentially containing HIV may be made available to exposed health-care workers. The efficacy of postexposure zidovudine has not yet been demonstrated through a research trial. Therapy should ideally begin as soon as possible and within 24 hours after exposure (Beninger & Cooper, 1991). This should be coupled with services such as risk assessment, an explanation of risks, benefits and alternatives, counseling and education for at least the exposed worker, and their family if possible and desirable. Such services are not yet widely in place (Cohen et al., 1992).

Hepatitis B and Tuberculosis.   Heightened interest in infectious diseases and occupational risk has also renewed concern about hepatitis and tuberculosis (TB), both associated with persons who are HIV-infected (Centers for Disease Control, 1989b; O'Brien & Bartlett, 1992). HBV is primarily transmitted sexually, but the parenteral route, including accidental needlestick injuries in occupational settings, also accounts for a significant number of infections annually (Centers for Disease Control, 1987). The Occupational Safety and Health Administration (OSHA) reports that HBV is the greatest bloodborne infection risk to health-care workers, a risk underscored by the fact that the incidence of reported clinical HBV has been increasing since 1978 (Centers for Disease Control, 1987). While this increase may be related to better casefinding, it more likely stems from changes in sexual and drug use behaviors. There are an estimated 300,000 cases of HBV annually in the United States, resulting in more than 10,000 hospitalizations; 250 deaths annually due to fulminant hepatitis; 4,000 deaths as a result of cirrhosis; and 800 deaths resulting from hepatitis-related primary cancer. As noted earlier, the risk of acquiring an HBV infection following needlestick injury far exceeds the risk of HIV infection under similar circumstances (Centers for Disease Control, 1987). Posttexposure programs for health-care workers are now mandatory, although the details of such programs, including recommended medical interventions, may vary somewhat among institutions (American Nurses Association, 1992; HIV exposure, 1991; Position statement, 1991).

As described in Chapter 1, tuberculosis has been on the increase in the United States since 1986 (Centers for Disease Control, 1991c), largely as a result of the increase of cases of HIV/AIDS and problems related to health-care access by persons living in poverty. About 90% of new TB cases arise from the estimated 10 million Americans infected with the organism causing TB (McKinney, 1992). In 1990, more than 25,000 cases were reported in the U.S., the steepest increase since 1953 (O'Brien & Bartlett, 1992). In 1991 in New York City, TB cases surged 30% among the homeless, drug users, and persons with AIDS (TB hits 500, 1992). One outgrowth of this epidemic was the reported TB infections among 500 of New York City's hospital workers, a harbinger, say experts, of future infections among health care workers in other urban settings (TB hits 500, 1992). A serious related concern has been the emergence of multidrug resistant strains of TB among HIV-infected persons (O'Brien & Bartlett, 1992), particularly among those who do not complete their treatment regimen.

Problems related to the linked HIV and TB epidemics have led the CDC (1989b) to advise that "all patients with HIV infection and undiagnosed pulmonary disease should be suspected of having TB, and appropriate precautions to prevent airborne transmission should be taken until TB is either diagnosed and treated or ruled out" (p. 8). Reduction of the risk of transmission of TB in occupational settings includes several recommendations: a) Placing of all patients suspected of having TB in acid-fast bacilli isolation until they are proven not to be infectious; b) instituting early and appropriate anti-TB therapy; c) advising known TB patients to cover the nose and mouth when coughing and sneezing; d) ensuring adequate ventilation (including determining where the patient's room is vented); e) properly wearing (both health-care workers and infected patients) disposable masks (particulate respirators); and f) appropriately using germicidal ultraviolet (UV) lamps (use of UV lamps should be considered only a supplement to adequate ventilation since long-term exposure to UV light may pose health hazards) (CDC, 1989b; Drug-resistant TB, 1992; O'Brien & Bartlett, 1992). Workers and students in health-care settings are also increasingly aware of the need to have tuberculin skin tests at regularly scheduled intervals 8–12 weeks following TB exposure (O'Brien, 1992). Efforts including several demonstration projects are now underway by the U.S. Public Health Service to improve programs which ensure that patients complete TB therapy. Legislation has been introduced in Congress to improve TB detection and prevention efforts over the next several years, with the ambitious goal of eliminating TB as a public health problem by 2010 (Coalition pushes, 1992).

OSHA Bloodborne Standard.   The renewed concerns around transmission of infectious diseases has produced changes in health education and practice to prevent occupationally acquired bloodborne infections. These concerns have also sparked an interest in research, testing, and development relative to barrier protection and medical devices which hold potential to decrease the risk of disease transmission (see, for example, Korniewicz, Kirwin, & Larson, 1991). Pressure from several sources has also resulted in the issuance, following several years of study and comment, of a bloodborne pathogen standard by the OSHA in late 1991. (Prior to 1988, compliance with CDC's universal precautions recommendations was not required.) This standard, a landmark in health-care occupational safety, aims to limit occupational exposure to blood and other potentially infectious materials and *mandates* a variety of safety measures in work settings, many of which had been previously implemented as a result of recommendations from the CDC. According to the U.S. Department of Labor (1991), this standard will protect 5.6 million workers (mostly employed in hospitals, nursing homes, and practitioners' offices) and prevent an estimated 9,200 infections and 200 associated deaths. Total annual costs of the standard are estimated by the Department of Labor (1991) at about $821 million, mostly for protective equipment. Key features of the OSHA standard are displayed in Table 16.1.

The HIV-infected Health-care Worker.   Fear of infection has also extended to health-care consumers, reaching a nadir when the Centers for Disease Control (1991a) invited public comment around a proposed policy for infected health-care workers, particularly those engaged in invasive procedures (see Chapter 12). As of late 1992, however, there has been only one documented case of transmission from an HIV-infected health care worker (a Florida dentist) to patients. While most researchers believe the dentist may have inadvertently infected five

Table 16.1 Key Provisions of OSHA Bloodborne Pathogens Standard

Purpose: Limits occupational exposure to blood and other potentially infectious materials.

Scope: Covers all employees who could be "reasonably anticipated" to come into contact with blood and other potentially infectious materials as a result of job performance.

Exposure Control Plan: Employees must identify in writing, tasks and procedures as well as job classifications where occupational exposure to blood occurs and specify procedures to evaluate exposures. Employees must have access to this plan which is to be updated at least annually.

Methods of Compliance: Requires universal precautions with emphasis upon engineering and work practice controls. Stresses handwashing and specifies procedures to minimize exposures.

Personal Protective Equipment: Employers must provide, at no cost to employees, personal protective equipment—e.g., gloves, gowns, masks.

Written Schedule for Cleaning: The standard requires a written schedule for cleaning equipment, including the method of decontamination, and method for cleaning following contact with potentially infectious material. Specifies methods for sharps disposal and for handling contaminated laundry.

HIV/HBV Research Laboratories/Production Facilities: Address special requirements for such facilities, including microbiological practices, exposure risk reduction, containment equipment, decontamination.

Hepatitis B Vaccination: Requires vaccinations be made available without charge to all employees with potential occupational exposure within ten working days following employment. Affected employees declining the vaccination must sign a declination form but may opt for the vaccine later. Booster doses, if recommended by the USPHS, must be offered without cost.

Post-Exposure Evaluation and Follow-Up: Specifies procedures which must be available to all employees who experience an exposure accident. Such procedures must be without cost to the employee—confidential medical examination, testing the exposure source if feasible, testing the employee's blood with consent, post-exposure prophylaxis, counseling, and illness evaluation. Any subsequent diagnoses must remain confidential.

Hazard Communication: Requires warning labels on regulated waste and other containers which store/transport potentially infectious materials. (Specimen/laundry labels are not required in facilities using universal precautions). Signs must be posted to identify restricted areas in research/production areas.

Information and Training: Requires training of employees initially upon assignment and annually. Specifies areas to be covered in such training with opportunities for questions and answers. Trainer must be knowledgeable in the subject matter.

Recordkeeping: Medical records of exposed employees must be maintained during employment plus 30 years. Other data related to employees must also be maintained. Training records must be maintained for 3 years. Employee medical records must be available to employee, others with the employee's written permission, OSHA and NIOSH.

Source: U.S. Department of Labor (1991). OSHA Bloodborne pathogens final standard: Summary of key provisions. Washington, DC: Author. A copy of the full text of the standard may be ordered by contacting the U.S. Department of Labor Publications Department at (202) 523-9667.

patients via a blood-to-blood route or through contaminated instruments, intentional infection theories have also been postulated (Ciesielski et al., 1992; Intentional infection, 1992). This case has stimulated much ongoing debate about patients' right to know their health-care workers' HIV status, and has resulted in calls to mandatorily test health providers for HIV (Gerberding, 1991) and to limit the practice of infected health-care workers, possibly to non-invasive patient encounters. The Florida case has also led to discussion among the professions about how to define an "invasive procedure." Most of the professional organizations have issued statements on HIV-infected health-care workers and students, including the American Dental Association, American Medical Association, American Nurses' Association, American Association of Colleges of Nursing, National League for Nursing, International Council of Nursing, American Hospital Association, and others.

Since 1990 at least 32 "look-back" studies of infected health-care workers and their patients have been conducted. More than 13,000 patients have been tested for HIV infection after treatment by 27 HIV-infected health-care workers and 75 patients were found to be HIV-seropositive. For 10 of the 75, other risk factors were identified, but determination of the infection source for the rest has not been made. This type of investigation is difficult because of several factors: The HIV status of the patients before exposure may be unknown, the degree of invasiveness of the procedure is not determined, other possible HIV exposures for the patient are not known, the adequacy of instrument sterilization and disinfection is unknown, the health-care worker's clinical history including the presence of dementia or skin lesions may not be known, and the HIV-genetic sequence testing for the relatedness of HIV strains is not always available or adequate (Chamberland & Bell, 1992; Danila, MacDonald, Rhame, Moen, Reier, Le Tourneau, et al., 1991; Taylor, 1992). Recent studies involving the use of DNA sequence analysis may provide new evidence to link transmission of HIV from infected providers to patients. Such evidence, if irrefutable, would undoubtedly raise to new levels public pressure to impose limitations on the professional activities of HIV-infected health-care workers. In regard to HBV, 29 dentists or surgeons are known to have transmitted HBV to patients (Chamberland & Bell, 1992). While the CDC has issued recommendations to prevent transmission of HIV and hepatitis B from health-care workers to patients (Centers for Disease Control, 1991b), no federal policy or legislation currently restricts the work of HIV-infected health-care workers. States therefore have been advised by the CDC to determine on a case-by-case basis whether infected health-care workers should restrict their practice (States to determine, 1992). The demand by some patients and their advocates that HIV-infected health-care workers, particularly those performing invasive procedures, reveal their HIV seropositive status is fraught with legal and ethical difficulties, and may involve both transmission and competency issues. Policy in this area must take into account scientific evidence regarding risk, risk perception, rights and obligations of health-care workers and regulatory agencies, and possible legal sequelae (Daniels, 1992a; Glantz, Mariner, & Annas, 1992). Illinois' Patient Notification Act, passed in late 1991, provides an example of one state's efforts to require HIV status disclosure. This law requires HIV-infected health-care workers and patients to inform each other of any possible exposure during an invasive procedure (Task Force, 1992). This act, hailed as one of the strictest disclosure measures in the nation, may not be implemented, however, because of ethical concerns. The Illinois law reinforces the tenet that policies aimed at HIV-seropositive health-care workers must rise to the challenge of "protect[ing] patients while respecting the privacy and livelihood of health care workers" (Lo & Steinbrook, 1992).

Once information about health-care workers' HIV status is provided to patients, infected health-care providers, regardless of whether they perform invasive procedures, will find that few patients seek out or accept their services (Daniels, 1992b). Moreover, while laws exist to protect handicapped workers, HIV-infected health-care workers, including those in good health, often find themselves unable to find employment. Current scientific evidence relative to the extremely small risk, if any, of HIV transmission from health-care workers to patient and ethical considerations suggest that the disclosure of the HIV-seropositive health-care workers' status to patients and practice restrictions, in most cases, are unwarranted. A variety of alternative approaches, suggested by experts (Centers for Disease Control, 1991c) and summarized in Table 16.2, provide options for policymakers to consider.

CONCLUSION

The battle to contain the HIV/AIDS epidemic is being waged on several fronts. While medical and scientific breakthroughs have improved the quality of life for some infected persons and hold promise in the future for an effective vaccine and/or cure, health-care givers, especially nurses, have borne the primary responsibility for the day-to-care comfort and care of those living with HIV/AIDS. This responsibility to care provides nurses a "privileged place" in the epidemic and at the same time challenges all health-care workers to examine their own motivations to care; to confront sometimes discomforting attitudes and behaviors in themselves and their colleagues; to encourage safe and responsible professional practice; and to champion the rights of those they would serve.

As the face of the epidemic changes to include more women and children, counter-transference issues will further challenge female providers to provide expert compassionate care and to examine the impact of the epidemic upon their personal lives. Significant numbers of health-care workers, including nurses, are HIV-infected. Concerns about risk and safety, of both health-care workers and consumers of health services, will drive future HIV/AIDS policy and challenge leaders to balance the rights of the individual health-care worker with public concerns.

Table 16.2 Recommendations Regarding HIV Seropositive Health Care Workers

- Health-care workers with identifiable risk(s) should be encouraged to seek anonymous HIV testing
- HIV seropositive health-care workers who perform "exposure-prone invasive procedures" (EPIP) should voluntarily submit to an expert panel. Standardized guidelines to assist expert panels in case-by-case deliberations should be determined, as should penalties for any violations of confidentiality
- Practice restrictions should not be placed on HIV+ health care workers who do not engage in EPIP
- Expedited reviews of dismissals of HIV+ health-care workers should be provided by appropriate government entities
- Hospitals should not be required to provide to the public information regarding employment of HIV/HBV+ health care workers
- Federal assistance should be provided to study, develop, implement, evaluate, and enforce effective infection control procedures
- Studies of adherence to universal precautions should be funded and conducted
- Inspection by regulatory agencies of health-care settings to enforce universal precautions should be stepped up
- Procedures (e.g., ""blind-field" manipulation of sharps) and equipment which increase risk of HIV/HBV transmission should be identified
- Data should be collected from carefully designed studies (prospective/ retrospective), using a variety of risk models, to determine the actual risk of infection from health-care worker to patient
- Studies and analyses regarding the cost/benefit ratio of any policies aimed at infected health-care workers should be performed prior to policy implementation
- HIV/HBV status should not be linked to licensure
- Statutes/regulations should be considered which limit malpractice insurance companies and professional practice committees from seeking information about health-care workers' HIV/HBV status
- An insurance pool/rehabilitation fund for infected health-care workers requiring counseling and retraining should be considered
- Accurate, responsible reporting by the news media should be encouraged
- Infection control content in the curricula of health professions schools should be evaluated and expanded

REFERENCES

American Nurses Association. (1988). Nursing and the human immunodeficiency virus: A guide to nursing's response to AIDS. Kansas City: Author.

American Nurses Association. (1992). *Compendium of HIV/AIDS positions, policies, and documents*. Washington, DC: Author.

Bachner, P. (1990). The epidemiology of fear. *Archives of Pathology and Laboratory Medicine, 114*, 319–323.

Baer, C., & Longo, M. (1989). Talking about it: Allaying staff concerns about AIDS patients. *Journal of Psychosocial Nursing, 27*(10), 30–32.

Beninger, P. R., & Cooper, E. C. (1991). Postexposure chemoprophylaxis: Approval criterial for clinical trials. *Journal of Acquired Immune Deficiency Syndromes, 4*, 513–515.

Benner, P., & Wrubel, J. (1989). *The primacy of caring: Stress and coping in health and illness.* Menlo Park, NJ: Addison-Wesley.

Bennett, J. (1987). Nurses talk about the challenge of AIDS. *American Journal of Nursing, 87,* 1150–1157.

Bosk, C., & Frader, J. (1990). AIDS and its impact on medical work: The culture and politics of the shop floor. *The Millbank Quarterly, 68* (Suppl. 2), 257–279.

Boston RNs win big AIDS insurance payout. (1992, June). *American Journal of Nursing, 92,* 79.

Breault, A., & Polifroni, E. C. (1992). Caring for people with AIDS: Nurses' attitudes and feelings. *Journal of Advanced Nursing, 17*(1), 21–27.

Burtis, R., & Evangelisti, J. (1992, May/June). "Will universal precautions protect me?": A look at staff nurses' attitudes. *Nursing Outlook, 39,* 133–138.

Centers for Disease Control. (1989a). Guidelines for prevention of transmission of human immunodeficiency virus and hepatitis B virus to health care and public safety workers. *Morbidity and Mortality Weekly Report, 38* (Suppl. 6), 5–6.

Centers for Disease Control. (1991a). Proceedings of open meeting on the risks of transmission of bloodborne pathogens to patients during invasive procedures. Atlanta: Author.

Centers for Disease Control. (1987). *Protection against occupational exposure to hepatitis B virus (HBV) and Human immunodeficiency virus (HIV).* Atlanta: Author.

Centers for Disease Control. (1989b). *TB/HIV: The Connection: What health care workers should know.* Atlanta: Author.

Centers for Disease Control. (1991b). Recommendations for preventing transmission of human immunodeficiency virus and hepatitis B virus to patients during exposure-prone invasive procedures. *Morbidity and Mortality Weekly Report, 40* (RR-8), 1–8.

Centers for Disease Control. (1985). Recommendations for protection against viral hepatitis. *Morbidity and Mortality Weekly Report, 34,* 313–324, 329–335.

Centers for Disease Control. (1991c). Tuberculosis morbidity in the United States: Final Data. *Morbidity and Mortality Weekly Report, 40* (SS-3), 23–27.

Chamberland, M. E., & Bell, D. M. (1992). HIV transmission from health care worker to patient: what is the risk? *Annals of Internal Medicine, 116,* 871–873.

Ciesielski, C., Marianos, D., Ou, C-Y, Dumbaugh, R., Witte, J., & Berkelman, R. et al. (1992). Transmission of human immunodeficiency virus in a dental practice. *Annals of Internal Medicine, 116,* 798–805.

Coalition Pushes for Massive Increases for Federal T.B. Funds (1992, August). *Nation's Health, 1,* 1, 16.

Cohen, F. L., Ferrans, C. E., & Dudas, S. (1992). [AIDS policies and procedures in U.S. hospitals: A national survey]. Unpublished data.

Daniels, N. (1992a). HIV-infected health care professionals: Public threat or public sacrifice. *The Milbank Quarterly, 70*(1), 3–42.

Daniels, N. (1992b). HIV-infected professions, patient rights, and the "switching dilemma." *Journal of the American Medical Association, 267*(10), 1368–1370.

Danila, R., MacDonal, K., Rhame, F., Moen, M., Reier, D., & LeTourneau. J., et al. (1991). A look-back investigation of patients of an HIV-infected physician. *New England Journal of Medicine, 325*(2), 1406–1411.

Durham, J., & Cohen, F. (1991). *The Person With AIDS: Nursing Perspectives* (2nd ed.). New York: Springer.

Drug-resistant TB emerging as threat (1992). *HIV/AIDS Prevention, 3*(1), 1–3.

Fahrner, R., & Gerberding, J. (1991). Risk of HIV infection in health care workers. In P. Volberding and M. Jacobson (Eds.), *AIDS Clinical Review* (pp. 215–225). NY: Marcel Dekker.

Flaskerud, J. (1991). A psychoeducational model for changing nurses' AIDS knowledge, attitudes, and practices. *Journal of Continuing Education in Nursing, 22*(6), 237–243.

Fox, R., Aiken, L., & Messikomer, C. (1990). The culture of caring: AIDS and the nursing profession. *Milbank Quarterly, 68* (Suppl. 2), 226–256.

Ganciclovir: Handle with care. (1992, May). *American Journal of Nursing, 92*, 16.

Gebbie, C. (1990). Current and future impact of HIV on nursing. In T. Phillips and D. Bloch (Eds.), *Nursing and the HIV epidemic: A national action agenda* (pp. 21–29). Washington, DC: U.S. Department of Health and Human Services.

Gerberding, J. (1991). Expected costs of implementing a mandatory human immunodeficiency virus and hepatitis B virus testing and restriction program for healthcare workers performing invasive procedures. *Infection Control, 12*(7), 443–447.

Gerberding, J., Bryant-LeBlanc, C., Nelson, K., Moss, A., Osmond, D., & Chambers, H. (1987). Risk of transmitting the human immunodeficiency virus infection, cytomegalovirus, and Hepatitis B virus to health care workers exposed to patients with AIDS and AIDS-related conditions. *Journal of Infectious Diseases, 156*, 1–8.

Gerbert, B. (1987). AIDS and infection control in dental practice: Dentists' attitudes, knowledge and behavior. *Journal of the American Dental Association, 114*, 311–314.

Glantz, L., Mariner, W., & Annas, G. (1992). Risky business: Setting public health policy for HIV-infected health care professionals. *The Milbank Quarterly, 70*(1), 43–79.

Gordin, F., Willoughby, A., Levine, A., Gurel, L., & Neill, K. (1987). Knowledge of AIDS among hospital workers: Behavioral correlates and consequences. *AIDS, 1*, 183–188.

Grady, C. (1989). Acquired immunodeficiency syndrome: The impact on professional nursing practice. *Cancer Nursing, 12*(1), 1–9.

HIV exposure demands immediate action. (1991). *American Nurse, 23*(10), 25.

Intentional infection theories continue. (1992, July 13). *ADA News*, 9.

Jemmott, J., Freileicher, J., & Jemmott, L. (1992). Perceived risk of infection and attitudes toward risk groups: Determinants of nurses' behavioral intentions regarding AIDS patients. *Research in Nursing and Health, 15*, 295–301.

Kelly, J. A., St. Lawrence, J. S., Smith, S. Jr., Hood, H. V., & Cook, D. J. (1987). Stigmatization of AIDS patients by physicians. *American Journal of Public Health, 77*, 789–791.

Korniewicz, D., Kirwin, M., & Larson, E. (1991). Do your gloves fit the task? *American Journal of Nursing, 91*, 38–40.

Larson, E. (1988). Nursing research and AIDS. *Nursing Research, 37*, 60–62.

Lo, B., & Steinbrook, R. (1992). Health care workers infected with the human immunodeficiency virus. *Journal of the American Medical Association, 267*(8), 1100–1105.

Marcus, R., & CDC Cooperative Needlestick Surveillance Group. (1988). Surveillance of health care workers exposed to blood from patients infected with the human immunodeficiency virus. *New England Journal of Medicine, 319*, 1118–1123.

McKinney, W., & Young, M. (1990). The cumulative probability of occupationally-acquired HIV infection: The risks of repeated exposures during a surgical career. *Infection Control and Hospital Epidemiology, 11*(5), 243–247.

McNabb, K., & Keller, M. (1991). Nurses' risk taking regarding HIV transmission in the workplace. *Western Journal of Nursing Research, 13*(6), 732–745.

Morse, J., Bottorff, J., Neander, W., & Solberg, S. (1991). Comparative analysis of conceptualizations and theories of caring. *Image, 23*(2), 119–126.

Nokes, K. (1992). Experiences of health care providers in administering aerosolized pentamadine treatments. *AIDS Patient Care, 6*(3), 126–129.

O'Brien. L., & Bartlett, K. (1992). TB plus HIV spell trouble. *American Journal of Nursing, 92*, 28–34.

Occupational risk for HIV infection. (1992). *Dental Asepsis Review* (Indiana University), *13*(4), 1.

Position statement on personnel policies and HIV in the workplace. *American Nurse, 23*(1), 24.

Scherer, Y. K., Haughey, B. P., & Wu, Y. W. (1989). AIDS: What are nurses' concerns? *Clinical Nurse Specialist, 3*(1), 48–54.

Schneiderman, L., & Kaplan, R. (1992). Fear of dying and HIV infection vs hepatitis B infection. *American Journal of Public Health, 82*, 584–586.

Selby, T. (1989). Nurses rise to challenge of AIDS epidemic. *American Nurse, 21*(6), 1, 8.

Smyser, M. S., Bryce, J., & Joseph, J. G. (1990). AIDS-related knowledge, attitudes, and precautionary behaviors among emergency medical professionals. *Public Health Reports, 105*, 496–504.

Somogyi, A. A., Watson-Abady, J. A., & Mandel, F. S. (1990). Attitudes toward the care of patients with acquired immunodeficiency syndrome. A survey of community internists. *Archives of Surgery, 125*, 50–53.

States to determine policies on HIV-positive health workers. (1992, June 17). *The Indianapolis Star*, A-7.

Swanson, J., Chenitz, C., Zalar, M., & Stoll, P. (1990). A critical review of human immunodeficiency virus infection—and acquired immunodeficiency virus infection-related research: The knowledge, attitudes, and practice of nurses. *Journal of Professional Nursing, 6*, 341–355.

Task force may topple Illinois law. (1992, July 13). *ADA News*, 8.

Taylor, R. (1992). Tracking health worker-to-patient HIV-1 transmission. *Journal of NIH Research, 4* (7), 39–42.

TB hits 500 NYC hospital workers; city strains to control outbreaks. (1992). *American Journal of Nursing, 92*, 103, 107.

United States Department of Labor (Office of Information). (1991). *Labor News* (News Release via Electronic Bulletin Board).

Young, E. W., Koch, P. B., & Preston, D. B. (1989). AIDS and homosexuality: A longitudinal study of knowledge and attitude change among rural nurses. *Public Health Nursing, 6*(4), 189–196.

Wallack, J. (1989). AIDS anxiety among health care professionals. *Hospital and Community Psychiatry, 40*, 507–510.

Wormser & Joline, C. (1989). Would you eat cookies prepared by an AIDS patient? Attitudes about AIDS. *Postgraduate Medicine, 86*, 174, passim.

Index

Abortion, 107, 110–111
Abstinence, 66, 177–178
Acquired immunodeficiency
    syndrome, *see* AIDS
Activists, 259–260
Acyclovir, 19, 200
Adolescents
    age distribution and AIDS, 163–
        165
    athletics and, 161–163
    clinical manifestations in, 195–196
    condom use by, 160, 170–172
    definition of, 156
    in developing countries, 274
    education programs for, 175–182
    epidemiology of HIV infection and
        AIDS, 156–169
    exposure categories, 163–167
    gay, 161, 165
    HIV seroprevalence in, 158
    natural history of HIV, 194
    peer pressure, 165
    physical maturity of, 161, 170–171,
        174
    prevention of HIV in, 170–188
    racial/ethnic distribution, 157
    risk behaviors, 156, 159, 170–174,
        180
    runaways, 161
    schools and, 175–179
    sexual behavior in, 170–172
    sexually transmitted diseases in,
        160
    sports and, 161–163
    statistics/patterns in, 156–157
    transmission, 159–161
Adoption, 223
Advocacy, 231, 233
African-American population, *see*
    Minorities
African countries
    blood transfusions in, 150
    cultural practices in, 271–272
    economic factors in, 265–267
    education prevention programs, 275–
        277
    mortality rates, 265
    prevalence in, 3
    sexual activity in, 269–270
    sexually transmitted diseases in,
        269–270
    statistics/patterns in, 9–10, 47
    transmission, 9–10, 264, 274
AIDS *see also* HIV infection and
    specific topics
    Africa, 47
    age, 44–45, 137–140
    classification, 5–7
    clinical manifestations
        in children, 189–207
        general, 14–21
        in women, 83–103
    definition, 5–8
    etiology, 3–4
    epidemiology, 3–14, 43–59, 137–
        255, 156–169
    exposure categories, 10–13, 49–56,
        142–152, 163–167